Lymphokines and the Immune Response

Editor

Stanley Cohen, M.D.

Chairman of Pathology and Laboratory Medicine
Hahnemann University School of Medicine
Philadelphia, Pennsylvania

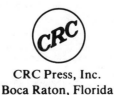

CRC Press, Inc.
Boca Raton, Florida

Library of Congress Cataloging-in-Publication Data

Lymphokines and the immune response / editor, Stanley Cohen.
   p.   cm.
   Includes bibliographies and index.
   ISBN 0-8493-6427-2
   1. Lymphokines--Physiological effect. I. Cohen, Stanley, 1937-
   [DNLM: 1. Immunity, Cellular. 2. Lymphokines. QW 568 L9857]
QR185.8L93L966   1990
616.07'.95—dc20   89-24022 CIP
DNLM/DLC
for Library of Congress

Direct all inquires to CRC Press, Inc., 2000 Corporate Blvd., N.W., Boca Raton, Florida, 33431.

© 1990 by CRC Press, Inc.

International Standard Book Number 0-8493-6427-2

Library of Congress Card Number 89-24022
Printed in the United States

PREFACE

The lymphokine concept grew out of initial attempts to understand certain kinds of immunity to infection in which antibody did not appear to play a role. These cell-mediated or delayed hypersensitivity reactions were found to be associated with soluble, lymphocyte-derived mediators that influenced the behavior of macrophages. The first such factor was macrophage migration inhibition factor (MIF), described by David and by Bennett and Bloom. At about the same time, a second mediator, now known as interferon gamma (IFN-γ) was described by Wheelock.

Shortly thereafter it became apparent that lymphocyte-derived soluble factors played a role in inductive as well as effector events in immune reactions. A whole range of antigen-specific and antigen-nonspecific helper and suppressor factors were described. This set of hormone-like polypeptides was defined as "lymphokines" by Dumonde. Finally, it became obvious that the afferent and efferent lymphokines were merely one manifestation of a larger family of biologically active macromolecules that could be derived from many different cell sources. The name "cytokine" was given to this family by Cohen and Bigazzi following the demonstration that viral infection of nonlymphoid cells led to the production, not only of IFN, but of a variety of chemotactic and migration inhibitory substances similar to those produced by antigen-activated T cells. Another important group of cytokines are the macrophage-derived factors, or monokines.

The central dilemma of lymphokine research was that for many years, they could only be detected in *in vitro* systems, and could only be assayed in terms of *in vitro* biological reactions. The recent demonstration of various *in vivo* roles of lymphokines, and the preparation of polyclonal and monoclonal antibodies to these, helped establish the field on a firm scientific basis. More recently, the application of modern protein purification strategies and molecular biological techniques has led to the availability of many lymphokines in a chemically pure form.

A great deal of interest has been generated in the use of lymphokines, not only as probes of mechanisms of immune responses, but also as therapeutic agents. We are only at the beginning of this exciting stage of lymphokine research. Current studies on structure-function relationships, ligand-receptor interactions, and intracellular mechanisms of action will pave the way for more effective use of these important biologic mediators.

This volume addresses these aspects of modern lymphokine research in detail, beginning with the ways in which lymphokines play a role in the activation of the immune response, and concluding with their participation in various facets of host defense. Although specific chapters have been devoted only to interleukins 1 and 2, tumor necrosis factor, lymphotoxin, and the colony stimulating factors, many of the other mediators are covered in the various chapters dealing with mechanisms of action and cytokine effects. Additionally, there is a discussion of the role of lymphokines in tumor immunity. Finally, an attempt is made to demonstrate that lymphokines and cytokines are involved in a variety of "nonimmunologic" physiologic responses such as reparative reactions involving fibrosis and angiogenesis. Together, these chapters provide a broad overview of the current understanding of the molecular basis of action of these factors, and of their various effects in health and disease.

THE EDITOR

Stanley Cohen, M.D., is Chairman of Pathology and Laboratory Medicine at the Hahnemann University School of Medicine, Philadelphia, Pennsylvania.

Dr. Cohen graduated in 1957 from Columbia College, New York, with a B.A. degree ("Highest Honors" and "Distinction in Chemistry") and obtained his M.D. degree in 1961 from the Columbia University College of Physicians and Surgeons, New York. His postdoctoral training in pathology and immunology was at Harvard and New York Universities.

Dr. Cohen is a member of the American Society for Clinical Investigation, American Association of Pathologists, American Association of Immunologists, Pluto Club, New York Academy of Sciences, Reticuloendothelial Society, Canadian Society of Immunology, New England Society of Pathologists, Clinical Immunology Society, and Sigma Xi. He co-chaired the first five International Lymphokine Workshops, the Congress on Research in Lymphokines and Cytokines, the Congress on Cytokine Research, and two Gordon Conferences in Molecular Pathology. He is a member of the immunopathology subcommittee of the American Board of Pathology. He is Associate Editor-in-Chief of *Clinical Immunology and Immunopathology* and Co-Editor-in-Chief of the *Journal of Experimental Pathology*. He is on the Editorial Boards of *Human Pathology, Cellular Immunology, Journal of Theoretical Biology, International Reviews of Cytology,* and *Receptors in Biology and Medicine.*

Among other awards, Dr. Cohen has received the Kinne Award, the Borden Award, the Parke-Davis Award in Experimental Pathology, and an N.I.H. Outstanding Investigator Award. He has published over 160 research papers and has edited 9 books. He has presented over 40 invited lectures at national and international meetings. His current major research interests relate to lymphokines and cytokines in aging and neoplastic diseases, with special attention to intracellular signal pathways leading to DNA replication following cell activation for proliferation. An additional interest is in the modification of the functional activity of tumor cells.

CONTRIBUTORS

Bruce Beutler, M.D.,
Assistant Investigator
Howard Hughes Medical Institute
Dallas, Texas

John C. Cambier, Ph.D.
Associate Professor
Department of Microbiology
University of Colorado School of Medicine
Denver, Colorado

Anthony Cerami, Ph.D.
Professor and Head
Department of Medical Biochemistry
Rockefeller University
New York, New York

Marion C. Cohen, Ph.D.
Associate Professor
Department of Microbiology
Hahnemann University School of Medicine
Philadelphia, Pennsylvania

Stanley Cohen, M.D.
Professor and Chairman
Department of Pathology
  and Laboratory Medicine
Hahnemann University School of Medicine
Philadelphia, Pennsylvania

Robert E. Cone, Ph.D.
Professor
Department of Pathology
University of Connecticut Health Center
Farmington, Connecticut

Charles A. Dinarello, M.D.
Associate Professor
Departments of Medicine and Pediatrics
Tufts University School of Medicine
Boston, Massachusetts

Scott K. Durum, Ph.D.
Senior Staff Fellow
Laboratory of Molecular Immunology
National Cancer Institute
National Institutes of Health
Frederick, Maryland

William L. Farrar, Ph.D.,
Section Head, Cytokinic Mechanisms
Laboratory of Molecular Immunoregulation
National Cancer Institute
National Institutes of Health
Frederick Cancer Research Facility
Frederick, Maryland

Douglas K. Ferris, Ph.D.
Scientist I
National Cancer Institute
National Institutes of Health
Frederick Cancer Research Facility
Frederick, Maryland

Frank W. Fitch, Ph.D.
Director
Ben May Laboratory for Cancer Research
University of Chicago
Chicago, Illinois

Kerin Fresa, Ph.D.
Assistant Professor
Department of Pathology and
  Laboratory Medicine
Hahnemann University School of Medicine
Philadelphia, Pennsylvania

Nicholas Martin Gough, Ph.D.
Cancer Research Unit
Walter and Eliza Hall Institute of
  Medical Research
Parkville, Victoria, Australia

Meera Hameed, M.D.
Research Associate
Department of Pathology and
  Laboratory Medicine
Hahnemann University School of Medicine
Philadelphia, Pennsylvania

Annick Harel-Bellan, Ph.D.
Senior Scientist
Laboratorie d'Immunologie
Batiment de Recherches
Villejuif, France

Louis B. Justement, Ph.D.
Postdoctoral Fellow
Department of Medicine
National Jewish Center
Denver, Colorado

Anne Kelso, Ph.D.
Research Fellow
Cancer Research Unit
Walter and Eliza Hall Institute
Parkville, Victoria, Australia

Joseph H. Korn, M.D.
Associate Professor of Medicine
Division of Rheumatic Diseases
University of Connecticut School of Medicine
Farmington, Connecticut

James T. Kurnick, M. D.
Associate Professor
Department of Pathology
Harvard Medical School
Massachusetts General Hospital
Boston, Massachusetts

John J. Marchalonis, Ph.D.
Professor and Chairman
Department of Microbiology and Immunology
University of Arizona
Tucson, Arizona

Robert T. McCluskey, M.D.
Benjamin Castleman Professor of Pathology
Department of Pathology
Harvard Medical School
Boston, Massachusetts

Donald Metcalf, M.D.
Research Professor of Cancer Biology
Cancer Research Unit
Walter and Eliza Hall Institute
Parkville, Victoria, Australia

Ruth Neta, Ph.D.
Senior Investigator
Department of Experimental Hematology
Armed Forces Radiobiology
    Research Institute
Bethesda, Maryland

Joost J. Oppenheim, M. D.
Chief
Laboratory of Molecular Immunoregulation
National Cancer Institute
National Institutes of Health
Frederick Cancer Research Facility
Frederick, Maryland

Gillis Otten, M.S.
Research Assistant
Committee on Immunology
University of Chicago
Chicago, Illinois

Theresa H. Piela, Ph.D.
Research Associate
Department of Medicine
University of Connecticut School of Medicine
Farmington, Connecticut

Michael B. Prystowsky, Ph.D.
Assistant Professor
Department of Pathology
University of Pennsylvania
Philadephia, Pennsylvania

Daniel E. Sabath, M.D., Ph.D.
Resident and Postdoctoral Fellow
Department of Laboratory Medicine
University of Washington
Seattle, Washington

TABLE OF CONTENTS

Chapter 1

PERSPECTIVES ON CELL MEDIATED IMMUNITY *IN VIVO*

James T. Kurnick and Robert T. McCluskey

TABLE OF CONTENTS

I. INTRODUCTION

Early knowledge of cellular immunity came in large part from studies of delayed type hypersensitivity (DTH) reactions in the skin, and for many decades the DTH reaction was the main measure of cellular immunity. A second major form of cell-mediated reaction, T lymphocyte mediated cytolysis, was discovered in the 1960s through *in vitro* studies designed to elucidate mechanisms of allograft rejection. We begin with a review of these two prototypic reactions and then discuss other manifestations of T cell-mediated immunity. We review what has been learned about cell-mediated reactions through the use of newer methods for analysis of cells in tissue infiltrates, namely *in situ* staining with monoclonal antibodies, and studies of T cells propagated from inflamed tissues, including investigation of T cell receptor gene rearrangement as a means of assessing clonality of propagated T lymphocytes.

II. GENERAL DESCRIPTION OF DTH REACTIONS

DTH reactions, which are generally elicited in the skin, are characterized grossly by slowly developing erythema, induration, and in severe cases, necrosis. The microscopic and ultrastructural features of DTH reactions have been carefully studied by Dvorak and associates,[1] who have recently reviewed this subject. We concentrate on mechanisms involved and the nature and interaction of cells in the infiltrate. Based on *in vivo* observations, the events involved in the classical DTH reaction are believed to follow a fairly well-characterized path.

The development of DTH to a particular antigen requires appropriate immunization. Under natural conditions DTH develops against a variety of microbial antigens, probably as the result of local infection. Experimentally, reactivity can also be induced against soluble protein antigens by local injections of antigens in adjuvants (usually complete Freund's adjuvant). Intravenous injections are generally ineffective and indeed often induce tolerance. Appropriate exposure to an antigen leads to expansion of specifically sensitized T lymphocytes, a process that occurs principally in lymph nodes draining the site of antigen inoculation. It is axiomatic that the lymphocytes that mediate DTH reactions are T cells; the most direct evidence for this belief is that transfer of T cells, but not of B cells or serum, from sensitized donors to normal syngeneic recipients results in DTH reactions at sites of antigen injection. Most of the T cells responsible for DTH reactions have the CD4+ phenotype;[2] however, since cells of the CD8+ phenotype can also mediate DTH reactions,[3] and since it appears that not all of the hetergeneous class of CD4+ T cells[4-6] produce DTH reactions, the functional designation Tdh is useful.

The cellular interactions involved in the proliferation of the Tdh cells are quite complex and not completely understood. In brief, antigen is processed and presented to CD4+ T cells by accessory antigen presenting cells. CD4+ T cells recognize nominal antigen only when presented on the accessory cell surface in association with MHC class II molecules. Knowledge of the signals, including IL-1 and IL-2 (interleukin-1 and -2), that lead to activation and expansion of the Tdh cells has been derived largely from *in vitro* studies and is reviewed elsewhere in this book.

After Tdh cells have been generated in large numbers in lymphoid tissue, some of them enter the circulation and are able to interact with antigen virtually anywhere in the host. Since DTH reactions can in some cases be elicited years after sensitization, it is reasonable to assume that long-lived recirculating memory T cells can initiate reactions. However, in reactions elicited shortly after immunization, recently divided large lymphocytes (lymphoblasts) probably trigger reactions.[7] Except when antigens are present on endothelial cells (as in allografts or perhaps certain viral infections), Tdh cells must emigrate from blood vessels to contact the triggering antigen. The mechanisms by which Tdh cells are caused initially to traverse blood vessels are not entirely clear; although random emigration of lymphocytes may occur normally to some extent, nonspecific inflammation induced by the trauma of injection, by the contact sensitizer, or by infection is probably involved.

In order to mediate a DTH reaction, the specifically sensitized Tdh cells must encounter the antigen in combination with class II MHC molecules on accessory cells. The Tdh cells are then activated and stimulated to produce and release a group of mediators (lymphokines), which result in an inflammatory reaction that generally reaches its peak within 1 or 2 d. The evidence for the role of lymphokines in DTH reactions *in vivo* has been reviewed.[8]

Perhaps the most satisfactory definition of the DTH reaction is an inflammatory reaction dependent upon certain kinds of lymphokines released from sensitized T lymphocytes following interaction with antigens. Under this definition, it is assumed that B cells, which are known to be capable of producing lymphokines, do not participate in cell mediated reactions *in vivo*, except in some cases through effects of antibodies, which may accompany and modify cell mediated reactions. The definition also excludes reactions that might be initiated by stimulation of T cells by factors other than antigen, such as lectins; whether, in fact, such reactions occur under natural conditions is not known. The definition does not exclude the participation in DTH reactions of mediators (cytokines) released from cells other than T cells, notably macrophages.

Once the DTH reaction begins to develop, a complex interplay of cells and mediators is set in motion, which serve to intensify the rate of emigration of various types of leukocytes, including lymphoblasts with a variety of antigen specificities. (The lymphocytes that emigrate at sites of cell mediated reactions have been variously referred to as large (recently divided) lymphocytes, lymphoblasts, or inflammatory lymphocytes; for convenience we use the term "lymphoblast", even though the cells may not possess all of the morphologic features that some require to so designate a cell.) Although the events that occur following the initial activation of Tdh cells by antigen can be labeled secondary mechanisms, the tremendous amplification that occurs can account for the difference between a trivial or an intense reaction.

The mechanisms that promote emigration of lymphocytes in delayed reactions (or other inflammatory reactions) are not entirely known; however, changes in endothelial cells that lead to adhesion of leukocytes are clearly important.[9] Since many of the studies related to adhesion of leukocytes have been performed in cell mediated reactions other than DTH, or in other forms of inflammatory reactions, this subject is discussed in a later section.

Changes in the microvasculature in DTH reactions are not only involved in leukocyte adhesion, but also lead to increased permeability, which results from the development of gaps between adjacent endothelial cells.[10] The responsible mediators are poorly defined. Other alterations in the microvasculature, which include hypertrophy and damage of endothelial cells, may contribute to the development of necrosis in severe DTH reactions.[1]

Following emigration of leukocytes, a variety of cytokines act to modify the cells in the infiltrate, especially macrophages, with respect to their motility and state of activation. Macrophage activating factors (MAF) result in an increase in the capacity of these cells to kill certain microorganisms, and this is the most important mechanism in resistance to intracellular pathogens such as *Mycobacteria, Brucella abortus,* and *Listeria monocytogenes.* Interferon-γ (IFN-γ) can cause macrophage activation and thus is one form of MAF. There is evidence that the lymphokines that lead to macrophage activation may differ from those that provide help to B cells,[4] a process which also involves intimate physical contact between T and B cells. Lymphokines that inhibit macrophage motility or cause macrophage aggregation *in vitro* may have similar effects *in vivo,* although direct evidence for this is not available.[8]

A prominent feature of DTH reactions is extravascular fibrin deposition, which accounts for the characteristic induration of these reactions. Fibrin accumulation depends on increased vascular permeability and on factors that lead to clotting of fibrinogen. The mechanisms and consequences of fibrin deposition in DTH reactions have recently been reviewed.[1] We will only note that fibrin deposition may influence the migration of cells in the infiltrate[11] and that fibrinopeptides may have important biologic effects, including inhibition of lymphocyte activation.[12] In addition, fibrin and associated fibronectin deposition may be involved in scar tissue formation, which occurs in some long-standing reactions.[13]

III. CELLULAR DIVERSITY OF DTH REACTIONS

An aspect of DTH reactions that is not sufficiently emphasized in the immunological literature is the diversity of the infiltrates in reactions elicited under various conditions. Although some of this may be due to the concurrent effects of other mechanisms, such as antibody mediated components, even apparently pure reactions exhibit variability. Species differences are important. In most species, including man, lymphocytes, or mononuclear phagocytes usually predominate, although small numbers of neutrophils are commonly found. Neutrophils can be especially numerous in early stages of tuberculin reactions. The mononuclear cells generally accumulate preferentially around small vessels (perivascular cuffs).[1] In mice, neutrophils are usually the most abundant type of cell in DTH reactions.[14] Even within a given species the composition of the infiltrate in DTH reactions varies considerably, depending on several factors, including the tissue involved, the time at which the reaction is studied, the method of immunization, and the physical state of the eliciting antigen. For example, the injection of an insoluble antigen in a sensitized host may result in a granulomatous lesion, characterized by nodular accumulation of epithelioid mononuclear phagocytes, with only scanty lymphocytes, whereas another reaction in the same animal elicited by a soluble form of the antigen may be characterized by a widespread infiltrate of lymphocytes, neutrophils, and macrophages.[15]

A type of reaction in man and guinea pigs that has generally been considered to be T cell mediated, and a variant of DTH, is characterized by basophil-rich infiltrates (cutaneous basophil hypersensitivity, CBH). It appears likely, however, that CBH reactions are heterogeneous and that some forms of CBH may not depend entirely on T cells, but also on antibodies.[16-18] CBH reactions differ from classical DTH reactions in respects other than the presence of numerous basophils; notably, they lack interstitial fibrin deposition and severe endothelial cell injury.[1]

Another type of reaction that is generally classified as a form of DTH is *contact sensitivity*, in which the immunogens consist of conjugates of small molecular weight substances with autologous proteins, formed after application of the sensitizer to the skin. It is, however, possible that contact reactions include a component mediated by cytolytic T cells directed against neoantigens on epidermal cells.[19,20] The distribution of infiltrating cells in contact reactions differs from that of DTH reactions, which reflects the sites of maximal antigen concentration. Thus, in contact reactions infiltrates are more intense in the epidermis and upper dermis than in DTH reactions elicited by intradermal injection.

In most DTH reactions eosinophils are found only in small numbers, but in some circumstances they are numerous. Associated antibody-mediated mechanisms appear to account for eosinophil accumulation in some reactions, as for example in the "retest" reaction (elicited by reinjection of antigen at the skin site of an earlier DTH reaction). In this situation there is evidence that an interaction between a precursor (ECFp) and specific immune complexes generates a potent eosinophilic chemotactic factor (ECP).[21] The requirement that ECFp interact with immune complexes containing the same antigens as those triggering the lymphocytes is surprising. Cohen[8] has suggested that the ECFp is associated with anti-idiotypic activity.

In other reactions, lymphokines probably account for eosinophil accumulation, as in schistosome granulomas.[22] An eosinophil-stimulating lymphokine (HILDA) has also been recently reported as being produced in response to IL-2.[23] Since IL-2 participates in DTH reactions, it may play a role in eosinophil infiltration in certain reactions, possibly in association with an effect of immunoglobulin E (IgE).[24]

It seems likely that the diversity of DTH reactions occurs in part because various reactions are initiated by different subsets of T cells, in particular, subsets of CD4[+] T cells that produce different types of mediators.[4,5]

IV. REACTIONS MEDIATED BY CYTOLYTIC T CELLS

The second prototypic T cell reaction, T cell mediated cytolysis, has been investigated largely through *in vitro* studies, which were designed to elucidate mechanisms of allograft rejection or destruction of viral infected cells. The killing of a target cell by a cytolytic T cell requires close contact between the two cells. The binding of a cytolytic T cell to its target (a major histocompatibility complex (MHC) restricted event) stimulates the cytolytic activity of the cell.[25] Although the mechanism of lysis has not been fully elucidated, there is evidence that the T cells secrete cell membrane-damaging molecules, including a serine esterase[26] and a cytolytic pore forming protein (PFP/perforin).[27]

A recent investigation of the interactions between specific cytolytic T cells and target cells infected with lymphocytic choriomeningitis (LCM) virus revealed interdigiting connections between the two cells and evidence that the contents of granular inclusions are released by the cytolytic cell in contact with infected cells.[28] In addition to the production of cell membrane injury, cytolytic T cells also cause internal disintegration of the target cell through undetermined mechanisms.[28]

The human T cells that exert the strongest cytolytic effects are predominantly CD8[+], which recognize target cells bearing class I MHC antigens;[29] however, CD4[+] T cells can also exert cytolytic effects, but unlike CD8[+] cells, recognize target cells bearing class II MHC antigens.[30]

Although evidence of cytolytic T cell injury has been obtained largely from *in vitro* studies, there is no doubt that they also exert their effects *in vivo* and are particularly important in viral infections, allograft rejection, and possibly in resistance to tumors. The major events in the development of cytolytic T cell reactions *in vivo* appear to parallel those leading to DTH reactions, although the latter subject has been studied more thoroughly. Cytolytic T cells proliferate mainly in lymphoid tissue following appropriate exposure to antigen. Certain kinds of antigens are effective in stimulating cytolytic T cells, notably alloantigens or those expressed in association with class I MHC products on the surface of the usual types of target cells: allogeneic cells, viral infected cells, and tumor cells. The efficient generation of cytolytic T cells usually requires assistance from CD4[+] or analogous inducer T cells, but may also occur independently.[31,32]

Following proliferation of cytolytic T cells, they are released into the circulation and thus, like Tdh cells, can participate in a reaction anywhere in the body. Except in situations where endothelial cells are themselves targets, as in allografts or perhaps in certain viral infections, cytolytic T cells (like Tdh cells) must traverse blood vessels to encounter target cells. The mechanisms responsible for the emigration of cytolytic T cells are not entirely clear. It appears that an accompanying DTH reaction is often involved, as discussed later.

Once cytolytic T cells encounter target cells, they presumably produce injury through the same mechanisms that have been observed *in vitro*. Compelling evidence that cytolytic T cells can act alone to cause cell lysis *in vivo* has been obtained in studies of mice with LCM virus infection, and in particular in a model of hepatitis induced by a hepatotropic LCM virus.[33] The lesions were characterized by infiltration of lymphocytes and necrosis of hepatocytes. Cytolytic T cells could be recovered from infected livers. Analysis of experiments in which populations of Ly2[+] cytolytic cells were transferred into irradiated recipients indicated single hit kinetics of liver cell death and were consistent with the interpretation that the effector cells destroyed infected liver cells via direct contact rather than via soluble mediators. Immunohistochemical studies of the liver in human beings with chronic hepatitis B infection have also provided evidence for a direct cytolytic effect of T cells. Thus, CD8[+] cells predominate in areas of necrosis of liver cells, whereas both CD4[+] and CD8[+] cells are seen in portal areas.[34] It is also possible, however, that lymphokines released from cytolytic T cells may participate in tissue injury.

In addition, certain lymphokines released from cytolytic T cells may exert protective effects. Thus, Woan-Chen and McGregor[35] have reported that resistance to *Listeria monocytogenes* in the rat is transferable by OX8[+] cells (CD8[+] analogs), which do not directly kill the bacteria, but apparently activate macrophages to do so. Furthermore, there is evidence that murine Ly2[+] cells can produce a lymphokine that is cytotoxic for Gram negative organisms.[36]

Although destruction of viral infected cells generally serves a protective role, the models of LCM virus infection in mice have clearly demonstrated that cytolytic T cells can also be responsible for tissue injury that has no useful purpose. Thus, the LCM virus is not cytopathic and in the absence of LCM virus reactive cytolytic T cells the virus produces no damage.[37]

V. INTERACTIONS BETWEEN Tdh, OR T HELPER/INDUCER T CELLS, AND CYTOLYTIC T CELLS

We stated above that DTH may play a role in the emigration of cytolytic T cells. The basis for this statement comes largely from studies of allografts. Evidence that both DTH and cytolytic T cells participate in graft rejection has come from several sources, including the similarity of morphologic features in DTH and allografts,[1] analysis of the phenotype of the infiltrating cells[38] and of functional properties of T cells propagated from infiltrates,[39] as well as through transfer experiments. Endothelial cell changes similar to those seen in classical DTH reactions are seen in allografts, and these alterations are believed to be important in adhesion and subsequent emigration of leukocytes. Fairly direct evidence that cytolytic T cells directed against allogeneic cells can emigrate at sites of DTH reactions has been obtained by Prendergast,[40] who demonstrated that cells labeled *in situ* with ³H thymidine in lymph nodes draining a skin allograft emigrated into DTH reactions elicited with protein antigens at remote sites.

It is likely that a DTH component is also important in emigration of cytolytic T cells in reactions resulting from viral infections. The DTH component in allografts or viral infections may result not only from CD4[+] T cells (found in infiltrates of allografts and viral lesions, especially around blood vessels), but also from CD8[+] cells with reactivity toward viral or alloantigens. The interpretation that CD8[+] cells can function as Tdh cells is supported by several lines of evidence, including the findings that such cells can produce lymphokines *in vitro*,[41] and that clones of Ly2[+] cells capable of protecting mice against type A influenza virus can induce foot pad swelling when injected locally with live or attenuated virus.[3] Thus, even in situations where cytolytic T cells appear to reach target cells on their own (as in experiments in which transfer of clones of cytolytic T cells into immunoincompetent recipients confers protection against viral infection[42]), a DTH component may be involved. However, it has not been proved that emigration of cytolytic T cells always requires an accompanying DTH reaction. In contrast with the infiltrates of classical DTH reactions, CD8[+] cells generally outnumber CD4[+] cells in sites of viral infection; it may be that this results from greater local proliferation or survival of CD8[+] cells, since there is no evidence that T lymphocytes of a particular phenotype emigrate more efficiently than others.

Aside from the possiblity that DTH promotes emigration of cytolytic T cells, there are at least two other aspects of interactions between Tdh (or more broadly T cells with inducer/helper functions) and cytolytic T cells: the extent to which inducer cells are required for the expansion of cytolytic T cells[31,32] and the extent to which cytolytic T cells and DTH components provide effector mechanisms for the destruction of allografts, viral infected cells, or tumors. These issues have not always been considered separately, and in any case are not easy to unravel. Most attention has been focused on the participation of DTH and cytolytic T cells in the production of tissue injury, and in particular in allograft rejection. The relative importance of these two mechanisms in allograft rejection has been the subject of controversy and has recently been reviewed.[43] Without attempting to discuss all the evidence, we favor the conclusion that cytolytic T cells provide crucial effector mechanisms in most forms of allograft rejection, but that helper/inducer cells are required for the full development and function of the cytolytic T cells.[44]

Numerous transfer experiments have been performed in attempts to determine the role of individual cell types in allograft rejection. The demonstration that transfer of populations of T cells of the inducer/helper phenotype can induce rejection has been cited as crucial evidence that DTH is the responsible mechanism.[45] There are, however, difficulties in the interpretation of such studies, even when pure subsets or clones of cells are transferred. In particular, the transferred cells almost never act alone but lead to the participation of recipient cells in the reactions. For example, helper T cells may induce the formation of cytolytic T cells in syngeneic recipients or recruit other types of cells to sites of inflammation. To some extent, this problem can be avoided by the use of immunologically deficient recipients; however, even this approach may not suffice, because depletion of T cells is usually not complete. Thus, Le Francois and Bevan[46] have shown that the ability of Ly2[-] cells to mediate graft rejection involves the recruitment of Ly2[+] cells, even in irradiated bone marrow reconstituted hosts. Also, small numbers of Ly2[+] cells can resist destruction and expand *in vivo* even after strenuous attempts to deplete this subset prior to transfer.

Although most reactions in which cytolytic T cells are important (such as viral infection or allografts) may involve a DTH component, it is not known whether the converse occurs, namely that cytolytic T cells participate in classical DTH reactions, such as those elicited by soluble protein antigens. For one thing, it is not clear whether cytolytic T cells are usually generated by such antigens, and for another it is not obvious that there would be a suitable target cell in the reaction site, other perhaps than accessory cells bearing antigen.

VI. CELL MEDIATED REACTIONS COMBINED WITH ANTIBODY OR OTHER MECHANISMS

T cell reactions may take place in association with antibody mediated injury. Antibodies may produce immune complex injury, anaphylactic reactions (IgE mediated), or effects on cell surfaces, including antibody-dependent cell mediated cytotoxicity (ADCC). Small numbers of B cells and plasma cells are found in some cell mediated reactions, even in situations where there is no clear evidence of antibody mediated mechanisms. The B cells may function not only as antibody producing cells, but as antigen presenting cells. In some long-standing lesions in which cell mediated mechanisms participate, ectopic lymphoid tissue develops, with follicle and germinal center formation; obviously, this provides a setting for efficient local generation of effector and regulatory cells. (Even in infiltrates without lymphoid architecture, local proliferation of such cells may occur.) Some of the inflammation in cell mediated reactions may be secondary to destruction of tissue; in the final stages of allograft rejection, for example, numerous neutrophils often accumulate. Cells with natural killer (NK) activity frequently take part in T cell mediated reactions, especially those resulting from viral infections.[47] Varying combinations of cellular and antibody mechanisms probably occur in most naturally occurring immunopathological processes, including autoimmune diseases, as well as in allografts. This is not to say that all components are equally important; for example, T cells are almost always responsible for rejection of solid allografts, even though some plasma cells are often found in the infiltrate. In general, many immunogens elicit either a predominantly cellular or humoral response.

VII. MECHANISMS RESPONSIBLE FOR LEUKOCYTE EMIGRATION IN CELL MEDIATED REACTIONS

The first step in leukocyte emigration is adhesion to endothelial cells. Evidence that changes in endothelial cells are important in promoting adhesion in cell mediated or chronic inflammatory reactions has been obtained in a variety of ways. The endothelial cells of venules in DTH reactions, in allografts, and in certain chronic inflammatory sites, such as rheumatoid synovia, undergo a variety of changes (referred to as activation), including hypertrophy and increased development of biosynthetic organelles. As a result they come to resemble the high endothelial cells in venules (HEV) of lymph nodes.[1,9,10] Adhesion is thought to be an important factor in the physiological passage of lymphocytes into lymphoid tissue. Binding of lymphocytes to HEV in lymph nodes can be demonstrated in tissue sections, which presumably results from receptors for lymphocytes on the endothelial cells. It has also been shown that lymphocytes adhere in tissue sections to endothelial cells in rheumatoid synovia;[48] similar studies have apparently not been performed in DTH reactions. There is, however, evidence that mediators known to be involved in DTH reactions promote lymphocyte adhesion to endothelial cells. Thus, it has been shown that lymphocyte adhesion to cultured umbilical vein endothelial cell monolayers is enhanced by IFN-γ and IL-1.[49,50] Furthermore, IFN-γ, tumor necrosis factor (TNF), and IL-1 cause increased expression by endothelial cells of an antigen called ICAM-1,[10] which appears to be involved in lymphocyte adhesion, as judged by *in vitro* experiments. Another leukocyte adhesion molecule called E-LAM-1 can be induced by IL-1 and TNF.[10] Moreover, this antigen has been shown to be expressed on endothelial cells in DTH reactions in man.[51]

Further studies are needed to define precisely the endothelial cell receptors that may be involved in lymphocyte adhesion in inflammatory reactions, including DTH reactions. It is likely that at least some of the receptors are different from those in HEV in lymph nodes, since most of the lymphocytes that emigrate at sites of inflammation in various forms of cell mediated reaction (DTH, allografts, T cell mediated autoimmune diseases) are lymphoblasts,[8,52,53] whereas those that enter lymphoid tissue are small long-lived cells. In fact, Jalkanen et al.[48] have obtained evidence that binding of lymphocytes to endothelium in rheumatoid synovium is mediated by adhesion molecules that are distinct from those on lymph node HEV. Thus, a monoclonal antibody to receptors on HEV that blocks the adhesion of lymphocytes in lymph nodes fails to do so in rheumatoid synovial tissue.

Class II MHC antigens are another group of molecules that may be induced or increased on endothelial cells in some cell mediated reactions and lead to adhesion of lymphocytes. Pober et al.[54] have shown that IFN-γ can cause expression of these antigens on endothelial cells *in vitro*, and Masuyama et al.[55] have presented evidence that expression of HLA-DR on cultured endothelial cells leads to adhesion of lymphocytes. Fibronectin, which is known to accumulate on endothelial cells in DTH reactions, may also promote adhesion of leukocytes.[56]

Certain antigens that are involved in leukocyte adhesion are expressed not on endothelial cells, but on leukocytes. One antigen in this group is called the lymphocyte function-associated molecule, LFA-1.[57] (Despite it name, LFA-1 is found on all types of leukocytes, with the exception of some macrophages.) A monoclonal antibody to LFA-1 inhibits a variety of T cell functions, including T cell binding to endothelial cells in culture.[9] Furthermore, activation of T cells by phorbol esters causes increased adhesion of lymphocytes to cultured endothelial cells and this increase can be inhibited by antibodies to LFA;[58] in contrast, these antibodies have little effect on the binding enhancement mediated by IL-1 or lipopolysaccharide (LPS). The authors suggested that increased adhesion of activated lymphocytes accounts, in part, for the emigration of lymphoblasts in cell mediated reactions.[58]

After they adhere to endothelium, lymphocytes may proceed by random motion to find their way between endothelial cells and emigrate. In addition, chemotactic factors probably contribute to lymphocyte emigration,[59] and, of course, chemotactic factors are thought to be involved in the emigration of monocytes and granulocytes in DTH reactions.[8] Some of these factors have been defined in functional assays and have been only partially characterized.[8]

Another mechanism that may contribute to the accumulation of leukocytes in DTH reactions is an increase in certain types of circulating leukocytes, especially those with increased adhesion molecules, resulting from release of cells from the bone marrow via mediators such as IL-2, colony stimulating factors (CSFs), and interferons (IFNs).[60]

VIII. INCREASED ENDOTHELIAL EXPRESSION OF CLASS II MHC MOLECULES: A POSSIBLE MECHANISM FOR ANTIGEN PRESENTATION

The appearance or increased expression of class II MHC molecules on endothelial cells may lead not only to lymphocyte adhesion in some cell mediated reactions, but possibly also to antigen presentation. (In man endothelial cells in many vessels normally express MHC class II antigens; in other species in which the phenomenon has been studied, this is generally not found.)

Expression of class II MHC molecules on endothelial cells *in vivo* has been described in DTH reactions and in the T cell mediated autoimmune models of experimental allergic encephalomyelitis (EAE)[61,62] and uveitis.[63] Sobel et al.[61] have performed careful studies on this phenomenon in guinea pigs developing EAE following immunization with myelin basic protein. They found increased expression of class II MHC antigens (and fibronectin) on the lumenal surface of endothelial cells in vessels in the CNS, but not in other tissues. Surprisingly, this preceded histologically detectable inflammation; nevertheless it seems likely that the effect was mediated by a few lymphocytes that emigrated and interacted with myelin basic protein, with the release of lymphokines, in particular IFN-γ.

The possibility that increased expression of class II MHC molecules may result in the ability of endothelial cells to present antigens to adherent lymphocytes is supported by the observation that endothelial cells from the CNS of mice with EAE are able to present myelin protein to lymphocytes *in vitro*.[64] For this to occur *in vivo* it would be necessary for antigen to be located on the endothelial cell surface; in this regard viral antigens have been found on endothelial cells in the brains of ferrets with encephalitis resulting from measles virus.[65]

IX. SPECIFICITY OF THE T CELLS IN CELL MEDIATED REACTIONS

It is clear that specifically sensitized T cells must enter tissue at sites of antigenic challenge in order to initiate T cell reactions. Despite extensive studies there is uncertainty concerning the question as to how many of the cells in the infiltrate of fully developed lesions are specifically sensitized to the eliciting antigen. Early experiments were designed to determine what proportion of cells in DTH reactions produced by passive transfer were of donor or recipient origin.[66] Studies in guinea pigs showed that when donor cells were labeled with ³H thymidine, only small numbers of labeled cells were found in reactions in the recipients.[66] Conversely, when prospective recipient guinea pigs were given repeated injections of ³H thymidine for several days prior to transfer of unlabeled lymph node cells from sensitized donors, the great majority (up to 90%) of the infiltrating mononuclear cells were labeled. The latter results clearly showed that the majority of infiltrating cells were not specifically sensitized. However, since many of the labeled cells were mononuclear phagocytes, the results left unanswered the question whether a substantial proportion of the lymphocytes in the infiltrate were specifically sensitized.

Several studies have been performed to determine if there is preferential migration of lymphocytes from donors sensitized to a particular antigen into reactions elicited by that antigen, using different forms of cell mediated reactions, including allografts,[38,39] DTH reactions,[66,67] and two types of T cell mediated autoimmune diseases, adrenalitis and encephalitis.[69] The general design of most experiments was as follows. Recipients were given labeled lymph nodes cells from donors immunized to one antigen and unlabeled cells from donors sensitized to a different antigen. By morphologic criteria most of the labeled cells appeared to be lymphocytes.[68] Reactions were elicited at separate sites in the recipients with each antigen and the infiltrates were studied for labeled cells. In most such studies, approximately equal numbers of labeled cells were found at each site. In at least one study, however, slight preferential accumulation of lymphocytes from sensitized donors in relevant sites was noted.[70] Even if the latter observation is valid, however, it is clear that lymphocytes of various specificities emigrate at sites of cell mediated reactions and the percentage of specifically sensitized cells is probably very small.

What could the consequences of having T cells at an inflammatory site where no specific antigen is present? For at least several days IL-2 responsive cells could persist and release lymphokines, thus potentiating the reaction. Eventually, however, such cells would disappear, whereas cells reactive with an antigen in the site could survive and be stimulated further. In this regard, it is important to note that the transfer studies were designed to measure the cells *arriving* at the lesion and not to assess the possibility that proliferation of specific T cells, driven by antigen present at the site, might expand their numbers locally. This question is addressed in a later section of this chapter, where studies of cells isolated from inflamed tissue are described.

The question as to how many of the lymphocytes in a reaction are specifically sensitized to the eliciting antigen is perhaps not of overriding importance, in view of the remarkable amplification of effects that occur following interaction of a few sensitized cells with antigen.

X. DOWN REGULATION OF CELL MEDIATED REACTIONS: ROLE OF LOSS OF ANTIGEN AND OF SUPPRESSOR CELLS

Most early experimental studies of cell mediated reactions dealt with the way in which they develop; however, more recently attention has also been paid to factors responsible for their disappearance.

DTH reactions elicited by injections of soluble protein antigens fade quickly and disappear within a few days. Loss of antigen from the site can eventually cause the reaction to regress. Antigen may be lost by diffusion or by phagocytosis and degradation, especially after combination with antibodies. When antigen is no longer present, the inductive phase of the response, which is required to activate the Tdh cells, is lost. As shown *in vitro*, activated T lymphocytes are dependent upon IL-2 for survival.[71] Since IL-2 has a very short half-life *in vivo*,[72] the supply of this lymphokine in a cell mediated reaction is dependent upon continued (although perhaps intermittent) production. In sites with persistent antigenic stimulation, activated lymphocytes may lead to prolonged production of IL-2. Examples of antigens that may persist for prolonged periods or indefinitely include autologous antigens, allografts, products of microbes that cannot be eradicated, and certain nondegradable antigens. However, many microbial or other foreign proteins will eventually disappear.

Athough "deactivation" of lymphocytes following antigen loss may lead to regression of cell mediated reactions, there is also evidence that active suppressor mechanisms are important. Most attention has been directed at suppressor T cells. The phenomenon of T cell suppression of cell mediated reactivity has been convincingly demonstrated in experiments in which transfer of certain populations of T cells to syngeneic recipients prevents the development of a variety of reactions, including DTH and contact reactions,[73] autoimmune diseases,[74] or schistosome granulomatous reactions.[75] There is also evidence that suppressor T cells are at least partially responsible for the regression of schistosome granulomas[75] and for the diminished likelihood, as time goes on, that allografts in partially immunosuppressed hosts will be rejected.[76] It has, however, been difficult to characterize or isolate the cells responsible for suppression, in part because of problems in interpretation of transfer studies, as discussed earlier. Subsets of inducer and effector suppressor T cells have been described.[4-6,73] In mice, complex interactions have been defined between various subsets of suppressor cells, which interact with one another through idiotypic-anti-idiotypic networks.[73] In experimental studies, the most compelling evidence for suppressor function has been obtained through transfer studies. In man, identification of cells with suppressor function is limited to *in vitro* assays.

Numerous efforts have been made to find phenotypic characteristics that would permit identification of cells with suppressor function. It appears that most antigen-specific effector cells are CD8[+]; it is not generally possible, however, to distinguish cytotoxic from suppressor cells within the CD8[+] population, although it has been claimed this may be achievable through the use of selected monoclonal antibodies, such as Leu 15.[77] There are no widely accepted clusters of differentiation antigens that uniquely define effector suppressor T cells. The status of I-J, which was long thought to be a marker of murine suppressor cells, is at present uncertain.[78] Evidence has been obtained through transfer experiments that clones of T cells may exhibit either suppressor or helper function, depending on the the conditions of the experiment, including the number of cells transferred.[79] If this observation is valid and occurs under other circumstances, it would mean that identification of a cell type with suppressor function in one assay would not be sufficient evidence to exclude other potential functions for that cell. In addition, cells other than T cells, in particular mononuclear phagocytes, may be involved in suppression.[80]

Evidence for a role of suppressor T cells present within inflammatory infiltrates has been obtained in studies of lepromatous leprosy. In this condition there is deficient or absent T cell reactivity to leprae bacilli and lack of granuloma formation. The infiltrates contain relatively few T cells and most of these are CD8[+]. Clones of CD8[+] cells derived from the skin lesions of lepromatous leprosy can suppress the response of CD4[+] T cells to *Mycoplasma leprae*.[81,82] It is reasonable to assume that this type of suppressor function contributes to the paucity of CD4[+] T cells in lepromatous infiltrates, possibly through interference with proliferation of CD4[+] T cells or through their destruction.

Not only has it been difficult to identify cells responsible for suppression, but also to define the mediators involved. Although several suppressor factors have been described, none has been isolated and fully characterized. Undoubtedly, the down-regulation of the immune response is as complex as the induction phase and much more information is needed to elucidate the mechanisms involved.

XI. ANALYSIS OF CELL MEDIATED REACTIONS IN MAN

In many human diseases in which there is reason to implicate immunologic mechanisms, lesions with lymphocytic infiltrates are seen. Although this finding suggests a role of cell mediated mechanisms, further evidence is needed. Obviously, transfer experiments, which have provided crucial evidence in experimental models for the importance of T cells, cannot be performed in man. Three approaches that have been taken to obtain evidence of a role of T cells in human disease are (1) demonstration of *in vitro* correlates of cell mediated immunity (for example, lymphokine production) following interaction of the patient's lymphocytes with putative pathogenic antigens,[83] (2) analysis of the phenotype of infiltrating cells in tissue sections by immunoperoxidase techniques with monoclonal antibodies,[84] and (3) studies of functional properties of cells obtained or propagated from lesions. We now discuss the second and third approaches.

XII. ANALYSIS OF INFILTRATING CELLS BY IMMUNOHISTOCHEMICAL TECHNIQUES

The use of monoclonal antibodies and immunoperoxidase techniques can provide information about the phenotype of mononuclear cells in inflammatory infiltrates.[84] The finding of large numbers of T cells in a lesion, especially cells with activation markers (IL-2 receptor, transferrin receptor, HLA-DR) suggests that the cells are playing an important role, probably in response to an antigen present at the site. Identification of T cell subsets can give further insight into the nature of the reaction. Studies of classical DTH reactions have shown that CD4+ cells are the predominant type of T cell,[85] so that the finding of a preponderance of CD4+ T cells in an infiltrate can be taken as evidence of DTH, especially if there also numerous macrophages. Furthermore, since most nucleated cells bear class I MHC antigens and are targets for CD8+ cell cytolysis, lesions with CD8+ cells in juxtaposition to parenchymal cells undergoing necrosis may be considered as cytolytic T cell reactions; this interpretation is particularly credible in settings such as viral infections[86] or allografts[87] since there is experimental evidence of the role of cytolytic T cells in such reactions.

An example of how analysis of the phenotypes and distribution of infiltrating lymphocytes can reveal evidence for the participation of DTH and cytolytic components in human lesions is provided by studies of allografts. Both CD4+ and CD8+ cells are found in rejecting allografts, and CD8+ cells are often more numerous. Bhan et al.[88] studied skin allografts in nonimmunosuppressed human volunteers and found a predominance of CD4+ T cells in perivascular cuffs (consistent with a DTH component) and a preponderance of CD8+ cells in association with the epidermis and hair follicles (consistent with direct killing of these cells). Similarly, in human renal allografts undergoing rejection, CD4+ cells appear to be more numerous in perivascular aggregates than in peritubular infiltrates and also appear to be especially numerous early in rejection.[89]

Although such interpretations may be valid in general, they cannot be considered conclusive and do not provide a complete picture of cellular events in an inflammatory reaction because of several considerations, some of which have already been discussed. Individual monoclonal antibodies do not adequately discriminate among functional subsets; for example, antibodies that recognize "helper/inducer" T cells also react with some mononuclear phagocytes.[90] Moreover, CD4+ T cells have diverse functions, which include not only the initiation of DTH reactions, but also the induction of suppressor and cytotoxic cells, or, the provision of help in antibody production. In addition, CD4$^+$ T cells can manifest cytotoxic activity against cells bearing certain antigens in association with class II MHC products[30] and can probably act as suppressor effector cells. Similarly, CD8$^+$ cells have diverse functions, including cytolytic effects,[91] suppression,[91] or even initiation of DTH reactions.[3] As discussed later, double positive CD4$^+$/CD8$^+$ cells can be recovered from some infiltrates;[38] unless double staining is performed (which to date has been technically difficult), such cells would be counted as either CD4$^+$ or CD8$^+$ cells in tissue sections. Furthermore, unless repeated observations are made, only a static picture is obtained. Finally, no information is obtained through the use of monoclonal antibodies about the antigen reactivity of the T cells.

XIII. ANALYSIS OF ANTIGEN SPECIFICITY OF T CELLS IN HUMAN INFLAMMATORY INFILTRATES

An approach used some years ago to detect antigen reactive cells in infiltrates was to prepare cells in suspension from large specimens and study the cells *in vitro*. Rejected human renal allografts were investigated in this manner and some of the isolated cells were demonstrated to exhibit "specific" cytotoxicity for donor cells or proliferative responses to donor antigens.[92,93] A major problem with this approach is that large amounts of tissue are required to prepare adequate numbers of cells. A method that makes it possible to obtain large numbers of T cells from small specimens is described next.

XIV. CULTIVATION OF LYMPHOCYTES FROM TISSUE INFILTRATES IN IL-2: USE IN ISOLATION OF ANTIGEN REACTIVE T CELLS

Several years ago methods were developed in this laboratory for the propagation of T lymphocytes from tissue specimens with lymphocytic infiltrates, using IL-2-containing media.[39] The propagated cells can be studied for specific antigen reactivity through measurement of proliferative responses, lymphokine production, or cytotoxic activity.

The approach was based on the finding that IL-2 (formerly known as T cell growth factor) could be used to propagate T lymphocytes. IL-2 reacts preferentially with activated T lymphocytes that express high affinity receptors for this lymphokine.[94] In many inflammatory reactions lymphocytes with "activation" markers, notably class II MHC antigens or IL-2 receptors,[87] have been found; however, it has not always been possible to demonstrate IL-2 receptors on T cells in specimens from which T cells can be grown in IL-2-containing media. This discrepancy is probably due in large part to the fall in IL-2 receptor density (as shown with anti-TAC) before complete loss of IL-2 responsiveness.[95]

The culture method is as follows. Specimens of tissue obtained at surgery are cut into fragments smaller than 1 mm, and are incubated in IL-2-containing medium. Since only very small amounts of tissue are required, preparation of histologic sections for diagnostic purposes is not interfered with. Infiltrating cells begin to migrate from the tissue (Figure 1) within a few days. With the use of heavily infiltrated tissue as many as 10 million cells can be propagated from a cubic millimeter of tissue within 7 to 10 d.

In contrast with what occurs in cultures of lymphocytes in suspension, where IL-2 receptors are usually lost within 1 or 2 weeks, lymphocytes associated with tissue fragments may retain IL-2 responsiveness for more than 3 months. The reason for this is unknown, but it is probable that the continued presence of antigen in tissue plays some role. Even in the environment of tissue, however, lymphocytes eventually become unresponsive to IL-2. Responsiveness of antigen specific lymphocytes can be restored by stimulation with antigen. Stimulation of lymphocytes with a broad range of specificities can be accomplished with polyclonal T cell activators, such as phytohemagglutinin (PHA) or anti-CD3 antibodies.[96,97]

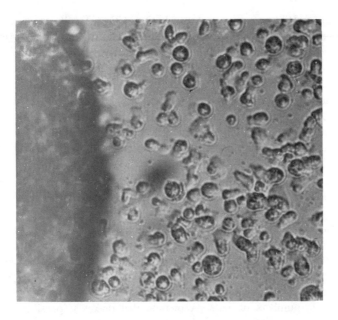

FIGURE 1.   Propagation of activated T lymphocytes from inflamed tissue in IL-2 culture. Three days after establishing culture of allograft biopsy tissue in L-2, extruded mononuclear cells can be seen adjacent to the tissue fragment. As shown by phenotypic analysis the majority of the cells are mature T lymphocytes.

Through the combined use of IL-2 and periodic stimulation with polyclonal activators it is possible to expand cells indefinitely.

There are several limitations to the study of lymphocytes propagated from tissues. First, in order to test for antigen reactivity, relevant antigen(s) must be known (or at least suspected) and available. Second, even though the surface phenotypes of the propagated cells are comparable to the cells found in the tissue,[38] it is not known to what extent the specificities of the populations of cells that grow are representative of those in the infiltrate. Third, the studies can obviously only deal with the cells that grow in IL-2 and cannot provide insight into the contribution of other cells, such as B cells or macrophages, or into the complex interactions among various cell types in the infiltrates.

The method of propagation of T cells in IL-2 has been used to study lymphocytes derived from allografts, tumors, infectious diseases, and autoimmune diseases, both in man and in experimental models.

XV. LYMPHOCYTES PROPAGATED FROM RENAL ALLOGRAFTS

Our initial studies of lymphocytes propagated from tissue dealt with human renal allografts.[38,98] We used biopsy specimens obtained to evaluate rejection or other causes of renal functional impairment. Similar studies have dealt with liver,[99] heart,[100] and heart-lung allografts.[101]

We obtained the following results with renal allografts:[38,39,98]

1. Large numbers of donor reactive T cells were grown from the tissue. In confirmation of other studies, similarly reactive T cells could not be cultured in IL-2 from peripheral blood. These findings indicate that activated alloreactive T cells are concentrated to some degree in the graft.

2. Both CD4$^+$ and CD8$^+$ cells were propagated; in general, the proportion of each type was similar to that found in tissue sections by immunohistochemical procedures.

3. Pure populations of CD8$^+$ cells, which were obtained from the culture by cell sorting, were enriched for cytotoxic activity and were responsive to donor antigens in secondary mixed lymphocyte (MLR) proliferation assays, which indicates the presence of so-called helper-independent cytotoxic cells.

4. Sorted pure CD4$^+$ lymphocytes were largely devoid of cytotoxic activity, but did respond in proliferative assays to donor antigens.

5. Small numbers of CD4$^+$/CD8$^+$ (double positive) lymphocytes were detected and sorted by flow cytometry, using double staining techniques. These cells were CD3$^+$ and were shown to have rearranged T cell β-chain antigen receptor genes. They did not exhibit cytotoxic effects or proliferative responses to donor cells. The CD4$^+$/CD8$^+$ phenotype suggests such cells are immature.

In addition to studies of T cell populations obtained by cell sorting, clones of cells were prepared from some renal allograft specimens.[98] Although most of the results with cloned cells paralleled those obtained with cells prepared by cell sorting, some additional findings were made. Both CD4$^+$ and CD8$^+$ clones but no CD4$^+$/CD8$^+$ clones were isolated. As expected, most of the CD8$^+$ clones but no CD4$^+$/CD8$^+$ clones were isolated. As expected, most of the CD8$^+$ cells were highly cytotoxic for donor cells. In addition, all CD8$^+$ cells were capable of lysing either donor targets, an NK target (the K562 cell line), or both. Since K562 cells lack class I MHC antigens,[102] their interaction with CD8$^+$ cells must occur independently of the MHC-restricted T cell antigen receptor. As might have been predicted from cell sorting experiments, many of the donor-specific cytotoxic CD8$^+$ cells were able to proliferate in response to donor lymphocytes. Among the CD4$^+$ clones, most showed several clones exhibited both cytotoxic and proliferative activities.

Taken together, the results of studies on populations obtained by cell sorting and by cloning support the interpretation (discussed earlier) that both antigen-specific CD4$^+$ and CD8$^+$ cells participate in the rejection of renal allografts. CD8$^+$ cells appear to provide most of the cytotoxic activity against donor cells. CD4$^+$ cells exhibit proliferative responses but less cytolytic activity against donor cells; they may function as inducers of cytotoxic CD8$^+$ cells (although, as noted, some CD8$^+$ cells may proliferate without help from CD4$^+$ cells) or as initiators of DTH reactions.

What information do the studies on IL-2 propagated lymphocytes provide about the percentages of specifically sensitized lymphocytes in the infiltrates of renal allografts? Clearly, the findings show that specifically reactive cells are present in greater concentrations in the tissue than in the blood. Beyond that, in two clonings,[98] it was found that 67% of IL-2 responsive clones prepared after 14 d of culture were donor reactive. It may be asked whether donor reactive cells grow more rapidly than other T cells in the infiltrate, especially since donor tissue is present in the culture. In another experiment, however, cloning was performed using PHA expansion 24 h after initiation of the cultures, and approximately 50% of the clones were found to be donor reactive. In this experiment, care was taken to use irradiated antigen presenting cells from a third individual who shared no known HLA antigens with the allograft donor; thus, the high percentage of donor reactive cells was not merely the result of a secondary MLR *in vitro*. Although precise percentages cannot be determined, the findings provide impressive evidence for the presence of appreciable numbers of specifically sensitized cells in the graft.

As discussed earlier, a number of transfer experiments have failed to provide evidence of preferential emigration of sensitized cells in cell mediated reactions. These experiments were designed to measure cells emigrating at the inflamed site, however, and did not measure the effects of local proliferation of sensitized cells in the presence of the relevant antigen.

Thus, the findings with propagated cells and in transfer studies are not necessarily contradictory.

XVI. TUMOR INFILTRATING LYMPHOCYTES

The role of the immune response in containment of tumors has stimulated the imagination and frustrated the hopes of immunologists for many years. Early experimental studies showed that rejection of transplanted tumors is often associated with mononuclear cell infiltration.[103] Although many of the early studies dealt with allogeneic tumors whose destruction resulted from allograft rejection, it was learned in the 1950s that inbred strains of mice were capable of rejecting certain syngeneic or autologous tumors against which they had previously been immunized. These and subsequent experiments led to the concept that effective tumor immunity depends on recognition of tumor-associated antigens on the surface of neoplastic cells. The antigen need not be unique for tumors, but would have to be concentrated on the cells in order to lead to selective tumor destruction. With certain experimental tumors it has been shown that transfer of T cells can retard tumor growth;[104] as with allografts, there is evidence that both DTH and cytolytic T cell components are involved.

The relevance of these experimental studies to neoplasms that arise spontaneously is not clear. Obviously, malignant tumors are generally not destroyed by the immune response. Nevertheless, experimental studies indicate that T cell immune reactions occurring at the tumor site may be capable of retarding tumor growth or even eliminating certain tumors. We focus our futher discussion on the nature and possible role of lymphocytes found at human tumor sites.

In many forms of human nonlymphoid malignant tumors histologic examination reveals mononuclear cells infiltrates adjacent to or invading the tumor mass. Many of the mononuclear cells appear to be lymphocytes. A few neoplasms, notably seminomas and medullary breast carcinomas, consistently show intense infiltration, but with most types of tumors the intensity varies considerably from one patient to another, or even in different sites in the same patients. Numerous attempts have been made to correlate the behavior of tumors with the degree of lymphocytic infiltration; although some findings suggest that an intense lymphocytic infiltrate is associated with a relatively favorable prognosis, with most tumors the results have not been consistent. Melanomas are one form of neoplasm in which there is compelling evidence that intense lymphocytic infiltration is associated with a favorable prognosis.[105]

In vitro studies of lymphocytes obtained from tumor sites have also supported the notion that an immune response can help restrain certain neoplasms. Vanky et al.[106] studied the ability of lymphocytes derived from lung cancers to kill autologous tumor cells and concluded that those few patients whose lymphocytes reacted with their own tumors had a relatively favorable prognosis. With the recognition that soluble factors control the growth, differentiation, and activation of lymphocytes, further studies were performed which showed that the cocultivation of tumor with autologous lymphocytes (especially in the presence of added IL-2) could lead to an enhanced mixed tumor-lymphocyte reaction and generation of specific cytotoxic T lymphocytes.[107] Such findings argue in favor of the immune system's intrinisic ability to mount a response to the tumor, perhaps as the result of lymphokine activating signals (such as IL-2).

Why does the generation of effective cytolytic lymphocytes generally fail to occur *in vivo*? Several factors have been reported to hamper the immune response to tumors. For one thing, many tumor cells may lack autoimmunogenic antigens. Furthermore, potentially immunogenic antigens may be masked by "blocking" antibodies.[108] Even when tumor-associated antigens are "recognized", tumor cells may fail to trigger T cell activation. For example, if the antigens are not "processed" by antigen presenting cells, induction of IL-2 may not occur owing to a lack of IL-1 and a failure in the expansion of lymphocytes capable of recognizing tumor cells will result.[109] Furthermore, tumors may secrete nonspecific suppressor factors, which inhibit mixed tumor-lymphocyte reaction *in vitro* and result in immunosuppression *in vivo,* as shown by loss of previous DTH reactivity. Such factors have been described in sera and ascitic fluid, as well as in the culture medium from tumors carried *in vitro.*[110]

The combination of the observations that some tumors contain cytotoxic lymphocytes, and that IL-2 enhances the responsiveness of lymphocytes to tumors, led to attempts to isolate and propagate tumor-infiltrating lymphocytes in IL-2. We showed that the culture of lymphocyte-containing tumor fragments in IL-2 leads to the outgrowth of activated T lymphocytes.[111] In our subsequent studies of over 50 tumors, failure to obtain outgrowth of T lymphocytes occurred with only one specimen, a recently irradiated tumor mass; however, the rate at which lymphocytes could be propagated has varied greatly among different specimens and has depended, at least in part, on the intensity of the infiltrate.

Among T cells propagated from lung tumors the CD8[+] subset usually predominated. The lymphocytes were active in cytotoxicity assays against the NK target K562 cell line. The lymphocytes were also able to produce IL-2 and IFN-γ when stimulated with PHA. Limited studies have been performed to detect cytolytic activity of the propagated lymphocytes against tumor cells. Using a small cell carcinoma cell line, it was not possible to demonstrate lytic activity by lymphocytes derived from any of six lung tumors. In one case, however, in which autologous adenocarcinoma tumor cells were propagated *in vitro,* it was found that the lymphocytes showed cytolytic activity against the autologous tumor. Despite this, the tumor cells did not induce proliferation or lymphokine production by the autologous lymphocytes, which indicates that certain activation pathways were not triggered by the tumor.[111]

Any discussion of IL-2 activation of lymphocytes involved in tumor reactivity would be remiss in not mentioning the ability of this lymphokine to induce a group of broadly reactive cytotoxic cells referred to as lymphokine activated killer (LAK) cells.[112] It does not appear that LAK cells represent a single cell lineage, but rather a group of lymphocytes with cytotoxic activity against a variety of cell types, including tumor cells;[113] in this respect they resemble cells with NK activity. Like cells with NK activity, LAK cells can somehow discriminate between normal and malignant cells. It is not known what receptors or target antigens are involved in LAK activity; however, both the susceptibility to lysis of the K562 target, which does not express MHC antigens, and the ability of CD3-negative cells to lyse tumor targets emphasize the need to invoke recognition systems in addition to the MHC-restricted T cell antigen receptor. These considerations do not eliminate the possibility that cytolytic T lymphocytes are included in LAK populations since, as noted above, such cells can exhibit both MHC-restricted and LAK/NK lytic capacities.[98]

Tumor infiltrating lymphocytes propagated in IL-2 have recently been used therapeutically in conjunction with IL-2. Some tumors, notably melanoma and renal cell carcinomas, have responded to therapy with IL-2 and LAK[114] or tumor infiltrating lymphocytes,[115] with appreciable reduction of tumor mass; however, the specific *in vivo* activities of the various cell types and lymphokines injected or induced remain undeciphered. Of note is that activated T lymphocytes may not traffic appropriately *in vivo*; thus, studies in animals[116] and man[117] indicate that the majority of systemically transferred lymphocytes accumulate in the lungs, liver, and spleen and do not concentrate in tumor sites. Nevertheless, significant tumor reduction *in vivo* has been noted both in mice[117] and men treated with IL-2 propagated tumor infiltrating cells.[115,118] It is possible that a few cells reach the tumor site and produce effects through recruitment of host cells. In cases of cutaneous melanomas undergoing regression following transfer of tumor infiltrating lymphocytes, we have observed intense mononuclear cell infiltrates, with predominance of T lymphocytes; in this situation most of the infiltrating lymphocytes are almost certainly recruited in the host. A marked vasculitis in some tumors following transfer of tumor infiltrating cells suggests that a vascular target may be important in tumor rejection, as in some forms of allograft rejection.[115]

XVII. EXPERIMENTAL PYELONEPHRITIS

The method of *in vitro* cultivation of infiltrating lymphocytes has also been used to study T cell reactivity in a model of ascending pyelonephritis in rats induced with *Escherichia coli*[119] or *Pseudomonas aeruginosa*. Large numbers of T cells appeared in the renal infiltrate after several days. Immunohistochemical studies showed a predominance of cells with the inducer/helper phenotype (W3/25), although cells with the cytotoxic suppressor phenotype (OX8) were also found. The IL-2 responsive T cells propagated from day 8 pyelonephritic lesions were enriched for W3/25$^+$ T cells and showed a proliferative response to *E. coli*, but not to unrelated organisms. It is reasonable to assume that the W3/25$^+$ T cells in the infiltrate function to help in the production of antibodies against *E. coli* (which would be beneficial) or to induce a DTH reaction (which would probably serve no protective purpose and might be harmful). Obviously, both mechanisms might occur. Some of the lymphocytes, especially OX8$^+$ cells, may also function to mediate killing of the invading bacteria through a recently described mechanism. Markham et al.[36] have reported that murine Ly1$^-$, 2$^+$ I-J$^+$ T cells can kill Gram negative bacteria, apparently through the action of a lymphokine.

XVIII. AUTOIMMUNITY: THYROIDITIS, DIABETES MELLITUS

IL-2 has also been used successfully to propagate activated T lymphocytes from specimens of Grave's disease and Hashimoto's thyroiditis.[120,121] The lymphocytes were shown to react with thyroglobulin and/or autologous thyroid epithelial cells. Exposure of cultured thyroid epithelial cells to IFN-γ greatly enhances the stimulatory capacity of the cells, probably due to enhanced induction of class II antigens.[122]

In the nonobese diabetic mouse, inflamed islets contain activated T-lymphocytes which can be transferred into prediabetic animals to induce an accelerated diabetic state. Both CD4$^+$ and CD8$^+$ cells are required to induce diabetes in these mice.[123]

XIX. ARTHRITIS: T CELL ANTIGEN RECEPTOR GENE REARRANGEMENT AS A MEANS TO ASSESS CLONALITY OF TISSUE INFILTRATING LYMPHOCYTES

Examination of T cell antigen receptor gene rearrangement offers another means by which T cells propagated from tissue infiltrates can be examined. Southern blot analysis with cDNA probes for the receptor gene makes it possible to detect clones of T cells, provided sufficient numbers of the lymphocytes belong to a given clone.[124] We have used this approach to investigate T cells in rheumatoid synovia.

Rheumatoid arthritis is an important disease in which immunologic mechanisms appear to play a role, although the nature of the immune events and pathogenic antigens remain unknown. There is a growing belief that T cells are of importance. Rheumatoid synovial membranes are characterized by infiltrates of lymphocytes, including numerous activated CD4$^+$ T cells.[125,126] It is likely that some of these provide help for the production of anti-IgG antibodies, but the antigen reactivity of other T cells is unknown. We undertook studies to determine if T cells derived from rheumatoid synovia and propagated in IL-2 were oligoclonal. The possibility that there may be limited diversity in the immune response to antigens that are important in rheumatoid arthritis is suggested by evidence that anti-IgG (rheumatoid factor) antibodies may have a restricted heterogeneity.[127] Moreover, there is

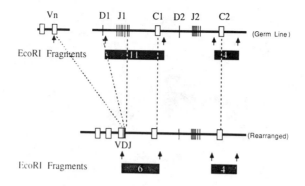

FIGURE 2. Schematic of T cell antigen receptor β gene rearrangement. In the upper scheme, the germline pattern of the β-chain of the T cell antigen receptor is shown as a set of V region genes (Vn) distant from the D, J, and C region genes. If the germline gene is cut with EcoR1 restriction endonuclease and blotted with a probe for the C region of the β-chain (hybridizes with both $C_\beta 1$ and $C_\beta 2$ regions) two fragments are generated at 11 and 4 kb; these correspond to restriction sites, including the $C_\beta 1$ region (11 kb fragment) and $C_\beta 2$ region (4 kb fragment). In a mature T lymphocyte the rearranged β-chain gene shows the V region gene now adjacent to the D, J, and C regions with resultant loss of the restriction site near D1. Instead of the 11 kb fragment a new fragment size is generated (6 kb in this example) while the $C_\beta 2$ fragment (at 4 kb) is unchanged. The use of different V, D, or J region segments results in different size fragments, which replace the 11 kb germline pattern.

evidence that the T cell response is often characterized by recognition of relatively few epitopes, even in complex antigens, in contrast to most B cell responses.[128]

The basis for detection of rearrangements of the T cell antigen receptor β-chain gene complex is as follows.[129] When the restriction endonuclease, EcoR1, is used to digest germline DNA, which is then electrophoresed, blot transferred, and hybridized with a Cβ probe, two fragments are revealed (11 and 4.2 kb), which correspond to Cβ1 and Cβ2 (see Figure 2). A mature T lymphocyte has both copies (maternal and paternal) of the β-chain rearranged; as a result, the 11 kb band is lost; the 4.2 kb band is unchanged. In the case of a highly heterogeneous population of T lymphocytes, in which there are many different β-chain rearrangements, only the 4.2 kb band is detected (see Figure 3); the 11 kb band is replaced by a homogeneous smear resulting from the rearrangement of many different genes.[130] However, if the population of cells contains a clone that accounts for more than 5% of the cells with rearrangement of the V-D-J segment, to Cβ1, a new band can be detected. Other endonucleases, such as HindIII, which cut at different nucleotide sequences, can be used to detect additional rearrangements.

T cells were propagated from synovial specimens obtained at synovectomy or joint replacement.[131] We studied specimens from patients with a clinical diagnosis of rheumatoid arthritis or osteoarthritis; however, one specimen from a patient clinically diagnosed as osteoarthritis showed an inflammatory reaction consistent with rheumatoid arthritis. EcoR1 digests of DNA from lymphocytes propagated from 13 of 14 synovial specimens (11 from patients with rheumatoid arthritis and 2 with osteoarthritis) revealed loss of the 11 kb germline band and the appearance of 1 to 3 new rearranged bands. The remaining specimen (from a patient with osteoarthritis) contained only the residual 4.2 kb band. HindIII digests demonstrated additional rearranged bands in some samples.

The results indicate that the IL-2 responsive T cells propagated from chronically inflamed

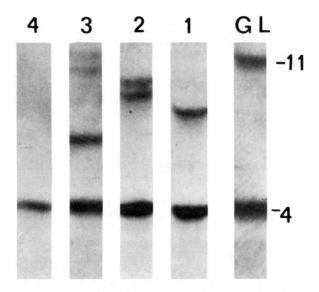

FIGURE 3.   Southern blot of synovial T lymphocytes hybridized with
C_β probe. An EcoR1 digest of DNA from hepatocytes (GL = germline), or samples of T lymphocytes propagated from inflamed synovia
(lanes 1-4). The GL pattern shows both 11 and 4 kb fragments corresponding to the $C_\beta 1$ and $C_\beta 2$ regions, while lane 1 shows a population
containing a dominant clone which gives rise to a newly rearranged
band smaller than the 11 kb germline band. Lane 2 shows a pattern
with two new rearranged bands, which either correspond to a single
dominant clone in which there is an expressed and nonexpressed rearrangement, or reflects two different clones in which there are deletions
of the nonexpressed β-chain genes. Lane 3 shows three new bands
(two faint and one strong) in which there must be at least two dominant
clones (one that shows both expressed and nonexpressed rearrangements, and a second which shows only one rearrangement), or perhaps
three different "dominant" clones. Lane 4 shows a "polyclonal" population of T lymphocytes in which the 11 kb band is lost and no distinct
band is present in its place. This is the pattern seen when no population
with greater than 5% of the cultured cells is present as a clone. (Blots
courtesy of Dr. Ivan Stamenkovic.)

synovia are characterized by the presence of a few "dominant clones". We use the term
"dominant" since many other clones are probably present among the propagated cells, but
because each of these nondominant clones is represented by so few copies, rearrangement
of their T cell receptor genes results in no distinct bands.

In those samples in which three rearranged bands were detected it appears that more
than one dominant clone was present. Two rearranged bands could represent two clones; it
is also possible, however, that two bands represent a productive and nonproductive rearrangement of a single clone, since only one allele appears to be expressed in a given cell.[132]
Ongoing studies using V region probes indicate that at least some of the dominant bands
are associated with productive rearrangements which contain the V-D-J-C segments.

In the 14 samples examined no consistent restriction fragment size was noted in different
patients; this does not provide evidence as to whether the dominant clones obtained from
various patients are reactive with the same or different antigens. On the one hand, T
lymphocytes may use different C_β gene segments for the recognition of a given antigen,
and on the other hand T lymphocytes with different antigen specificities sometimes utilize
the same V_β gene segment.[133] It is noteworthy that in one instance where two synovial

samples were obtained from two joints from the same patient, the EcoR1 digested DNA showed the same rearranged bands.

There are two general interpretations of the finding that T cells propagated from rheumatoid synovia are oligo- or monoclonal. One is that the results reflect an *in vitro* artifact, due to rapid outgrowth of a limited number of cells. However, there is evidence that the culture conditions used do not automatically select for subsets of lymphocytes with potential for unusually rapid growth. Thus, T lymphocytes isolated from the peripheral blood and stimulated with a variety of polyclonal activators or specific antigens *in vitro* before propagation in IL-2 failed to give rise to dominant clones even after more than 3 months in culture. The second possibility is that the clones detected *in vitro* are present as dominant clones in the synovial infiltrates. Direct evidence for the *in vivo* presence of these "dominant" clones might be obtained by immunohistochemical studies, using anticlonotypic antibodies prepared against cultured clones. Another approach would be to study DNA of lymphocytes obtained directly from synovial tissue for rearrangements of β-chain genes; so far we have not been able to obtain sufficient tissue to perform such studies.

If the synovial infiltrates *in situ* indeed contain very few dominant clones, and if these are antigen reactive rather than immunoregulatory cells, the findings would indicate that most of the activated T cells in the infiltrate recognize a small number of antigenic determinants. As noted earlier, T cells, which recognize linear peptide sequences on antigens, may react with a relatively limited number of epitopes, even on complex exongeous antigens such as ovalbumin.[128] Perhaps in general, the T cell repertoire would be even more limited for autologous than exogenous antigens. Whatever the diversity of response to the antigens that might be involved initially, there might be selection forces favoring the development of dominant clones in rheumatoid synovia and perhaps in other chronic inflammatory reactions. Weiss et al.[134,135] have reported the findings that some clinically benign skin lesions contain dominant T lymphocyte clonal rearrangements and have taken this as evidence of a lymphoproliferative disorder; however, our findings indicate that the demonstration of dominant T cell clones cannot be taken as conclusive evidence of T cell malignancy.

XX. CONCLUDING REMARKS

We have discussed the events and mechanisms of cell mediated reactions *in vivo*. Early studies revealed that reactions are triggered by the interaction of a small number of specifically sensitized T cells and antigen. This crucial antigen-specific step leads to the activation of T cells, with production and release of lymphokines and a remarkable amplication of the reaction, with recruitment of a wide variety of leukocytes. Recent development of knowledge of lymphokines and monokines, and in particular the availability of recombinant products, has facilitated investigation of their role *in vivo*. Yet it is clear that dissection of events occurring *in vivo* is remarkably difficult, since one cytokine may induce the formation or suppression of other cytokines. Furthermore, as with many biological systems, the role of one lymphokine that ordinarily predominates in a certain type of reaction can be replaced by alternative pathways.

There are similar difficulties in the analysis of the complex interactions between cells that occur in cell mediated reactions, which may depend not only on cytokines but also on direct cell contact. The availability of "pure" populations of T cells (including T cell subsets) has helped define their role *in vivo*; nevertheless, as we have discussed, transfer studies are difficult to interpret because of recruitment of host cells into the reaction.

The use of recently developed monoclonal antibodies with immunoperoxidase techniques has made it possible to identify various types of lymphocytes and other mononuclear cells in tissue sections and has helped clarify reactions *in vivo*. However, there are two serious limitations to these studies: (1) phenotypes of T cells that can be identified with currently available antibodies do not adequately define function and (2) there is no information about the antigen reactivity of the T cells. Since antigen initiates and in some conditions perpetuates cell mediated reactions, this limitation is crucial.

Progress in immunohistochemical studies should be forthcoming with the use of monoclonal antibodies that recognize functional subsets within the CD8$^+$ and CD4$^+$ T cell populations. For example, CD4$^+$ T cells can be divided into 2H4$^+$ and 4B4$^+$ subsets, which function as inducers of CD8$^+$ suppressor cells[6] or as inducers of helper cells, respectively.[136] However, since the 2H4 and 4B4 antigens are not restricted to CD4$^+$ T cells, double staining techniuqes will be required to identify individual cells within infiltrates. In addition, the development of new technologies, including *in situ* molecular hybridization with probes for transcribed messenger RNA, should allow detection of activation markers and individual lymphokines in tissue-infiltrating lymphocytes.

The development of methods for propagation of activated T cells from tissue specimens (even from small biopsies) in IL-2-containing media has provided a means to obtain sufficient T cells to permit study of their antigen reactivities *in vitro*. Using this approach evidence has been obtained for the presence of appreciable numbers of specifically sensitized cells in several reactions as, for example, donor reactive T cells in renal allografts. The findings suggest that there is considerable local concentration of specifically sensitized cells, which probably results from local proliferation (since reactions are apparently triggered by very small numbers of such cells).

Obviously, to study cultivated cells for antigen specificity, relevant antigens must be used. In several important chronic diseases in which T cells are thought to play a crucial role, knowledge of pathogenic antigens is lacking. An example is rheumatoid arthritis; although this is widely believed to be an autoimmune disease, relevant autologous antigens have not been identified (anti-IgG and antinuclear antibodies are often found, but these are probably not crucial to the development of the principal lesion, synovitis). A method that may help characterize T cells in such conditions, although it will not directly lead to identification of antigen specificities, is examination of rearrangements of T cell antigen receptor genes. This approach has revealed dominant clones among T cells cultivated from rheumatoid synovia. The full significance of this finding remains to be investigated, but it raises the possibility that down-regulation of the dominant clones might ameliorate the damage they may mediate. The possibility that there is limited heterogeneity of the T cell response in many inflammatory disease processes suggests a role for clonally directed immunoregulatory intervention.

On a more general note, progress in basic immunology will undoubtedly lead to a more complete understanding of cell mediated reactions *in vivo*. Of particular importance may be the further unravelling at the molecular level of the nature of the interactions between the T cell antigen receptor complex and the processed antigen-Ia complex, and of interactions between cells and lymphokines.

REFERENCES

1. **Dvorak, H. F., Galli, S. J., and Dvorak, A. M.,** Cellular and vascular manifestations of cell-mediated immunity, *Hum. Pathol.,* 17, 122, 1986.
2. **Scheynius, A., Klareskog, L., and Forsum, U.,** *In situ* identification of T lymphocyte subsets and HLA-DR expressing cells in the human skin tuberculin reaction, *Clin. Exp. Immunol.,* 49, 325, 1982.
3. **Lin, Y. L. and Askonas, B. A.,** Biological properties of an influenza A virus-specific killer T cell clone. Inhibition of virus replication *in vivo* and induction of delayed-type hypersensitivity reactions, *J. Exp. Med.,* 154, 225, 1981.

4. **Killar, L., MacDonald, G., West, J., Woods, A., and Bottomly, A.,** Cloned, Ia-restricted T cells that do not produce interleukin 4(IL 4)/B cell stimulatory factor 1(BSF-1) fail to help antigen-specific B cells, *J. Immunol.,* 138, 1674, 1987.

5. **Mosmann, T. R., Cherwinski, H., Bond, M. W., Giedlin, M. A., and Coffman, R. L.,** Two types of murine helper T cell clone. I. Definition according to profiles of lymphokine activities and secreted proteins, *J. Immunol.,* 136, 2348, 1986.

6. **Morimoto, C., Letvin, N. L., Distaso, J. A., Aldrich, W. R., and Schlossman, S. F.,** The isolation and characterization of the human suppressor inducer T cell subset, *J. Immunol.,* 134, 1508, 1985.

7. **McCluskey, R. T. and Leber, P. D.,** Cell mediated reactions *in vivo,* in *Mechanisms of Cell-Mediated Immunity,* McCluskey, R. T. and Cohen, S., Eds., John Wiley & Sons, New York, 1974, 1.

8. **Cohen, S.,** Physiologic and pathologic manifestations of lymphokine action, *Hum. pathol.,* 17, 112, 1986.

9. **Cotran, R. S. and Pober, J. S.,** Effects of cytokines on vascular endothelium: their role in vascular and immune injury, *Kidney Int.,* 35, 969, 1989.

10. **Cavender, D., Haskard, D., Yu, C. L., Iguchi, T., Miossec, P., Oppenheimer-Marks, N., and Ziff, M.,** Pathways to chronic inflammation in rheumatoid synovitis, *Fed. Proc.,* 46, 113, 1987.

11. **Godfrey, H. P., Angadi, C. V., Haak-Frendscho, M., and Kaplan, A. P.,** Concurrent production of macrophage agglutination factor and factor VII by antigen-stimulated human peripheral blood mononuclear cells, *Immunology,* 57, 77, 1986.

12. **Edgington, T. S., Curtiss, L. K., and Plow, E. F.,** A linkage between the hemostatic and immune systems embodied in the fibrinolytic release of lymphocyte suppressive peptides, *J. Immunol.,* 134, 471, 1985.

13. **Clark, R. A., DellaPelle, P., Manseau, E., Lanigan, J. M., Dvorak, H. F., and Colvin, R. B.,** Blood vessel fibronectin increases in conjunction with endothelial cell proliferation and capillary in growth during wound healing, *J. Invest. Dermatol.,* 79, 269, 1982.

14. **Sy, M. S., Schneeberger, E., McCluskey, R., Greene, M. I., Rosenberg, R. D., and Benacerraf, B.,** Inhibition of delayed-type hypersensitivity by heparin depleted of anti-coagulant activity, *Cell. Immunol.,* 82, 23, 1983.

15. **Unanue, E. R. and Bennacerraf, B.,** Immunological events in experimental hypersensitivity granulomas, *Am. J. Pathol.,* 71, 379, 1973.

16. **Stashenko, P. P., Bhan, A. K., Schlossman, S. F., and McCluskey, R. T.,** Local transfer of delayed hypersensitivity and cutaneous basophil hypersensitivity, *J. Immunol.,* 119, 1987, 1977.

17. **Sobel, R. A., Hanzakos, J. L.,Blanchette, B. W., Williams, A. M.,** Dellapelle, P., and Colvin, R. B., Anti-T cell monoclonal antibodies *in vivo.* I. Inhibition of delayed hypersensitivity but not cutaneous basophil hypersensitivity reactions, *J. Immunol.,* 138, 2500, 1987.

18. **Askenase, P. W.,** Cutaneous basophil hypersensitivity in contact-sensitized guinea pigs. I. Transfer with immune serume, *J. Exp. Med.,* 138, 1144, 1973.

19. **Tamaki, K., Fujiwara, H., Levy, R. B., Shearer, G. M., and Katz, S. I.,** Hapten specific TNP-reactive cytotoxic effector cells using epidermal cells as targets, *J. Invest. Dermatol.,* 77, 225, 1981.

20. **Sunday, M. E. and Dorf, M. E.,** Hapten-specific T cell response to 4-hydroxy-3-nitrophenyl acetyl. X. Characterization of distinct T cell subsets mediating cutaneous sensitivity responses, *J. Immunol.,* 127, 766, 1981.

21. **Cohen, S. and Ward, P. A.,** *In vitro* and *in vivo* activity of a lymphocyte and immune complex-dependent chemotactic factor for eosinophils, *J. Exp. Med.,* 133, 133, 1971.

22. **Colley, D. G.,** Eosinophils and immune mechanisms, *J. Immunol.,* 110, 1419, 1973.

23. **Moreau, J. F., Bonneville, M., Peyrat, M. A., Jacques, Y., and Souillou, J. P.,** Capacity of alloreactive human T clones to produce factor(s) inducing proliferation of the IL3-dependent DA-1 murine cell line. I. Evidence that this production is under IL2 control, *Ann. Inst. Pasteur Immunol.,* 137, 25, 1986.

24. **Kradin, R. L., Kurnick, J. T., Preffer, F. I., Dubinett, S. M., Dickersin, G. R., Millin, J., Pinto, C., and Boyle, L. A.,** The induction of immediate hypersensitivity skin test reponses in cancer patients receiving adoptive transfers of autologous tumor-infiltrating lymphocytes and recombinant IL 2, *Clin. Immunol. Immunopathol.,* 50, 184, 1989.

25. **Kranz, D. M., Pasternack, M. S., and Eisen, H. N.,** Recognition and lysis of target cells by cytotoxic T lymphocytes, *Fed. Proc.,* 46, 309, 1987.

26. **Pasternack, M. S. and Eisen, H. N.,** A novel serine esterase expressed by cytotoxic T lympocytes, *Nature,* 314, 743, 1985.

27. **Young, J. D. E., Damiano, A., DiNome, M. A., Leong, L. G., and Cohn, Z. A.,** Dissociation of membrane binding and lytic activities of the lymphocyte pore-forming protein (perforin), *J. Exp. Med.,* 165, 1371, 1987.

28. **Patterson, S., Byrne, J. A., Lampert, P. W., and Oldstone, M. B. A.,** Morphologic analysis of the interactions between lymphocytic choriomeningitis virus-specific cloned cytotoxic T cells and virus infected targets, *Lab. Invest.,* 57, 29, 1987.

29. **Meuer, S. C., Schlossman, S. F., and Reinherz, E. L.,** Clonal analysis of human cytotoxic T lymphocyte: T4 and T8 effector TR cells recognize products of different major histocompatibility regions, *Proc. Natl. Acad. Sci. U.S.A.,* 79, 4385, 1982.

30. **Krensky, A. M., Clayberger, C., Reiss, C. S., Strominger, J. L., Burakoff, S. J.,** Specificity of OKT4+ cytotoxic T lymphocyte clones, *J. Immunol.,* 129, 2001, 1982.

31. **von Boehmer, H., Kisielow, P., Leiserson, W., and Haas, W.,** Lyt-2 cell-independent functions of Lyt-2+ cells stimulated with antigen or concanavalin A, *J. Immunol.,* 133, 59, 1984.

32. **Buller, R. M. L., Holmes, K. L., Hugin, A., Frederickson, T. N. and Morse, H. C.,** III, Induction of cytotoxic T cell responses *in vivo* in the absence of CD4 helper cells, *Nature,* 328, 77, 1987.

33. **Zinkernagel, R. M., Haenseler, W., Leist, T., Cerny, M., Hengartner, H., and Althage, A.,** T cell-mediated hepatitis in mice infected with lymphocytic chorimeningitis virus, *J. Exp. Med.,* 164, 1075, 1986.

34. **Paronetto, F.,** Cell-mediated immunity in liver disease, *Hum. Pathol.,* 17, 168, 1986.

35. **Woan-Chen, M. and McGregor, D. D.,** The mediators of acquired resistance to listeria monocytogenes are contained within a population of cytotoxic T cells, *Cell Immunol.,* 87, 538, 1984.

36. **Markham, R. B., Pier, G. B., Goellner, J. J., and Mizel, S. B.,** *In vitro* T cell-mediated killing of *Pseudomonas aeruginosa.* II. The role of macrophages and T cell subsets in T cell killing, *J. Immunol.,* 134, 4112, 1985.

37. **Zinkernagel, R. M., Pfau, C. J., Hengartner, H., and Althage, A.,** A model for MHC-disease associations: susceptibility to murine lymphocytic choriomeningitis maps to class I MHC genes and correlates with LCMV-specific cytotoxic T cell activity, *Nature,* 316, 814, 1985.

38. **Preffer, F. I., Colvin, R. B., Leary, C. P., Boyle, L. A., Tuazon, T. A., Lazarovitis, A. I., Cosimi, A. B., and Kurnick, J. T.,** Two-color flow cytometry and functional analysis of lymphocytes cultured from human renal allografts: identification of Leu-2+3+ subpopulation, *J. Immunol.,* 137, 2823, 1986.

39. **Mayer, T. G., Fuller, A. A., Lazarovitis, A. I., Boyle, L. A., and Kurnick, J. T.,** Characterization of *in-vivo*-activated allospecific T lymphocytes propagated from human renal allograft biopsies undergoing rejection, *J. Immunol.,* 134, 258, 1985.

40. **Prendergast, R. A.,** Cellular immunity in the homograft reaction, *J. Exp. Med.,* 119, 377, 1964.

41. **Amento, E. P., Bhalla, A. K., Kurnick, J. T., Kradin, R., Clemens, T. L., Holick, S. A., Holick, M. F., and Krane, S. M.,** 25-Dihydroxyvitamin D3 induces maturation of the human monocyte cell line, U937, and in association with a factor from human T lymphocytes, augments production of the monokine, mononuclear cell factor, *J. Clin. Invest.,* 132, 2244, 1984.

42. **Burakoff, S. J.,** Cell-mediated cytology: an overview, *Fed. Proc.,* 46, 307, 1987.

43. **Steinmuller, D.,** Which T cells mediate allograft rejection, *Transplantation,* 40, 571, 1985.

44. **Rosenberg, A. S., Mizuochi, T., Sharrow, S., and Singer, A.,** Phenotype, Specificity and function of T cell subsets and T cell interactions involved in skin allograft rejection, *J. Exp. Med.,* 165, 1296, 1987.

45. **Loveland, B. E., Hogarth, P. M., Ceredig, R., and McKenzie, I. F. C.,** Cells mediating graft rejection in the mouse. I. Lyt-1 cells mediate skin graft rejection, *J. Exp. Med.,* 153, 1044, 1981.

46. **Le Francois, L. and Bevan, M. J.,** A reexamination of the role of LyT-2-positive T cells in murine skin graft rejection, *J. Exp. Med.,* 159, 57, 1984.

47. **Allen, J. E., Doherty, P. C., and Allan, J. E.,** Natural killer cells contribute to inflammation but do not appear to be essential for the induction of clinical lymphocytic choriomeningitis, *Scand. J. Immunol.,* 24, 153, 1986.

48. **Jalkanen, S., Steere, A. C., Fox, R. I., and Butcher, E. C.,** A distinct endothelial cell recognition system that controls lymphocyte traffic into inflamed synovium, *Science,* 233, 556, 1986.

49. **Pober, J. S., Gimbrone, M. A., Jr., Lapierre, L. A., Mendrick, D. L., Fiers, W., Rothlein, R., Springer, T. A.,** Overlapping patterns of activation of human endothelial cells by interleukin 1, tumor necrosis factor, and immune interferon, *J. Immunol.,* 137, 1893, 1986.

50. **Cavender, D., Haskard, D., Foster, N., and Ziff, M.,** Superinduction of T lymphocyte endothelial cell (EC) binding by treatment of EC with interleukin 1 and protein synthesis inhibitors, *J. Immunol.,* 138, 2149, 1987.

51. **Cotran, R. S., Gimbrone, M. A., Bevilacqua, M. P., Mendrick, D. L., and Pober, J. S.,** Induction and detection of a human endothelial activation antigen *in vivo, J. Exp. Med.,* 164, 661, 1986.

52. **Werdelin, O. and McCluskey, R. T.,** The nature of the specificity of mononuclear cells in experimental autoimmune inflammation and the mechanisms leading to their accumulation, *J. Exp. Med.,* 133, 1242, 1971.

53. **Asherson, G. L. and Allwood, G. G.,** Inflammatory lymphoid cells: cells in immunized lymph nodes that move to sites of inflammations, *Immunology,* 22, 493, 1972.

54. **Pober, J. S., Ginbrone, M. A., Jr., Cotran, R. S., Reiss, C. S., Burakoff, S. J., Fiers, W., and Ault, K. A.,** Ia expression by vascular endothelium is induced by activated T cells and by human gamma interferon, *J. Exp. Med.,* 157, 1339, 1983.

55. **Masuyama, J., Minato, N., and Kano, S.,** Mechanisms of lymphocyte adhesion to human vascular endothelial cells in culture, *J. Clin. Invest.,* 77, 1596, 1986.

56. **Clark, R. A., Horsburgh, C. R., Hoffman, A. A., Dvorak, H. F., Mosesson, M. W., and Colvin, R. B.,** Fibronectin deposition in delayed-type hypersensitivity. Reactions of normals and a patient with afibrinogenemia, *J. Clin. Invest.,* 74, 1011, 1984.

57. **Springer, T. A., Dustin, M. L., Kishimoto, T. K., and Marlin, S. D.,** The lymphocyte function associated LFA-1, CD2, and LFA-3 molecules: cell adhesion receptors of the immune system, *Annu. Rev. Immunol.,* 5, 223, 1987.

58. **Haskard, D., Cavender, D., and Ziff, M.,** Phorbol ester-stimulated T lymphocytes show enhanced adhesion to human endothelial cell monolayers, *J. Immunol.,* 137, 1429, 1986.

59. **Mibu, Y., Shimokaway, Y., and Hayashi, H.,** Lymphocyte chemotaxis in inflammation. X. Heterogeneity of chemotactic responsiveness in human T subsets towards lymphocyte chemotactic factors from delayed hypersensitivity reaction site, *Immunology,* 55, 473, 1985.

60. **Verma, D. S., Johnston, D. A., and McCredie, K. B.,** Evidence for the separate human T-lymphocyte subpopulations that collaborate with autologous monocyte/macrophages in the elaboration of colony-stimulating activity and those that suppress this collaboration, *Blood,* 62, 1088, 1983.

61. **Sobel, R. A., Blanchette, B. W., Bhan, A. K., and Colvin, R. B.,** The immunopathology of experimental allergic encephalomyelitis. II. Endothelial cell Ia increases prior to inflammatory cell infiltration, *J. Immunol.,* 132, 2402, 1984.

62. **Sobel, R. A., Natale, J. M., and Schneeberger, E. E.,** The immunopathology of acute experimental allergic encephalomyelitis. IV. An ultrastructural immunocytochemical study of class II major histocompatibility complex molecule (Ia) expression, *J. Neurol. Exp. Neurol.,* 46, 239, 1987.

63. **Fujikawa, S. L., Chi-Chao, C., McAllister, C., Gery, I., Hooks, J. J., Detrick, B., and Nussenblatt, R. B.,** Retinal vascular endothelium expresses fibronectin and class II histocompatibility complex antigens in experimental autoimmune uveitis, *Cell. Immunol.,* 106, 139, 1987.

64. **McCarron, R. M., Kempski, O., Spatz, M., and McFarlin, D. E.,** Presentation of myelin basic protein by murine cerebral vascular endothelial cells, *J. Immunol.,* 134, 3100, 1985.

65. **Wisniewski, H. M., Brown, H. R., and Thormar, H.,** Pathogenesis of viral eneephalitis: demonstration of viral antigen(s) in the brain endothelium, *Acta Neuropathol. (Berlin),* 60, 107, 1983.

66. **McCluskey, R. T., Benacerraf, B., and McCluskey, J. W.,** Studies on the specificity of the cellular infiltrate in delayed hypersensitivity reactions, *J. Immunol.,* 90, 466, 1963.

67. **Cohen, S., McCluskey, R. T., and Benacerraf, B.,** Studies on the specificity of the cellular infiltrate of delayed hypersensitivity reactions, *J. Immunol.,* 98, 269, 1967.

68. **Werdelin, O., Wick, G., and McCluskey, R. T.,** The fate of newly formed lymphocytes migrating from an antigen-stimulated lymph node in rats with allergic adrenalitis, *Lab. Invest.,* 25, 279, 1971.

69. **Werdelin, O. and McCluskey, R. T.,** The nature and the specificity of mononuclear cells in experimental autoimmune inflammation and mechanisms leading to their accumulation, *J. Exp. Med.,* 133, 1242, 1971.

70. **Najarian, J. S. and Feldman, J. D.,** Specificity of passively transferred delayed hypersensitivity, *J. Exp. Med.,* 118, 341, 1963.

71. **Smith, K. A.,** T-cell growth factor, *Immunol. Rev.,* 51, 337, 1980.

72. **Cheever, M. A. and Greenberg, P. D.,** *In vivo* administration of interleukin 2, *Contemp. Topics Molec. Immunol.,* 10, 263, 1985.

73. **Greene, M. I., Schatten, S., and Bromber, J. S.,** Delayed hypersensitivity, in *Fundamental Immunology,* Paul, W. E., Ed., Raven Press, New York, 1984, 685.

74. **Kelly, C. J., Clayman, M. D., and Neilson, E. G.,** Immunoregulation in experimental interstitial nephritis: immunization with renal tubular antigen in incomplete Freund's adjuvant induces major histocompatibility complex-restricted, OX8+ suppressor T cells which are antigen-specific and inhibit the expression of disease, *J. Immunol.,* 136, 903, 1986.

75. **Warren, K. S.,** The secret of the immunopathogenesis of schistosomiasis: *in vivo* models, *Immunol. Rev.,* 61, 189, 1982.

76. **Reed, E., Hardy, M., Benvenisty, A., Lattes, C., Brensilver, J., McCabe, R., Reemstma, K., King, D. W., and Suciu-Foca, N.,** Effect of antiidiotypic antibodies to HLA on graft survival in renal-allograft recipients, *N. Engl. J. Med.,* 316, 1450, 1987.

77. **Landay, A., Gartland, G. L., and Clement, L. T.,** Characterization of a phenotypically distinct subpopulation of Leu 2+ cells that suppress T cell proliferative responses, *J. Immunol.,* 131, 2757, 1983.

78. **Klein, J., Ikezawa, Z., and Nagy, Z. A.,** From LDH-B to J: an involuntary trip, *Immunol. Rev.,* 83, 79, 1985.

79. **Howie, S. E., Ross, J. A., Norval, M., and Maingay, J. P.,** *In vivo* modulation of antigen presentation generates Ts rather than TDH in HSV-1 infection, *Immunology,* 60, 419, 1987.

80. **Spina, C. A., Dorey, F., Vescera, C., Brosman, S., and Fahey, J. L.,** Depression of the generation of cell-mediated cytotoxicity by macrophage-like suppressor cells in bladder carcinoma patients, *Cancer Res.,* 41, 4324, 1981.

81. **Modlin, R. L., Kato, H., Mehra, V., Nelson, E. E., Xu-dong, F., Rea, T. H., Pattengale, P. K., and Bloom, B. R.,** Genetically restricted suppressor T cell clones derived from lepromatous leprosy lesions, *Nature,* 322, 459, 1986.

82. **Ottenhoff, T. H. M., Elferink, D. G., Klatser, P. R., and deVries, R. R. P.,** Cloned suppressor T cells from a lepromatous leprosy patient suppress *Mycobacterium leprae* reactive helper T cells, *Nature,* 322, 462, 1986.

83. **Rocklin, R. E., Lewis, E. J., and David, J. R.,** *In vitro* evidence for cellular hypersensitivity to glomerular basement membrane antigens in human glomerulonephritis, *N. Engl. J. Med.,* 283, 497, 1970.

84. **Bhan, A. K.,** Applications of monoclonal antibodies to tissue diagnosis, in *Advances in Immunohisto-chemistry,* DeLellis, R. A., Ed., Masson Publishing, New York, 1984, 1.

85. **Platt, J. L., Grant, B. W., Eddy, A. A., and Michael, A. F.,** Immune cell populations in cutaneous delayed type hypersensitivity, *J. Exp. Med.,* 158, 1227, 1983.

86. **Paronetto, F.,** Cell-mediated immunity in liver disease, *Hum. Pathol.,* 17, 168, 1986.

87. **Tuazon, T. V., Schneeberger, E. E., Bhan, A. K., McCluskey, R. T., Cosimi, A. B., Schooley, R. T., Rubin, R. H., and Colvin, R. B.,** Mononuclear cells in acute allograft glomerulopathy, *Am. J. Pathol.,* 129, 119, 1987.

88. **Bhan, A. K., Mihm, M. C., and Dvorak, H. F.,** T cell subsets in allograft rejections: *in situ* characterization of T cell subsets in human skin allografts by the use of monoclonal antibodies, *J. Immunol.,* 129, 1578, 1982.

89. **Bhan, A. K., Colvin, R. B., Cosimi, A. B., and McCluskey, R. T.,** Nature of cellular infiltrate in renal allograft rejection, *Kidney Int.,* 21, 293, 1982.

90. **Moscicki, R. A., Amento, E. P., Krane, S. M., Kurnick, J. T., and Colvin, R. B.,** Modulation of surface antigens of human monocyte cell line, U937, during incubation with T lymphocyte-conditioned medium. Detection of T4 antigen and its presence on normal blood monocytes, *J. Immunol.,* 131, 743, 1983.

91. **Reinherz, E. L. and Schlossman, S. F.,** The differentiation and function of human T lymphocytes, *Cell,* 19, 8219, 1980.

92. **Tilney, N. L., Garovoy, M. R., Busch, G. J., Strom, T. B., Graves, M. J., and Carpenter, C. B.,** Rejected human renal allografts. Recovery and characteristics of infiltrating cells and antibody, *Transplantation,* 28, 421, 1979.

93. **von Willebrand, E. and Hayry, P.,** Composition and *in vitro* cytotoxicity of cellular infiltrates in rejecting human kidney allografts, *Cell. Immunol.,* 41, 358, 1978.

94. **Leonard, W. J., Depper, J. M., Robb, R. J., Waldman, T. A., and Greene, W. C.,** Characterization of the human receptor for T-cell growth factor, *Proc. Natl. Acad. Sci. U.S.A.,* 80, 6957, 1983.

95. **Bich-Thuy, L. T., Dukovich, M., Peffer, N. J., Fauci, A. S., Kehrl, J. H., and Greene, W. C.,** Direct activation of human resting T cells by IL 2: the role of an IL 2 receptor distinct from the TAC protein, *J. Immunol.,* 139, 1550, 1987.

96. **Kurnick, J. T., Gronvik, K. O., Kimura, A. K., Lindblom, J. B., Skoog, V. T., Sjoberg, O., and Wigzell, H.,** Long-term growth *in vitro* of human T cell blasts with maintenance of specificity and function, *J. Immunol.,* 122, 1255, 1978.

97. **Liu, M. A., Kranz, D. M., Kurnick, J. T., Boyle, L. A., Levy, R., and Eisen, H. N.,** Anti-T3 containing heterobifunctional antibodies mediate cytotoxic T cell cytolysis of human tumor cell line, *Proc. Natl. Acad. Sci. U.S.A.,* 82, 8648, 1985.

98. **Stegagno, M., Boyle, L. A., Preffer, F. I., Leary, C. P., Colvin, R. B., Cosimi, A. B., and Kurnick, J. T.,** Functional analysis of T cell subsets and clones in human renal allograft rejection, *Transplant. Proc.,* 19, 394, 1987.

99. **Fung, J. J., Zeevi, A., Starzl, T. E., Demetris, J., Iwatsuki, S., and Duquesnoy, R. J.,** Functional characterization of infiltrating T lymphocytes in human hepatic allografts, *Hum. Immunol.,* 16, 182, 1986.

100. **Zeevi, A., Fung, J., Zerbe, T. R., Kaufman, C., Rabin, B. S., Griffith, B. P., Hardesty, R. L., and Duquesnoy, R. J.,** Allospecificity of activated T cells grown from endomyocardial biopsies from heart transplant patients, *Transplantation,* 41, 620, 1986.

101. **Fung, J. J., Zeevi, A., Kaufman, C., Paradis, I. L., Dauber, J. H., Hardesty, R. L., Griffith, B., and Duquesnoy, R. J.,** Interactions between bronchoalveolar lymphocytes and macrophages in heart-lung transplant recipients, *Hum. Immunol.,* 14, 287, 1985.

102. **Roberts, T. E., Shipton, U., and Moore, M.,** Role of MHC class-I antigens and the CD3 complex in the lysis of autologous human tumours by T-cell clones, *Int. J. Cancer,* 39, 436, 1987.

103. **McCluskey, R. T. and Bhan, A. K.,** Cell-mediated reactions *in vivo,* in *Mechanisms of Tumor Immunity,* Green, I., Cohen, S., and McCluskey, R. T., Eds., John Wiley & Sons, New York, 1975, 1.

104. **Bhan, A. K., Perry, L. L., Cantor, H., McCluskey, R. T., Benacerraf, B., and Greene, M. I.,** The role of T cell sets in the rejection of a methylcholanthrene-induced sarcoma in syngeneic mice, *Am. J. Pathol.,* 102, 20, 1981.

105. **Day, C. L., Lew, R. A., Mihm, M. C., et al.,** A multivariate analysis of prognostic factors for melanoma patients with lesions $\geqslant$ 3.65 mm in thickness, *Ann. Surg.,* 195, 44, 1982.

106. **Vanky, F., Peterffy, A., Book, K., Willems, J., Klein, E., and Klein, G.,** Correlation between lymphocyte-mediated auto-tumor reactivities and the clinical course. II. Evaluation of 69 patients with lung carcinoma, *Cancer Immunol. Immunother.,* 16, 17, 1983.

107. **Knuth, A., Danowski, B., Oettgen, H. F., and Old, L. J.,** T-cell-mediated cytotoxicity against autologous malignant melanoma: analysis with interleukin 2-dependent T-cell cultures, *Proc. Natl. Acad. Sci. U.S.A.,* 81, 3511, 1984.

108. **Hellstrom, K. E. and Hellstrom, I.,** Lymphocyte-mediated cytotoxicity and blocking serum activity to tumor antigens, *Adv. Immunol.,* 18, 209, 1974.

109. **Talmage, D. W., Woolnough, J. A., Hemmingsen, H., Lopez, L., and Lafferty, K. J.,** Activation of cytotoxic T cells by nonstimulating tumor cells and spleen cell factor(s), *Proc. Natl. Acad. Sci. U.S.A.,* 74, 4610, 1977.

110. **Medoff, J. R., Clack, V. D., and Roche, J. K.,** Characterization of an immunosuppressive factor from malignant ascites that resembles a factor induced *in vitro* by carcinoembryonic antigen, *J. Immunol.,* 137, 2057, 1986.

111. **Kurnick, J. T., Kradin, A., Blumberg, J., Schneeberger, E. E., and Boyle, L. A.,** Functional characterization of T lymphocytes propagated from human lung carcinomas, *Clin. Immunol. Immunopathol.,* 38, 367, 1986.

112. **Grimm, E. A., Mazumder, A., Zhang, H. Z., and Rosenberg, S. A.,** Lymphokine activated killer cell phenomenon. Lysis of natural killer-resistant fresh solid tumor cells by interleukin 2 activated autologous human peripheral blood lymphocytes, *J. Exp. Med.,* 155, 1823, 1982.

113. **Lanier, L. L. and Phillips, J. H.,** Evidence for three types of human cytotoxic lymphocytes, *Immunol. Today,* 7, 5, 1986.

114. **Rosenberg, S. A., Lotze, M. T., Muul, L. M., et al.,** Observations on the systemic administration of autologous lymphokine-activated killer cells and recombinant interleukin 2 to patients with metastatic cancer, *N. Eng. J. Med.,* 313, 1485, 1985.

115. **Kradin, R., Dubinett, S., Mullin, J., Boyle, L., Strauss, H. W., Bourgoin, P. M., Preffer, F. I., and Kurnick, J.,** Treatment of patients with advanced cancer using tumor-infiltrating lymphocytes and interleukin 2, *Transplant. Proc.,* 20, 336, 1988.

116. **Lotze, M. T., Line, B. R., Mathisen, D. J., and Rosenberg, S. A.,** The *in vivo* distribution of autologous human and murine lymphoid cells grown in T cell growth factor (TCGF). Implications for the adoptive immunotherapy of tumors, *J. Immunol.,* 125, 1487, 1980.

117. **Rosenberg, S. A., Speiss, P., and Lafreniere, R.,** A new approach to the adoptive therapy of cancer with tumor-infiltrating lymphocytes, *Science,* 233, 1318, 1986.

118. **Kradin, R. L., Boyle, L. A., Preffer, F. I., Callahan, R. J., Barlai-Kovach, M., Strauss, H. W., Dubinett, S., and Kurnick, J. T.,** Tumor-derived interleukin 2-dependent lymphocytes in adoptive immunotherapy of lung cancer, *Cancer Immunol. Immunother.,* 24, 76, 1987.

119. **Kurnick, J. T., McCluskey, R. T., Bhan, A. K., Wright, K. A., Wilkinson, R., and Rubin, R.,** Bacteria-specific T lymphocytes in experimental pyelonephritis, *J. Immunol.,* 141, 3220, 1988.

120. **Londei, M., Bottazzo, G. F., and Feldmann, M.,** Human T-cell clones from autoimmune thyroid glands: specific recognition of autologous thyroid cells, *Science,* 228, 85, 1985.

121. **Weetman, A. P., Volkman, D. J., Burman, K. D., Margolick, J. B., Petrick, P., Weintraub, B. D., and Fauci, A. S.,** The production and characterization of thyroid-derived T-cell lines in Graves' disease and Hashimoto's thyroiditis, *Clin. Immunol. Immunopathol.,* 39, 139, 1986.

122. **Weetman, A. P., Volkman, D. J., Burman, K. D., Gerrard, T. L., and Fauci, A. S.,** The *in vitro* regulation of human thyrocyte HLA-DR antigen expression, *J. Clin. Endocrinol. Metab.,* 61, 817, 1985.

123. **Miller, B. J., Appel, M. C., O'Neil, J. J., and Wicker, L. S.,** Both the Lyt-2$^+$ and L3T4$^+$ T cell subsets are required for the transfer of diabetes in nonobese diabetic mice, *J. Immunol.,* 140, 52, 1988.

124. **Minden, M. D., Toyonaga, B., Ha, K., Yanagi, Y., Chin, B., Gelfand, E., and Mak, T. W.,** Somatic rearrangement of T-cell antigen receptor gene in human T-cell malignancies, *Proc. Natl. Acad. Sci. U.S.A.,* 82, 1224, 1985.

125. **Frre, O., Thoen, J., Lewa, T., Bobloug, J. H., Mellbye, O. J., Natvig, J. B., Pahle, J., and Solheim, B. G.,** *In situ* characterization of mononuclear cells in rheumatoid tissues, using monoclonal antibodies. No reduction of T8-positive cells or augmentation in T4-positive cells, *Scand. J. Immunol.,* 16, 315, 1982.

126. **Poulter, L. W., Duke, O., Panayi, G. S., Hobbs, S., Raferty, M. J., and Janossy, G.,** Activated T lymphocytes of the synovial membrane in rheumatoid arthritis and other arthropathies, *Scand. J. Immunol.,* 22, 683, 1985.

127. **Jirik, F. R., Sorge, J., Fong, S., Heitzmann, J. G., Curd, J. G., Chen, P. P., Goldfien, R., and Carson, D. A.,** Cloning and sequence determination of a human rheumatoid factor light-chain gene, *Proc. Natl. Acad. Sci. U.S.A.,* 83, 2195, 1986.

128. **Shimonkevitz, R., Colon, S., Kappler, J. W., Marrack, P., and Grey, H. M.,** Antigen recognition by H-2 restricted T cells. II. A tryptic ovalbumin peptide that substitutes for processed antigen, *J. Immunol.,* 133, 2067, 1984.
129. **Yanagi, Y., Yoshikai, Y., Leggett, K., Clark, S. P., Alekasander, L., and Mak, T. W.,** A human T cell-specific cDNA clone encodes a protein having extensive homology to immunoglobulin chains, *Nature,* 308, 145, 1984.
130. **Flug, F., Pelicci, P. G., Bonetti, F., Knowles, D. M., and Dala-Favera, R.,** T-cell receptor gene rearrangements as markers of lineage and clonality in T-cell neoplasms, *Proc. Natl. Acad. Sci. U.S.A.,* 83, 3460, 1985.
131. **Stamenkovic, I., Stegagno, M., Wright, K. A., Krane, S. M., Amento, E. P., Colvin, R. B., Duquesnoy, R. J., and Kurnick, J. T.,** Clonal dominance among T lymphocyte infiltrates in arthritis, *Proc. Natl. Acad. Sci. U.S.A.,* 85, 1179, 1988.
132. **Hochgeschwender, U., Simon, H. G., Weltzien, H. U., Bartels, F., Becker, A., and Epplen, J. T.,** Dominance of one T-cell receptor in the H-2K sup b/TNP response, *Nature,* 326, 307, 1987.
133. **Goverman, J., Minard, K., Shastri, N., Hunkapiller, T., Hansburg, D., Sercarz, E., and Hood, L.,** Rearranged beta T cell receptor genes in a helper T cell clone specific for lysozyme: no correlation between V beta and MHC restriction, *Cell,* 40, 859, 1985.
134. **Weiss, L. M., Wood, G. S., Ellisen, L. W., Reynolds, T. C., and Sklar, J.,** Clonal T-cell populations in *Pityriasis lichenoides et Varioliformis acuta* (Mucha-Habermann disease), *Am. J. Pathol.,* 126, 417, 1987.
135. **Weiss, L. M., Wood, G. S., Trela, M. J., Warnke, R. A., and Sklar, J.,** Evidence for a lymphoproliferative etiology in a clinically benign disease, *N. Engl. J. Med.,* 315, 475, 1986.
136. **Morimoto, C., Letvin, N. L., Boyd, A. W., Hagan, M., Brown, H. M., Kornacki, M. M., Schlossman, S. F.,** The isolation and characterization of the human helper inducer T cell subset, *J. Immunol.,* 134, 3762, 1985.

Chapter 2

THE CYTOKINE CONCEPT: HISTORICAL PERSPECTIVES AND CURRENT STATUS OF THE CLONED CYTOKINES

Ruth Neta, Joost J. Oppenheim, and Scott K. Durum

TABLE OF CONTENTS

I. INTRODUCTION

A considerable number of peptides have now been identified that act as intercellular signals during the course of immunological responses. These peptides are termed "cytokines" and they elicit and regulate local and systemic inflammatory reactions. Although the existence of such regulatory peptides was predicted over 40 years ago,[1] only the advent of sophisticated tissue culture technology has permitted their detection by a variety of *in vitro* bioassays. With recent developments in biochemical and recombinant-DNA technology, these peptides have become available in sufficient quantities to be recognized as legitimate, important, and interesting entities with practical therapeutic potential. In this chapter we review the historical development of the concept that the immune system interacts with itself and with nonimmune tissues by means of a variety of endogenous peptide signals, and describe a number of the experimental observations that have converted this concept into a paradigm. We also briefly introduce those cytokines which have been cloned and discuss the challenges and issues that confront this burgeoning research field.

II. HISTORICAL PERSPECTIVE

The cytokine concept has evolved in a stepwise fashion. Perhaps the first observation implicating their action was made by Metchnikfoff,[2] who in the 1880s postulated that acquired resistance to infectious agents results from "the perfecting of the phagocytic and digestive power of the leukocytes". We now attribute much of this immune activation of phagocytic cells to the action of cytokines.

In 1932, Rich and Lewis[3] observed that cells from splenic explants of tuberculous animals were immobilized following exposure to specific mycobacterial antigens. This effect was attributed to toxicity, i.e, antigen was thought to be killing sensitized cells, and this explanation was invoked to account for the presence of necrosis in delayed hypersensitivity skin reactions. The above interpretation and their belief that "lymphocytes are phlegmatic observers of the vigorous activity of phagocytes" dissuaded Arnold Rich and other investigators for the next 25 years from further exploration of the inhibition of splenic cell migration.

In retrospect, it becomes clear that several other lines of investigation contributed to the elucidation of Rich and Lewis' observation and to the subsequent discovery of lymphocyte-elaborated soluble mediators, the lymphokines. Probably the most significant development during this period was the improvement of tissue culture methodology, due to the availability of antibiotics which permitted long-term maintenance of lymphoid cells in culture. This allowed for analysis of antigen-cell interaction in culture and revealed the stimulatory effect of antigens on lymphoid cells.[4]

The second line of investigation, conducted in the late 1950s and early 1960s focused on the role of specifically sensitized cells in acquired immunity. Several types of experiments were conducted. In one approach, use was made of the newly developed radiolabeled compound, tritiated thymidine. Transfer of labeled cells from sensitized donors to normal recipients provided evidence that only a small fraction of cells at sites of dermal delayed hypersensitivity reactions were derived from specifically sensitized donors. However, the bulk of inflammatory cells unexpectedly consisted of recipient macrophages derived from rapidly dividing precursors.[5] Other elegant studies conducted by Mackaness[6] demonstrated that when immunized animals were subsequently challenged with the immunizing antigen, their macrophages became activated and they became resistant to antigenically unrelated pathogens. Thus, both specific and nonspecific resistance was dependent upon the activation of macrophages. Consequently, the paradigm of immunologic specificity was modified to include participation of large numbers of recruited, nonsensitized, inflammatory cell types.

Another line of investigation, conducted by Svejcar and Johanovsky, utilized co-cultures of splenic explants from sensitized and normal animals in the presence of specific antigen. They showed that cell migration in both explants was inhibited, leading them to postulate the presence of a soluble mediator.[7] The existence of such a soluble mediator was demonstrated convincingly by David et al.[8] and by Bloom and Bennett.[9] Their work established that exposure of specifically sensitized lymphocytes to antigen resulted in the release into culture supernatants of a soluble mediator that inhibited the migration of normal macrophages. This migration inhibitory factor (MIF) acted nonspecifically and was distinct from lymphocyte-derived antibodies. Consequently, this discovery shattered the basic premise that lymphocyte responses to antigens are limited to the production of specific antibodies.

The discovery of MIF initiated an intensive search for other mediators. It was soon shown that supernatants from antigen-stimulated lymphocytes contained factors which could account for the morphological changes seen in delayed hypersensitivity reactions *in vivo*. The recruitment of the mononuclear cellular infiltrate was attributed to the action of lymphocyte-derived chemotactic factor (CF),[10] MIF and macrophage aggregation factor (MAgF),[11] the necrotic centers to the cytodestructive activity of lymphotoxin (LT),[12,13] and the presence of lymphoblasts and frequent mitotic figures to the presence of lymphocyte-derived mitogenic factors (LMF).[14] Indeed, the *in vitro* production of these factors could be correlated with the presence of *in vivo* cell-mediated immunity. The lymphocyte derived factors were termed "lymphokines" by Dumonde et al.[15] Detection of macrophage activating factor (MAF)[16] and interferon (IFN)[17] served to explain the basis for acquired resistance to infectious organisms. Discovery of these lymphokines revolutionized the concept of mechanisms underlying "cell mediated" immunity.

The lymphokine concept provided a basis for immunologically mediated inflammatory reactions, such as rejection of solid tissue grafts, organ-specific autoimmune reactions, acquired resistance to intracellular infections, and delayed-type hypersensitivity. It had previously been clearly established by Landsteiner and Chase[18] that specific immune reactivity in delayed-type hypersensitivity could be acquired by normal donors following the transfer of cells, but not of serum antibodies, from sensitized recipients. This dependence of immune reactivity on the whole living cell could now be envisioned as being mediated by lymphokines which were thought to recruit, activate, and retain leukocytes at inflammatory sites following antigen-specific initiation of this cascade.

That lymphokines indeed have this role was first demonstrated by Bennett and Bloom[19] who observed histological changes with the characteristics of delayed hypersensitivity following intradermal inoculation of lymphokine-containing supernatants. It was observed that intraperitoneal administration of partially purified preparations of MIF resulted in a macrophage disappearance reaction resembling that induced with specific antigen in sensitized animals.[20] Tumor necrosis developed after administration of lymphokine-containing supernatants into tumor sites. This activity was termed the tumor necrosis factor (TNF).[21] Conversely, lymphokines could also be detected in the circulation of sensitized animals following antigenic challenge, in patients or animals with lymphoproliferative diseases, as well as at the inflammatory site.[22] Although all the above reports confirmed that lymphokines are present and act in the body, the relative contribution of individual lymphokines remained undefined.

The discovery of lymphocyte-derived mitogenic factors led to studies of factors that regulate the activation of T- and B-lymphocytes. In the course of such an analysis, Gery and Waksman[23] observed that stimulated nonlymphocytic adherent cells also release a soluble mediator that augments the growth of lymphocytes, which they named the lymphocyte activating factor (LAF) (now interleukin 1). Furthermore, analysis of supernatants from cultured nonlymphoid cell types, such as fibroblasts, revealed them to be an additional source of factors with biological activities on lymphoid cells (e.g., MIF activity). These findings led Cohen et al.[24] in 1974 to propose the use of a more comprehensive term "cytokines" to comprise soluble factors with similar characteristics, produced by lymphoid as well as nonlymphoid cells.

During the 1970s, despite intensive efforts, little progress was made in defining these molecules biochemically. Instead, advances in tissue culture and bioassay methodology permitted further analysis of the effects of these factors on functions of different cells *in vitro*. By the late 1970s, more than 100 different biological activities had been described.[25] This overwhelmed and discouraged many immunologists and biochemists from pursuing the study of cytokines.

To distinguish the numerous cytokines from one another, a number of experimental approaches have been used. These included the production of T cell clones and T cell hybridomas in an effort to obtain preparations of single lymphokines released by T cell subsets. Notwithstanding the fact that cell lines generally produce a battery of lymphokines, certain lymphokines were successfully discriminated in this way. A more successful approach to dissecting the actions of different cytokines was based on the generation of specific antibodies against semipurified cytokine preparations. For example, antigenic differences distinguished several types of interferons, (IFNs) presently known as IFNs α, β, and γ. Furthermore, reports concerning multiple biological effects of IFNs were confirmed by the use of such antibodies; all three IFNs were shown to activate macrophages, natural killer (NK) cells, and cytotoxic T cells, as well as having antiproliferative activity on a variety of cell types.[26]

III. FROM CELLULAR IMMUNOLOGY TO BIOCHEMISTRY

The application of effective chromatography technology has led to the precise purification and definition of a number of the cytokines and has clearly established that some cytokines exhibit pleiotropic activities. For example, preparations of LAF purified to homogeneity had the same biochemical and biological characteristics as a B-cell activating factor (BAF), B-cell differentiating factor (BCDF), T-cell replacing factor (TRF), and mitogenic protein (MP). That one molecular entity exhibited all these diverse properties was confirmed by exchange of partially purified cytokines between different laboratories. To reflect the ability of this moiety to act as an intercellular signal between different populations of leukocytes, it was renamed interleukin-1 (IL-1).[27] Another group of lymphocyte-derived mitogenic activities, known as T-cell growth factor (TCGF), thymocyte mitogenic factor (TMF), killer cell helper factor (KHF), and secondary cytotoxic T-cell inducing factor (SCTF) were also shown to share biochemical properties and were, therefore, renamed interleukin-2 (IL-2).[27]

The purification of LAF/IL-1 was rapidly followed by yet another critical conceptual development. The biochemical similarity of IL-1 with macrophage/monocyte derived endogenous pyrogen (EP) led Rosenwasser et al.[28] to propose that EP was identical to LAF/IL-1: both had thymocyte stimulatory activity, and conversely, IL-1 was shown to exhibit EP activity. LAF/IL-1/EP was also shown to be identical with yet another activity known as leukocyte endogenous mediator (LEM). LEM had previously been demonstrated by Kampschmidt et al.[29] to induce a large number of events associated with inflammation, including neutrophilia and induction of *in vivo* acute phase protein production. LEM, EP, and IL-1 were indistinguishable in their biochemical and biological properties. The pleiotropic systemic effects on the CNS, bone marrow, and immune system of a mediator generated during infections, immunologic responses, and inflammatory conditions revealed a mechanism by which signals generated during an immune response could lead to a diversity of systemic inflammatory responses.

IL-1 is not the only cytokine with activities that extend beyond the immune and inflammatory systems. For example, colony-stimulating factors (CSF) are produced by a variety of cell types, including activated T cells. These factors induce hematopoietic progenitor

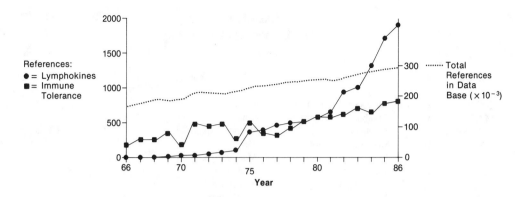

FIGURE 1. The growth of lymphokine research. Numbers of publications listed in *Index Medicus*.

cells to proliferate *in vitro*, producing colonies of myeloid, erythroid, and other lineages. Other lymphocyte-derived factors promote the growth and differentiation of mesenchymal cells; such factors include fibroblast activating factor (FAF), osteoclast activating factor (OAF), factors promoting angiogenesis (e.g., FAF, TNF, IL-1) and cartilage turnover (e.g, IL-1, TNF, TGFβ), and wound repair (e.g., FAF, TGF, IL-1).[31] Conversely, cytokines derived from nonlymphoid tissues regulate the growth and differentiation of T- and B-lymphocytes and provide the means by which host tissues can modulate specific immune responses.

Furthermore, a number of the cytokines can be produced by many tissues. For example, IL-1 is produced by a wide variety of cell types including epithelial cells, astrocytes, and mesenchymal cells as well as by reticulo-endothelial cells. Some CSF and TNF can be produced by endothelial cells and fibroblasts as well as by lymphoid cells. Thus, cytokines can function as bidirectional intercellular signals between immune and nonimmune systems. Injurious excitation of nonlymphoid tissues through the production of cytokines can marshall a variety of tissues, including the immune system, to contribute to the host response. Conversely, activation of the immune system generates lymphokines that enlist other organs such as the neuroendocrine and cardiovascular systems to participate in optimizing host defense.

One impact of the discovery of the pleiotropic effects of the cytokines has been to draw investigators from many other disciplines into the study of these mediators. The explosive growth of lymphokine research is illustrated in Figure 1, showing the numbers of annual publications keyed to the term lymphokine (a term used more frequently than cytokine). Beginning with a single reference in 1969 when the term was coined, the number grew to 1806 references in 1986. For comparison, Figure 1 shows references on another immunological subject, immune tolerance, whose growth parallels that of the biomedical literature as a whole.

IV. THE ERA OF MOLECULAR BIOLOGY

Gene cloning has provided the key technical advance responsible for this rapid acceleration in the cytokine research. At this point we will take our story of the cytokines from the historical perspective to the contemporary, with a discussion of the state of the art, the cloned cytokines, and how the availability of recombinant cytokines has extended and modified our concepts of cytokines.

The biological information obtained from cloning and expression established beyond doubt the identities of a number of distinct molecules. One could now be sure that many of the multiple activities attributed to a particular cytokine such as IL-1, for example, were

TABLE 1
The Cloned Cytokines

LK/MK	Mol wt (kDa)	Producers	Targets	Receptors (mol wt in kDa)
G-CSF	23	Fibroblast, macrophage	Hemato., stem	180
M-CSF	45	Fibroblast, macrophage	Mono., stem	165
GM-CSF	25	T, others	Hemato., stem, others	70 + 132
IFN-α	18	Macrophage, many	Many	120
IFN-γ	20	T, LGL	Macrophage, many	100
IL-1α	17	Macrophage, many	T, B, many	85
IL-1β	17	Macrophage, many	T, B, many	85
IL-2	15	T, LGL	T, B, other	55 + 75
IL-3	28	T	Hemato., stem	65
IL-4	20	T	T, B, mast, many	60
IL-5	18	T	B, T	?
IL-6	26	Fibroblast, T, other	B, preplasmacytoma, many	55 + 75 + 95
LT	25	T, other	Tumors, many	55 + 75 + 95
TNF	17	macrophage, other	Tumors, many	55 + 75 + 95
TGFβ	25	T, platelets, other	Connective tissue, T, macrophage	280 + 65 + 85

really due to a single moiety. On the other hand, cloning established that some of these activities were due to contaminants, as, for example, the recent identification of a unique (non-IL-1) chemotactic factor for neutrophils that had contaminated IL-1 preparations. Some cloned cytokines, such as TNF, were discovered to have many more activities than originally appreciated. The other great impact of cloning was to provide considerable quantities of pure cytokines, permitting studies of immunological, physiological, and therapeutic roles of cytokines.

V. PRESENT STATUS OF THE CLONED CYTOKINES

A number of cytokines, in fact all of the best studied ones, have now been cloned as cDNAs. Genomic organizations have been determined for several of the lymphokine genes. Recombinant proteins have been expressed for a number of the cytokine genes, and many are now commercially available. In the remainder of this chapter, the current state of cytokine research is summarized by briefly introducing each of the cloned cytokines in terms of cell sources, activities, interactions, and potential diagnostic and therapeutic applications (references are given only for the cloning; see following chapters for references to the original discovery of each cytokine). Table 1 indicates the current inventory of cloned cytokines and a number of their characteristics.

Granulocyte colony stimulating factor (G-CSF)[31,32] acts as a lineage specific factor *in vitro,* stimulating the growth and differentiation of polymorphonuclear neutrophilic granulocytes and their precursors; however, *in vivo* administration of G-CSF stimulates all the hematopoietic precursors either directly or indirectly. IL-1 and TNF can induce G-CSF production by endothelial cells and fibroblasts. Thus, infectious challenge and other immunostimulants can presumably signal the reticuloendothelial system and bone marrow stromal cells to produce G-CSF — this may account for the neutrophilia observed following such insults. The role of G-CSF in hematopoietic disorders remains to be established and the effect of pharmacological doses of G-CSF on restoration of impaired bone marrow functions is being explored.

Macrophage colony stimulating factor (M-CSF),[33] also known as CSF-1, is lineage specific both *in vito* and *in vitro,* stimulating predominantly phagocytic macrophages and their precursors. M-CSF, like G-CSF, is induced by IL-1 and TNF. Areas of current study include the role of M-CSF in the pathogenesis of disease and its therapeutic potential.

Granulocyte-macrophage colony stimulating factor (GM-CSF)[34] stimulates the *in vitro* growth and differentiation of hematopoietic stem cells predominantly into granulocytes and monocytes. GM-CSF also promotes the functional activities of the mature members of these lineages: it inhibits the migration of neutrophils and it activates macrophages to kill tumor cells. On the other hand, *in vivo* administration of GM-CSF has revealed pluripotent effects on all the other hematopoietic elements, including erythroid and megakaryocyte stem cells. This is presumably based on the capacity of GM-CSF to induce *in vivo* production of other as yet unidentified cytokines that stimulate these precursor cells. GM-CSF is produced not only by activated T lymphocytes, but also by endothelial cells and macrophages. Consequently, a variety of tissues can be stimulated to produce GM-CSF. Although GM-CSF is already being evaluated in phase I studies in man for its potential reconstitutive effects, its precise role in hematopoiesis and leukemogenesis are not clear as yet.

IFN-α and -β1. IFN-α1 was first cloned by Nagata et al.[35] and IFN-β1 by Taniguchi et al.[36] IFN-α is in general a product of leukocytes whereas IFN-β1 is produced by fibroblasts. From 14 to 16 different variants of IFN-α have been identified. They exhibit differences in amino acid sequence ranging from a single amino acid to over 70% of the residues; however, since these variants are generally thought to interact with the same cell surface receptor, they probably have the same biological activities. Recombinant IFN-α and IFN-β1 promote the antiviral state and have antiproliferative effects on the wide range of target cells that express receptors for IFN-α and -β1. In addition to inhibiting proliferation, IFN-α and -β1 promote the differentiation of a variety of target cells including muscle cells, myeloid and melanoma cells, natural killer lymphocytes, macrophages, and T and B lymphocytes. Thus, recombinant IFN-α and -β1 exhibit the effects of MIF and MAF on macrophages and promotes the maturation of macrophages and their expression of cell surface differentiation markers such as the receptors for the Fc portion of immunoglobulins (FcR), which facilitate macrophage functions such as phagocytosis of opsonized particles and antibody-dependent cellular cytotoxicity (ADCC). IFN-α and -β1 also augment the production of other cytokines such as IL-1 and TNF, the synthesis and secretion of proteolytic enzymes, and expression of class I MHC by macrophages. IFN-α and -β1 also interact with a number of other cytokines such as TNF and IL-1 in promoting cell differentiation, but antagonize the proliferative action of a number of growth factors, including the CSF. As a consequence of these effects, IFN-α and -β1 also modulate humoral and cellular immunity. The levels of IFN in various pathological states is being established and therapeutic efficacy in cancer and infectious diseases is being evaluated; hairy cell leukemia is now widely treated with IFN-α.

IFN-γ[37] also termed immune or type II IFN, is produced by several subsets of T cells as well as by large granular lymphocytes (LGL). Like the other IFNs, IFN-γ acts on many cell types to induce an antiviral state and promotes cell differentiation at the expense of cellular proliferation. Additionally, IFN-γ acts as a powerful macrophage activator and induces increased expression of cell membrane class II MHC antigens, e.g., Ia, on many cell types. The receptor for IFN-γ is distinct from that for IFN-γ and -β. IFN-γ also acts to augment the production of other cytokines such as IL-1 and TNF and thus participates in the lymphokine cascade.

IL-1, as discussed above, was independently discovered a number of times because it has a wide variety of biological activities. At least two distinct genes encode products with IL-1 activities; these have been termed IL-1α[38] and IL-1β;[39] they share the same biological activities and they apparently bind the same receptor, despite their limited homology (28% at the protein level). Il-1 is produced by many cell types, both inside and outside the immune system, and its effects are mediated in part by enhancing the production of many other cytokines. IL-1 also synergizes with a number of other cytokines involved in growth and differentiation. IL-1 is currently in the preclinical stage of evaluation and will shortly be examined for its restorative and reparative therapeutic effects.

IL-2[40] was originally discovered as a factor that would support long-term growth of human T cells. IL-2 is produced by several types of T cells and LGL following activation. Its effects, in addition to T cell growth, include activation of NK and lymphokine-activated killer (LAK) cells as well as cytotoxic T cells, macrophages, and promotion of B cell growth. The receptor for IL-2 has been cloned, including both the 55 kDa glycoprotein known as the TAc antigen;[41] and the second chain consisting of a 75-kDa protein that has not been cloned as yet. IL-2 also stimulates target cells to produce a battery of cytokines including IFN-α, TNF/LT, IL-1, and TGFβ which in turn can modulate immune and inflammatory reactions. Antitumor therapies in man are currently being developed based on IL-2 induction of LAK cells.

IL-3[42] has also been known as multi-CSF. Mouse IL-3 has been more thoroughly studied than its rather distantly related human counterpart. IL-3 is produced by activated helper T cells. Its actions include various growth and differentiation effects on all the hematopoietic precursor cells. IL-3 stimulates the growth of multilineage colonies from bone marrow stem cells including erythroid, granulocyte, macrophage, and megakaryocyte precursors. IL-3 is a particularly potent growth factor for mast cell precursors in bone marrow and mast cell lines.

IL-4[43] was previously known as BSF-1 and IgG1-inducing factor. It is a product of activated helper T cells. Originally, IL-4 was defined as a factor that acted on resting B cells, increasing their Ia expression and preparing them for membrane Ig cross-linking, which would in turn lead to proliferation and differentiation. Other activities now appreciated for this cytokine include macrophage activation and induction of class II MHC molecules, growth of some T cell and mast cell lines, promoting an isotype switch to IgE production by B cells, and as a cofactor in growth of hematopoietic cells from stem cells.

IL-5[44] is a term that has recently come into use to describe a factor formerly known as TRF and BCGF II. IL-5 is a factor produced by murine T cells that has activities on both B and T cells. It has both early and late effects on B cells. Early effects include inducing proliferation of B cells co-stimulated with dextran sulfate and it also increases proliferation of BCL1 tumor cells. Late effects include inducing secretion of IgM from *in vivo*-primed B cells, secretion of IgG from *in vivo*-primed secondary B cells, and IgM secretion from BCL1 tumor cells. IL-5 also promotes isotype switching to IgA production in B cells. Effects on T cells include promoting T cell proliferation and inducing development of cytotoxic T cells.

IL-6 was previously termed IFN-β2, B cell stimulating factor-2, and hepatocyte stimulating factor. As these many names imply, this cytokine represents a convergence of several independent lines of study. The earlier line of research involved analyzing lymphokines active on B cells and began in the early 1970s when it was recognized that T cells produced heterogeneous factors that induced B cells to proliferate and secrete Ig. One of the components of these supernatants (which also included IL-1, IL-4, and IL-5) was B-cell stimulating factor-2 (BSF-2),[45] also termed BCDF, which is a late acting factor that induces secretion of Ig but not proliferation of B cells. Another independent line of research identified and led to the cloning of a factor with the same predicted amino acid sequences that stimulated preplasmacytomas to proliferate — this was another property of BSF-2. Another group has established that the cDNA for hepatocyte stimulating factor (HSF), an activator of acute phase protein production, also coded for the same sequence. Finally, while the IFN (antiviral) activity of this molecule is doubtful, the putative antiviral property of a 26-kDa fibroblast-derived cytokine led to the independent cloning of the same molecule termed IFN-β2.[46] Thus, IFN-β2/BSF-2/HSF activities all appear to be attributable to the same cytokine, IL-6. As in the case for many of the broad spectrum cytokines, this molecule not only acts on a variety of target cells, but also is produced by a number of cell types including T and B lymphocytes, monocytes, fibroblasts, and myxoma cells. It is too early to have any information concerning the diagnostic and therapeutic potential of IL-6.

Lymphotoxin (LT)[47] and **tumor necrosis factor (TNF)**[48] are related cytokines that show only 28% protein homology but nevertheless bind to the same receptor on target cells. Consequently, LT and TNF display similar biological activities, therefore, were also named TNFβ and -α, respectively. Both LT and TNF were initially characterized as cytotoxic factors that could kill certain types of tumor cells. LT and TNF are preferentially expressed in different cell types, probably based on the differences in their promoters; LT was originally thought to be a T cell product, TNF a macrophage product, but this restriction is not absolute, and both cells can produce both products under certain conditions. TNF was also independently cloned and named "cachectin" based on its property of inducing cachexia *in vivo*; this results from inducing lipolysis in adipocytes, based on inhibition of lipoprotein lipase activity. In addition, recombinant TNF/LT, like IL-1, has been shown to have a broad spectrum of biological activities including activating angiogenesis, pyrogenicity, bone resorption, fibroplasia, and induction of acute phase protein production. IL-1 and TNF are often produced by the same cells in response to the same stimuli and have the same effect on target cells through distinct receptors. This apparent redundancy may actually be advantageous in that two signals would be required to achieve more marked (additive or synergistic) effects.

Transforming growth factor β (TGFβ)[49] was named on the basis of its ability to cause phenotypic transformation of rat fibroblasts. TGFβ is now known to be a multifunctional peptide with a wide range of regulatory effects on the many cell types that bear receptors for TGFβ. It is synthesized by many cell types: bone, T lymphocytes, and platelets are good sources. This panregulatory peptide promotes the growth and development of connective tissue, but has antiproliferative effects on keratinocytes, monkey kidney cells, hepatocytes, myeloid, and T and B lymphoid cells. TGFβ is especially active in antagonizing the mitogenic effects of other peptide growth factors, including IL-2. TGFβ is a late product of activated T cells and is a potent down-regulator of lymphocyte-mediated responses. However, the overall net effect of TGFβ is complicated by the fact that it promotes macrophage maturation and stimulates the production of such up-regulators of the immune response as IL-1. Like TGFβ, other mesenchymal cell growth factors such as platelet derived growth factor (PDGF), epidermal growth factor (EGF), and fibroblast growth factor (FGF) can regulate the production of a lymphokine, namely IFN-γ. Consequently, cytokines that are usually thought of as having activities restricted to connective tissues also can signal the immune system and promote host defenses.

The historical relationship of the contemporary cloned cytokines to their ancestral lymphokine activities is illustrated in Figure 2. It is ironic that some of the initially described lymphokines activities such as MIF and MAF are still not available in recombinant forms. Although IFN-α, -β, -γ and IL-4 are known to exhibit these activities, several investigators are pursuing the purification and cloning of unique lymphokines that are said to be responsible for these effects.

VI. CURRENT PERSPECTIVES AND CONCLUDING REMARKS

From the foregoing, it is apparent that the availability of recombinant cytokines has fueled progress in understanding the function of these regulatory factors. The cell sources of cytokines can now be identified at the mRNA level not only *in vitro,* but even in tissue sections using *in situ* hybridization. RIA and ELISA assays and bioassays can be developed to detect cytokines in normal as well as pathological conditions. Pharmacological doses of cytokines can be used for therapeutic purposes. The specific receptors for the various cytokines as well as their postreceptor transducing signals are now amenable to precise characterization.

However, many old and new issues remain difficult to resolve. The precise physiological

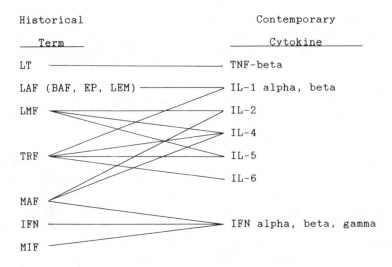

FIGURE 2.   Historical relationship of the lymphokines. The original terms for the crude lymphokine activities are shown in the left column. The contemporary terms for the cloned cytokines that comprised these activities are shown in the column on the right.

role of a given cytokine is difficult to define. Availability of cloned cytokines has revealed considerable duplication of biological activities by cytokine molecules that are biochemically quite distinct. The benefits of this apparent redundancy may be to maximize the efficiency of these cytokines through their synergistic interaction. The redundancy may also serve to minimize the incidence of deleterious deficiency states.

Cytokines can interact in a variety of ways: (1) one cytokine can induce production of another; (2) several different cytokines can be produced in coordinate fashion by the same cell; (3) one cytokine modulates the action of a second cytokine on the same target cell. The third interaction possibility, interaction at the target cell level, can occur by receptor modulation or by postreceptor events and can be agonistic or antagonistic, magnifying the potency and complexity of cytokine effects. We know too little of the postreceptor intracellular effects of the cytokines to understand the advantages to be gained from these interactions.

Those cytokines such as IL-1 and TNF that are active across species lines predictably show considerable interspecies structural homology. Other cytokines such as CSF and IFN, however, show restricted species specificity. The cross-reactive cytokines are therefore more evolutionarily conserved than the restricted cytokines. Species specificity of cytokines on the other hand, implies the coevolution of both the cytokines and their receptors. The causes for these divergent evolutionary patterns are intriguing and demand further study.

Although cytokines are assumed to contribute to host defense, the actual physiological and pathophysiological role of most of these factors is still a mystery. Some of them may play primary roles in development and reparative processes, for example, developmental roles for IL-1 detected in amniotic fluid and in developing brain have been suggested. Paradoxically, cytokines can also elicit serious deleterious responses in the host. TNF and IL-1 appear to mediate endotoxin shock. IFN-γ administration can lead to fatal autoimmune sequellae. Fatal infection of adult mice with lymphocytic choriomeningitis virus is directly attributable to the host's immune response and can be blocked by antibody to IFN. Generally, the deleterious effects of cytokines are seen only in cases of excessive challenge to the host resulting in coincidentally injurious host responses.

Progress has been slow in identifying cytokines that inhibit inflammatory processes. A few such mediators have been tentatively identified and their possible utility as negative feedback regulators for self-destructive inflammatory reactions needs more exploration. It is also certain that additional inhibitory as well as phlogistic cytokines are still to be identified which will play important roles in regulating the integrity of the host.

The interaction of immune and inflammatory processes with the neuroendocrine, connective tissue, hematopoietic, and cardiovascular systems is a growing area of study. Many of these interactions proceed via the regulatory action of cytokines. The recognition that lymphocytes are not the sole producers of such soluble factors has developed in parallel and contributed to the transformation of immunology from a science focused entirely on the lymphoid system to one which must integrate the immune system with other physiological systems that contribute to maintaining the integrity of the host.

ACKNOWLEDGMENTS

We thank Drs. Stephanie Vogel and Igal Gery for helpful comments on the manuscript and Roberta Unger for typing.

REFERENCES

1. **Menkin, V.**, Chemical basis of injury in inflammation, *Arch. Pathol.*, 36, 269, 1943.
2. **Metchnikoff, E.**, *Immunity in Infective Diseases*, Cambridge University Press, Cambridge, England, 1905.
3. **Rich, A. R. and Lewis, M. R.**, The nature of allergy in tuberculosis as revealed by tissue culture studies, *Bull. Johns Hopkins Hosp.*, 50, 115, 1932.
4. **Waksman, B. H. and Matoltsy, M.**, The effect of tuberculin on peritoneal exudate cells of sensitized guinea pigs in surviving cell culture, *J. Immunol.*, 81, 220, 1958.
5. **McCluskey, R. T., Benacerraf, B., and McCluskey, J. W.**, Studies on the specificity of the cellular infiltrate in delayed hypersensitivity reactions, *J. Immunol.*, 90, 466, 1963.
6. **Mackaness, G. B.**, The immunological basis of acquired cellular resistance, *J. Exp. Med.*, 120, 105, 1964.
7. **Svejcar, J. and Johanovsky, J.**, in *Proceedings of the Fifth European Congress of Allergy*, Schwabe, Basel, 1963, 375.
8. **David, J. R., Al-Askari, S., Lawrence, H. S., and Thomas, L.**, Delayed hypersensitivity *in vitro*. I. The specificity of inhibition of cell migration by antigens, *J. Immunol.*, 93, 264, 1964.
9. **Bloom, B. R. and Bennett, B.**, Mechanism of a reaction *in vitro* associated with delayed type hypersensitivity, *Science*, 153, 80, 1966.
10. **Ward, P. A., Remold, H. G., and David, J. R.**, Leukotactic factor produced by sensitized lymphocytes, *Science*, 163, 1079, 1969.
11. **Lolekha, S., Dray, S., and Gotoff, S. P.**, Macrophage aggregation *in vitro*. A correlate of delayed hypersensitivity, *J. Immunol.*, 104, 296, 1970.
12. **Ruddle, N. H. and Waksman, B. H.**, Cytotoxicity mediated by soluble antigen and lymphocytes in delayed hypersensitivity. III. Analysis of mechanism, *J. Exp. Med.*, 128, 1267, 1968.
13. **Kolb, W. P. and Granger, G. A.**, Lymphocyte *in vitro* cytotoxicity: characterization of human lymphotoxin, *Proc. Natl. Acad. Sci. U.S.A.*, 61, 1250, 1968.
14. **Kasakura, S. and Lowenstein, L.**, A factor stimulating DNA synthesis derived from the medium of leukocyte culture, *Nature*, 208, 734, 1965.
15. **Dumonde, D. C., Wolstencroft, R. A., Panayi, G. S., Matthew, M., Morley, J., and Howson, W. T.**, "Lymphokines": non-antibody mediators of cellular immunity generated by lymphocyte activation, *Nature*, 224, 38, 1969.
16. **Nathan, C. F., Karnovsky, M. L., and David, J. R.**, Alterations of macrophage functions by mediators from lymphocytes, *J. Exp. Med.*, 133, 1356, 1971.
17. **Green, J. A., Cooperband, S. R., and Kibnick, S.**, Immune specific induction of interferon production in cultures of human blood lymphocytes, *Science*, 164, 1415, 1969.
18. **Landsteiner, K. and Chase, M. W.**, Experiments on transfer of cutaneous sensitivity to simple compounds, *Proc. Soc. Exp. Biol. Med.*, 49, 688, 1942.
19. **Bennett, B. and Bloom, B. R.**, Reactions *in vivo* and *in vitro* produced by a soluble substance associated with delayed-type hypersensitivity, *Proc. Natl. Acad. Sci. U.S.A.*, 59, 756, 1968.

20. **Sonozaki, H. and Cohen, S.,** A macrophage disappearance reaction: mediation by a soluble lymphocyte derived factor, *Cell. Immunol.,* 2, 341, 1971.
21. **Carswell, E. A., Old, L. J., Kassel, R. L., Green, S., Fiore, N., and Williamson, G.,** An endotoxin induced serum factor that causes necrosis of tumors, *Proc. Natl. Acad. Sci. U.S.A.,* 72, 3666, 1975.
22. **Neta, R. and Salvin, S. B.,** Production of lymphokines *in vivo,* in *Lymphokines,* Vol. 2, Pick, E., Ed., Academic Press, New York, 1981, 295.
23. **Gery, I. and Waksman, B. H.,** Potentiation of the T-lymphocyte response to mitogens. II. The cellular source of the potentiating mediators, *J. Exp. Med.,* 136, 143, 1972.
24. **Cohen, S., Bigazzi, P. E., and Yoshida, T.,** Similarities of T cell function in cell-mediated immunity and antibody production, *Cell. Immunol.,* 12, 150, 1974.
25. **Waksman, B. H.,** Modulation of immunity by soluble mediators, *Pharmacol. Ther.,* 2A, 623, 1978.
26. **Vogel, S. and Friedman, R. M.,** Interferon and macrophages: activation and cell surface changes, in *Interferon: Interferons and the Immune System,* Vol. 2, Vilcek, J. and DeMayer, E., Eds., Elsevier, Amsterdam, 1984, 35.
27. **Aarden, L. A., et al.,** Revised nomenclature for antigen nonspecific T-cell proliferation and helper factors, *J. Immunol.,* 123, 2928, 1979.
28. **Rosenwasser, L. J., Dinarello, C. A., and Rosenthal, A. S.,** Adherent cell function in murine T-lymphocyte antigen recognition. IV. Enhancement of murine T-cell antigen recognition by human leukocytic pyrogen, *J. Exp. Med.,* 150, 709, 1979.
29. **Kampschmidt, R. F., Upchurch, H. F., Eddington, C. L., and Pulliam, L. A.,** Multiple biological activities of partially purified leukocytic endogenous mediator, *Am. J. Physiol.,* 224, 530, 1973.
30. **Ruscetti, F. W. and Chervenick, P. A.,** The release of colony stimulating activity from thymus derived lymphocytes, *J. Clin. Invest.,* 55, 520, 1975.
31. **Nakata, S., Tsuchiya, M., Asano, S., Kaziro, Y., Yamazaki, T., Yamamoto, O., Hirata, Y., Kubota, N., Oheda, M., Homura, H., and Ono, M.,** Molecular cloning and expression of cDNA for human granulocyte colony-stimulating factor, *Nature,* 319, 415, 1986.
32. **Souza, L. M., Boone, T. C., Gabrilove, J., Lai, P. H., Zsebo, J. M., Murdock, D. C., Chazin, V. R., et al.,** Recombinant human granulocyte colony-stimulating factor: effects on normal and leukemic myeloid cells, *Science,* 232, 61, 1986.
33. **Kawasaki, E. S., Ladner, M. B., Wang, A. M., Van Arsdell, J., Warren, M. K., Coyne, M. Y., Schweickart, V. L., Lee, M.-T., Wilson, K. J., Boosman, A., Stanley, E. R., Ralph, P., and Mark, D. F.,** Molecular cloning of a complementary DNA encoding human macrophage-specific colony-stimulating factor (CSF-1), *Science,* 230, 291, 1985.
34. **Gough, N. M., Gough, H., Metcalf, D., Kelson, A., Grail, V., Nicola, N. A., Burgess, A. W., and Dunn, A. R.,** Molecular cloning of cDNA encoding a murine hematopoietic growth regulator: granulocyte macrophage colony stimulating factor, *Nature,* 309, 763, 1984.
35. **Nagata, S., Taira, H., Hall, A., Johnsrud, H., Streuli, M., Escodi, J., Boll, W., Cantell, K., and Weissmann, C.,** Synthesis in *E. coli* of a polypeptide with human leukocyte interferon activity, *Nature,* 284, 316, 1980.
36. **Taniguchi, T., Ohno, S., Fujii-Kuriyama, Y., and Muratmatsu, M.,** The nucleotide sequence of human fibroblast interferon cDNA, *Gene,* 10, 11, 1980.
37. **Gray, P. W., Leung, D. W., Pennica, D., Yelverton, E., Najarian, R., Simonsen, C. C., Derynck, R., Sherwood, P. J., Wallace, D. M., Berger, S. L., Levinson, A. D., and Goeddel, D., V.,** Expression of human immune interferon cDNA in *E. coli* and monkey cells, *Nature,* 285, 503, 1982.
38. **Lomedico, P. T., Gubler, V., Hellman, C. P., Dukovich, M., Giri, J. G., Pan, Y., Collins, K., Semionow, R., Chua, A. O., and Mizel, S. B.,** Cloning and expression of murine interleukin-1 cDNA in *Escherichia coli, Nature,* 312, 458, 1984.
39. **Auron, P. E., Webb, A. C., Rosenwasser, L. J., Mucci, S. F., Rich, A., Wolff, S. M., and Dinarello, C. A.,** Nucleotide sequence of human monocyte interleukin 1 precursor cDNA, *Proc. Natl. Acad. Sci. U.S.A.,* 81, 7907, 1984.
40. **Taniguchi, T., Matsui, H., Fujita, T., Takaoka, C., Kashima, N., Yoshimoto, R., and Hamuro, J.,** Structure and expression of a cloned cDNA for human interleukin-2, *Nature,* 302, 305, 1983.
41. **Leonard, W. J., Depper, J. M., Crabtree, G. R., Rudikoff, S., Pumphrey, J., Robb, R. J., Kronke, M., Svetlik, P. B., Peffer, N. J., Waldmann, T. A., and Greene, W. C.,** Molecular cloning and expression of cDNAs for the human interleukin-2 receptor, *Nature,* 311, 626, 1984.
42. **Fung, M., Hapel, A. J., Ymer, S., Cohen, D. R., Johnson, R. M., Campbell, J. D., and Young, I. G.,** Molecular cloning of cDNA for murine interleukin-3, *Nature,* 307, 233, 1984.
43. **Noma, Y., Sideras, P., Naito, T., Bergstedt-Lindquist, S., Azuma, C., Severinson, E., Tanabe, T., Kinashi, T., Matsuda, F., Yaoita, Y., and Honjo, T.,** Cloning of cDNA encoding the murine IgG1 induction factor by a novel strategy using SP6 promoter, *Nature,* 319, 640, 1986.

44. **Kinashi, T., Harada, N., Severinson, E., Tanabe, T., Sideras, P., Konsihi, M., Azuma, C., Tominaga, A., Bergatedt-Lindqvist, S., Takahashi, M., Natsuda, F., Yaoita, Y., Takatsu, K., and Honjo, T.,** Cloning of complementary DNA encoding T-cell replacing factor and identity with B-cell growth factor II, *Nature,* 324, 70, 1986.

45. **Hirano, T., Yasukawa, K., Harada, H., Taga, T., Watanabe, Y., Matsuda, T., Kashiwamura, S., Nakajima, K., Koyama, K., Iwamatsu, A., Tsunasawa, S., Sakayama, F., Matsui, H., Takahara, Y., Taniguchi, T., and Kishimoto, T.,** Complementary DNA for a novel human interleukin (BSF-2) that induces B lymphocytes to produce immunoglobulin, *Nature,* 324, 73, 1986.

46. **Zilberstein, A., Ruggieri, R., Korn, J. H., and Revel, M.,** Structure and expression of cDNA and genes for human interferon-beta-2, a distinct species inducible by growth-stimulatory cytokines, *EMBO J.,* 5, 2529, 1986.

47. **Gray, P., Aggarwal, B. B., Benton, C. V., Bringman, T. S., Hensel, W. J., Jarrett, J. A., Leung, D. W., Moffet, B., Ng, P., Svedersky, L. P., Palladino, M. A., and Nedwin, G. R.,** Cloning and expression of cDNA for human lymphotoxin, a lymphokine with tumor necrosis activity, *Nature,* 312, 721, 1984.

48. **Pennica, D., Nedwin, G. E., Hayflick, J. S., Seeburg, P. H., Derynck, R., Palladino, M. A., Kohr, W. J., Aggarwal, B. B., and Goeddel, D. V.,** Human tumor necrosis factor: precursor structure, expression and homology to lymphotoxin, *Nature,* 312, 724, 1984.

49. **Derynck, R., Jarrett, J. A., Chen, E. Y., Eaton, D. H., Bell, J. R., Assoian, R. K., Roberts, A. B., Sporn, M. B., and Goeddel, D. V.,** Human transforming growth factor-B complementary DNA sequence and expression in normal and transformed cells, *Nature,* 316, 701, 1985.

Chapter 3

T CELL CLONES AS SOURCES OF LYMPHOKINES

Gillis Otten and Frank W. Fitch

TABLE OF CONTENTS

I. INTRODUCTION

A. GENERAL REMARKS

The impetus for cloning T lymphocytes originated from a realization that T lymphocytes are heterogeneous and that results obtained from experiments utilizing bulk, uncloned populations could not be interpreted easily. It was hoped that the nature and extent of T lymphocyte heterogeneity could be assessed by characterizing the heterogeneity of sets of T cell clones.[1] T cell clones have, in fact, contributed significantly to attempts to answer three fundamental questions:

1. What is the cellular and molecular basis for the specificity of T cell responses to antigens, and what is the means by which the repertoire of antigen specificities is generated?
2. How do T lymphocytes exert their effector functions?
3. What modes of intercellular communication and types of cell-cell interactions are used in the regulation of the immune system?

The recent identification of the T cell antigen receptor and enumeration of the mechanisms which create diversity in the repertoire of antigen receptor specificities[2] was absolutely dependent on the isolation and propagation *in vitro* of clonal populations of T cells. T cell clones have also played a critical role in the characterization of both effector and regulatory T cell functions.[3] The secretion of soluble "factors", termed lymphokines, appears to be a primary means by which T cells carry out their functions. Lymphokines are potent effector molecules — biologically active *in vitro* at picomolar to nanomolar concentrations — and the spectrum of described activities is broad.[4] Many different lymphokine activities may be contained in a single preparation of conditioned medium obtained from bulk populations of peripheral lymphoid cells stimulated *in vitro*. Thus, it has been the goal of immunologists to isolate, identify, and characterize the individual molecular species responsible for the various biological activities and to pinpoint their cellular sources. Rapid progress has been made recently in identifying and purifying lymphokines: several T cell-derived lymphokines have been obtained in pure, homogeneous form, and several lymphokine genes have been cloned.[5]

It is the goal of this review to describe how the use of homogeneous populations of cloned T cells has contributed to the identification and characterization of lymphokines and to the delineation of functionally distinct T cell subsets. In addition, cloned T cells are proving to be useful model systems for exploring the regulation of lymphokine secretion at both the cellular and molecular levels.

B. DEFINITION OF A T CELL CLONE

Clonal populations of T cells have been derived from three major sources: T cell tumors (thymomas, lymphomas, and leukemias) adapted to grow *in vitro*; hybridomas generated by fusion of normal T cells, isolated from peripheral lymphoid tissue, to an immortalized T cell line; and normal T cells propagated *in vitro* with the use of immunological stimuli and *not* deliberately immortalized through viral transformation or fusion to another cell.[1,3] Throughout this review "T cell clone" refers to these normal cells maintained *in vitro*.

In contrast to autonomously proliferating T cell tumor lines, normal T cell clones require specific growth factors and/or antigenic stimulation for growth. However, whether T cell clones are truly "normal" cannot be answered in the general case. Certainly, culture conditions have been defined under which T cell clones maintain a stable phenotype and antigen specificity, and such clones may have a phenotype and antigen reactivity similar to that of uncloned populations. It is unclear, however, whether a T cell clone with seemingly unusual properties truly represents a rare, but possibly important, subpopulation which exists *in vivo* or whether its properties were altered during culture. Variants do arise spontaneously *in vitro*[6] and a policy of regular subcloning and retesting of subclones can be useful in identifying variants. The causes of phenotypic variation may not be clear; however, karyotypic instability is of concern. Experience has shown that clones maintained by periodic restimulation with antigen can be karyotypically stable,[7,8] while clones grown only with a source of growth factors may develop karyotypic anomalies quickly.[7]

II. ENUMERATION AND CHARACTERIZATION OF LYMPHOKINES PRODUCED BY T CELL CLONES

A. ISOLATION OF LYMPHOKINE cDNAs FROM T CELL CLONES

The ability of T cell clones to secrete large amounts of lymphokines became apparent soon after techniques were developed for cloning and maintaining T cells *in vitro*.[1] Individual T cell clones, however, generally secrete more than one activity,[9] necessitating elaborate schemes for biochemical purification. There are many reports describing the purification and characterization of various lymphokines.[10,11] Not surprisingly, the degree of purification increases with the number of steps and the sophistication of the fractionation process while the recovery drops accordingly.[12] Biochemical approaches to isolating proteins with desired lymphokine activities have been superseded largely by molecular biological strategies for cloning lymphokine cDNAs and genes. Nevertheless, there is still a need for obtaining highly purified natural lymphokines in order that the bioactivities of natural and recombinant products may be compared.

Historically, lymphokines have been detected by measuring biological activity *in vitro*.[10,11] Several reports have documented that lymphokine bioassays may detect more than one molecular species.[12-15] Furthermore, inhibitory factors may obscure the presence of the lymphokine of interest.[16-18] Thus, attempts to use bioassays to enumerate T cell-derived lymphokines may yield incomplete or incorrect information. Currently, the best means for demonstrating that a specific lymphokine is made by a given T cell clone are to construct a cDNA library and to identify a cDNA clone for the relevant lymphokine or to measure hybridization of T cell-derived mRNA to a previously isolated cDNA probe. Both techniques have been used successfully.

Table 1 presents a list of lymphokines known to be synthesized by T cell clones, based on cDNA cloning or RNA hybridization. In many cases, homologous cDNAs or genes have been cloned from both human and murine sources; hence, it is possible to identify the lymphokines synthesized by either human or murine T cell clones. As illustrated in Table 1, T cell clones synthesize a wide variety of lymphokines, suggesting that *in vivo*, T cells are potential sources of these lymphokines. It is interesting to note that cloned T cells may secrete polypeptides not normally thought of as lymphokines. For example, Zurawski et al.[19] have isolated a cDNA clone for preproenkephalin from a concanavalin A (Con A)-activated murine T-helper (T_H) clone. Presumably preproenkephalin mRNA was functional since secreted [Met]enkephalin was detectable by radioimmunoassay.

A detailed account of lymphokine molecular biology is beyond the scope of this chapter, but is extensively reviewed elsewhere.[5,11] T cell clones have not been the only sources of lymphokine mRNAs for constructing cDNA libraries but nevertheless have been used in some innovative schemes for isolating lymphokine cDNAs, as described below.

Lacking protein or nucleotide sequence information or antilymphokine antibodies, several groups have developed expression systems for synthesizing *in vivo* or *in vitro/in vivo* biologically active proteins from cDNA clones. The pCD mammalian expression vector system was designed to allow synthesis and secretion of biologically active protein by COS monkey kidney cells transfected with pCD plasmids containing cDNA inserts.[20] Yokota et

TABLE 1
Lymphokines Synthesized by T Cells as Determined by cDNA Cloning or RNA Hybridization

Name (alternative name)	Acronym	Murine T cells	Human T cells	Ref.
Interleukin-1	IL-1	+	+	98, 99
Interleukin-2	IL-2	+	+	21, 93
Interleukin-3 (multilineage colony-stimulating factor, P cell-stimulating factor)	IL-3	+	?	93, 100
Interleukin-4 (B cell stimulatory factor-1, IgG$_1$ induction factor)	IL-4	+	+	23, 34, 35
Interleukin-5 (T cell replacing factor, B cell growth factor-II)	IL-5	+	?	26
Granulocyte-macrophage colony-stimulating factor	GM-CSF	+	+	101, 102
Gamma interferon (immune interferon)	IFN-γ	+	+	93, 96
Preproenkephalin		+	?	19

al.[21] constructed a pCD cDNA library using mRNA from a Con A-activated, interleukin-2 (IL-2)-secreting, murine T cell clone. COS cells were transfected with pooled cDNAs and later assayed for secretion of IL-2 bioactivity. After several rounds of subpooling and screening, specific cDNA clones were identified which coded for biologically active IL-2. This same group has used a similar approach to clone several other lymphokine cDNAs, including granulocyte-macrophage colony-stimulating factor (GM-CSF), IL-3, B cell-stimulatory factor-1 (BSF-1), and gamma interferon (IFN-γ).[22]

In another report, a combination of transcription *in vitro* with oocyte microinjection/translation was utilized to identify a cDNA clone for murine IgG$_1$ induction factor,[23] a B cell differentiation factor.[24,25] A murine T cell clone which secreted IgG$_1$ induction factor[24] was stimulated with Con A, and the extracted mRNA used to generate a pSP6K cDNA library. The pSP6K vector contains the SP6 promoter which allows high efficiency transcription *in vitro*.[23] Capped transcripts were injected into oocytes, and oocyte-conditioned medium was assayed for bioactive IgG$_1$ induction factor. Interestingly, this approach successfully identified cDNA clones for IgG$_1$ induction factor while a pCD cDNA library constructed from the same T cell clone was unsuccessfully screened by COS cell transfection. The same T cell clone was the source of a distinct cDNA clone coding for T-cell replacing factor (TRF), another B cell differentiation factor.[26]

B. LYMPHOKINES DERIVED FROM T CELL CLONES HAVE MULTIPLE BIOLOGICAL ACTIVITIES

Prystowsky et al.[9] described an alloreactive T cell clone, designated L2, which could be stimulated to secrete ten different lymphokine activities affecting at least five different cell types: T lymphocytes (IL-2), B lymphocytes (polyclonal B cell stimulating factor), hematopoietic cells (IL-3, GM-CSF), macrophages (IFN-γ), and fibroblasts (IFN-γ). Synthesis of IL-2, IL-3, and IFN-γ by L2 cells since has been confirmed by RNA hybridization.[27] In addition, GM-CSF and IL-3, secreted by L2 cells, were biochemically separable and antigenically distinct.[14]

Each T cell-derived lymphokine may have multiple biological effects, thus expanding the potential influence of a single T cell clone. The biological properties of individual lymphokines are discussed in detail in other chapters and hence are described here in brief. In addition to its well-established T cell growth factor activity,[28] IL-2 has been shown to regulate natural killer cell activity[29] and also to stimulate lymphokine-activated killer cells.[30] Some activated B cells also express high affinity receptors for IL-2 (IL-2R),[31] suggesting yet another function for IL-2. The multiple biological activities of IL-3 are well documented.[32] Briefly, murine IL-3 stimulates the growth of multiple hematopoietic lineages among bone marrow cells, causes the growth of mast cells, stimulates cells which have the potential to form erythroid bursts, stimulates 20α-hydroxysteroid dehydrogenase expression in *nu/nu* mouse spleen cell cultures, and induces expression of the Thy-1 antigen by cultured bone marrow cells. Due to its very recent identification,[33] the biological properties of human IL-3 have not been thoroughly characterized. The availability of cloned BSF-1[23,34,35] and TRF[26,36] should simplify the analysis of the rather confusing pathways of B cell proliferation and differentiation.[37] IFN-γ also has multiple biological effects ranging from enhancement of major histocompatibility complex (MHC) class I and class II antigens,[38] to activation of macrophage tumoricidal activity,[39] to antiviral activity.[40]

The actual effects of lymphokines secreted *in vivo* during the T cell immune response are not clear. In an attempt to simulate what may occur *in vivo* in the vicinity of antigen-activated T cells, Prystowsky et al.[41] cocultured bone marrow cells, responsive to IL-3 and to GM-CSF, with L2 cloned T_H cells in the presence of alloantigen. Titration of L2 cells indicated that as few as 100 L2 cells per microculture could stimulate bone marrow cell proliferation, but that growth factor activity could not be detected in culture supernatants. A similar coculture system was used to demonstrate that cloned T cells, present in very low numbers, could provide nonspecific help to B cells.[41] Thus, lymphokines may act *in vivo* at levels below those which are detectable in culture supernatants. It is not clear whether lymphokines act only locally or whether transport through the circulation would allow for a lymphokine to act at a site distant from the initial site of T cell reaction.

III. LYMPHOKINE EXPRESSION IN T CELL SUBSETS

Although many investigators have demonstrated that specific T cell clones could secrete one or more lymphokine activities, it was not known whether these clones were actually representative of T cells. Several attempts have been made to divide T cells into distinct subsets based on the types of lymphokines secreted.

Glasebrook and Fitch[42] described several murine alloreactive T cell clones, derived from secondary mixed lymphocyte culture (MLC), some of which proliferated vigorously to stimulation with alloantigen, in the absence of added growth factors. These clones were not cytolytic, but when stimulated with alloantigen, secreted a factor which amplified the proliferation of cultured cytolytic T cell (T_C) clones and also secreted factors which promoted polyclonal plaque-forming responses in B cells. The noncytolytic clones were thus considered to belong to the T_H subset. The T_C-amplifying factor was later shown to be IL-2.[6] The derived T_C clones did not proliferate in response to alloantigen alone and were apparently dependent on T_H-derived IL-2 for proliferation. Subsequently, T_H-independent T_C clones were described which proliferated in response to alloantigenic stimulation in the absence of exogenous IL-2, suggesting the existence of two T_C subsets.[43,44] At least some of the T_H-independent T_C clones secreted IL-2 when stimulated with alloantigens.[45,46]

Estimates of the frequency of IL-2 secreting, T_H-independent T_C vary significantly. In one report, a minimum estimate was made of 2 cells in 10,000 for the frequency of Lyt-2^+ T-precursor cells from the spleens of nonimmunized mice capable of generating IL-2-secreting progeny in MLC.[47] Among these same Lyt-2^+ cells, the frequency of T_C precursors was 25- to 50-fold higher, indicating that few Lyt-2^+ T_C precursors had the potential to develop into IL-2-secreting T cells. However, in another report, 38 of 46 (80%) H-2^d-reactive, short-term, cloned T_C secreted IL-2,[48] and Widmer et al.[46] reported a high frequency (70%) of H-1-reactive T_C capable of secreting IL-2. These reports all differ in both the mouse strain combinations used and in the culture conditions under which T_C clones were derived; hence, the critical parameters affecting the generation of T_H-independent T_C are unclear. Among human T cells, the frequency of IL-2-secreting CD8$^+$ (human homolog of murine Lyt-2[49]) T_C has not been determined; however, several IL-2-secreting human T_C have been described.[50]

In an extensive study of lymphokine secretion by functionally distinct T cell clones, Kelso and Glasebrook[45] measured secretion of macrophage-activating factor (MAF), colony-stimulating factor (CSF), IFN, and IL-2 by a panel of 64 alloreactive murine T cell clones. Clones were classified functionally and phenotypically as cytolytic (100% Lyt-2$^+$) or non-cytolytic (100% Lyt-2$^-$), and clones of either type could be found which secreted any, but not necessarily all, of the measured activities. There was not an absolute correlation between cytolytic potential and the types of lymphokines secreted, suggesting that T cells are quite heterogeneous; however, noncytolytic clones were more likely to secrete IL-2 and in general secreted higher titers of MAF, IFN, and CSF. Among cytolytic clones, IL-2 secretion was observed only among T_H-independent T_C clones.[45]

In more recent studies, a functional heterogeneity among L3T4$^+$, Lyt-2$^-$ murine T cell clones was discovered, based on the types of lymphokines secreted. Sideras et al.[24] measured the production of MAF, IL-2, and IgG$_1$ induction factor by T cells cloned from B6.C-H-2^{bm12} (bm12) anti-C57BL/6 (B6) secondary MLC. Although not shown specifically, it was suggested that such clones were not cytolytic. Two of three clones secreted IgG$_1$ induction factor but neither IL-2 nor MAF, while the third clone secreted MAF only. In another set of clones, derived by limiting-dilution, secretion of IL-2 and IgG$_1$ induction factor was mutually exclusive. A cDNA for IgG$_1$ induction factor was isolated recently from a cDNA library made from one of these clones.[23] This cDNA is apparently identical to a mouse BSF-1 cDNA,[34] and IL-4 has been proposed as the name for this lymphokine which has both BSF-1 and IgG$_1$ induction factor activities. The data of Sideras[24] suggested that such alloreactive T cells secreted either IL-2 or IL-4 but not both. Although the antigen-specificity of the clones was not stated it is presumed to be I-A^b, since the bm12 and B6 strains differ only in the I-A region of the MHC. Thus, it appears that T cells with similar antigen specificities can differ in the types of lymphokines secreted.

More extensive studies by Mosmann et al.[15] appeared to confirm the subdivision of murine L3T4$^+$, Lyt-2$^-$ clones based on secretion of IL-2 and IL-4. In addition, IFN-γ was secreted by IL-2-secreting clones and not by IL-4-secreting clones. This may be of functional significance since IFN-γ is antagonistic to the stimulatory effects of IL-4 on B cells.[16] The IL-2- and IL-4-secreting subsets were termed T_H1 and T_H2, respectively, because of their functional similarity to previously described helper cell subsets.[15] The relationship between these variously defined subsets has not been determined, however. The likelihood of isolating a T_H1 or T_H2 clone was influenced by the antigen used for immunization,[15] but the relationship between the functional phenotype of T_H cells and antigen specificity has not been characterized in detail. T_H1 clones were observed to grow more rapidly than T_H2 clones. Therefore, in terms of isolating clones with distinct functional phenotypes, it seems important to clone cells at an early stage before overgrowth by faster growing cells obscures the existence of other T cell subpopulations.

It is not certain that the division of T_H cells into T_H1 and T_H2 subpopulations will be observed in other species. In rats[51] and humans,[52] cell surface antigens homologous to mouse L3T4 serve to delineate a major fraction of T_H cells. The homologous human molecule has been termed CD4,[53] while the homologous rat T cell antigen has been referred to simply as T4. Functional heterogeneity among T4$^+$ peripheral rat T cells was noted, based on differential expression of the antigen defined by monoclonal antibody (mAb) OX-22,[54,55] which reacts with the high molecular weight form of the rat leukocyte-common antigen (L-CA).[54] OX-22$^+$ cells synthesized IL-2 *in vitro*, mediated graft vs. host (GvH) disease *in vivo*, and were a relatively poor source of B cell help. In contrast, OX-22⁻ cells were a potent source of B cell help, but were poor producers of IL-2 and did not cause GvH.[54,55] Similarly, when peripheral human T cells were fractionated by expression of the 2H4 antigen, the CD4⁺, 2H4⁻ subset was the more potent source of B cell help (in a pokeweed mitogen-driven, polyclonal Ig secretion assay *in vitro*), and proliferated more vigorously to stimulation *in vitro* with soluble antigens while the CD4⁺, 2H4⁺ subset was more responsive to Con A.[56] Interestingly, an anti-2H4 mAb precipitated high molecular weight bands (200, 220 kDa) from human T cells,[57] similar in size to the antigens precipitated by mAb OX-22 from rat T cells. It will, therefore, be of interest to study differential expression of the homologous antigens by murine T_H1 and T_H2 clones. It is of some importance to know whether human and rat T_H subsets, ad defined by their 2H4 or OX-22 phenotypes, differentially secrete IL-2, IL-4, and IFN-γ. A strong correlation between cell surface phenotype and the spectrum of lymphokines secreted by the T_H cells of these three species would be suggestive of a fundamental subdivision within the T_H subset.

IV. ACTIVATION AND REGULATION OF LYMPHOKINE GENES IN T CELL CLONES

A. STIMULI FOR LYMPHOKINE SECRETION
1. Antigen-Specific Stimulation of Lymphokine Production

Antigen-specific T cell activation cannot be studied easily in bulk T cell populations: few or no T cells may react with the antigen of interest, and cell-cell interactions are difficult to dissect. T cell clones represent, therefore, better systems for studying antigen-specific activation. The rules for antigen-stimulated lymphokine production by T cell clones are the same as for proliferation,[58] indicating that the T cell receptor for antigen (Ti) mediates both processes. This has been confirmed directly with anti-Ti mAb which stimulate both proliferation and lymphokine secretion;[50] however, depending on culture conditins and the lymphokine activity measured, it is possible to detect secretion of lymphokines without proliferation or proliferation without lymphokine production. For example, tritiated thymidine ([³H]TdR) uptake by cloned T cells shows a biphasic dependence on antigen concentration[59] or on the concentration of anti-Ti mAb,[60] such that above an optimal antigen or mAb concentration, [³H]TdR uptake may actually decrease as the stimulus concentration increases. In contrast, lymphokine secretion reaches and maintains plateau levels as the stimulus increases. The reduced [³H]TdR uptake observed with high levels of anti-Ti mAb appears to be a direct effect of Ti-anti-Ti binding and is not due to a soluble factor.[60] Prystowsky et al.[41] defined conditions for stimulating a T_H clone with antigen in such a way that [³H]TdR uptake and CSF secretion were observed but IL-2 was not detectable. The lack of detectable IL-2 activity could have been due to IL-2 consumption by the proliferating cloned T_H cells.

2. Polyclonal Activation

Lectins such as Con A and phytohemagglutinin (PHA) will stimulate lymphokine secretion by T cell clones in the absence of accessory cells.[9] However, the difficulty with using lectins to study lymphokine production comes from the fact that lectins bind to multiple membrane glycoproteins[61] whose relative importance to activation is unclear. It was demonstrated recently that lectin-stimulated lymphokine production by a T cell tumor line required the cell surface expression of a Ti/T3 complex.[62] It is not clear, however, whether this dependence indicates direct binding of lectin by Ti/T3. Other data suggest that PHA interacts with the CD2 (T11) T cell surface molecule;[63] hence the requirement for Ti/T3 may reflect the dependence of the CD2 activation pathway on Ti/T3.[64]

mAbs reactive with well-defined T cell surface molecules are of interest as polyclonal T cell activators. Both uncloned and cloned T cells can be activated to secrete lymphokines to proliferate using mAb reactive with CD2,[65] Tp44,[66,67] TAP,[68] Ly-6,[69] and Thy-1.[70-72] T cell clones have been used by several investigators to analyze transmembrane signaling and intracellular signal transduction by these activation molecules. How these structures function *in vivo* is not known. Except for CD2, which apparently binds to LFA-3 molecules found on the target cells and therefore may promote the adhesion of T cells to antigen-presenting cells,[73,74] the relevant ligands for these other T cell surface structures have not been identified.

3. IL-2 as a Stimulus or Costimulus of Lymphokine Secretion

Reports differ as to whether IL-2 by itself stimulates lymphokine secretion from T cells. In some reports, IL-2 was found to stimulate secretion of IFN-γ,[75-77] whereas in other cases it did not.[78] The heterogeneity of peripheral T cells and the low percentage of IL 2R$^+$ cells in healthy individuals limit the interpretation of data obtained from bulk populations. On the other hand, T cell clones are generally IL 2R^{+}[79] and, as homogeneous populations, are preferable to bulk populations for studying the effect of IL-2 on T cell secretion of lymphokines. Nevertheless, studies using various cloned populations have not produced any general rules because results have varied from clone to clone and range from direct stimulation by IL-2 to down-regulation by IL-2 of the response to antigen by T$_H$ clones. Examples are discussed below.

Howard et al.[80] studied the secretion of B cell growth factor-I (BCGF-I), a lymphokine which stimulates DNA synthesis in splenic B cells activated with suboptimal concentrations of anti-IgM antibodies. Uncloned or cloned, long-term ovalbumin (OVA)-reactive, murine T cell lines were induced to secrete BCGF-I by OVA plus syngeneic splenic accessory cells, or by IL-2 alone. Since the recently cloned IL-4 has BCGF-I activity,[34] it will be interesting to learn whether IL-2 induces IL-4 production. Such data would suggest possible interactions between T$_H$1 and T$_H$2 cells.

Kelso described L3T4$^+$, Lyt-2$^-$ and L3T4$^-$, Lyt-2$^+$ T cell clones which were induced by either Con A or IL-2 to secrete multi-CSF (IL-3) and GM-CSF.[81,82] However, compared to Con A, IL-2 preferentially caused GM-CSF secretion. Additional data were presented suggesting that IL-2 and Con A stimulated GM-CSF by different mechanisms, although IL-2 and Con A synergistically stimulated both multi-CSF and GM-CSF secretion.

Ythier et al.[83] described two human CD4$^+$ alloreactive T cell clones which secreted IL-2 and an IL-3-like activity (measured on a murine IL-3-sensitive cell line) when stimulated with alloantigen. The IL-3-like activity was also secreted when cloned T cells were stimulated with recombinant IL-2 (rIL-2) alone, and secretion was inhibited by mAb reactive with the IL-2R. Interestingly, anti-IL-2R mAb did not block alloantigen-stimulated secretion of IL-2, but did block secretion of the IL-3-like activity. These results suggest that antigen-stimulated secretion of IL-3-like activity involved an autocrine mechanism in which IL-2, secreted in response to alloantigen, acted on the cloned T cells to stimulate secretion of IL-3-like activity. It will be important to learn whether such an autocrine pathway occurs in other T cell clones. In addition, it remains to be shown that the IL-3-like activity was due to authentic human IL-3.[33]

The ability of a T cell clone to secrete lymphokines in response to IL-2 may also change during prolonged culture. A variant subclone of an alloreactive T$_C$ clone was isolated recently which, in contrast to the parent line, is induced by highly purified rIL-2 to secrete IFN-γ.[84] Both the parental and variant clones secrete IFN-γ in response to Con A. This variant phenotype appears to be rare among T$_C$, since the same preparation of rIL-2 does not cause a variety of other T$_C$ clones nor bulk populations of alloreactive T$_C$, derived from secondary MLC, to secrete IFN-γ. The mechanism by which IL-2 stimulates IFN production in this variant T$_C$ clone is under study.

Rather than directly stimulating secretion of lymphokines, IL-2 may only increase the level of lymphokines secreted in response to a second stimulus. By a mechanism that remains unknown, IL-2 increased both the rate and duration of MAF secretion in a large panel of alloreactive T_C and noncytolytic clones.[47] Since, in this study, all clones were IL-2-dependent for growth, the lymphokine-enhancing and growth-promoting effects of IL-2 could not be dissociated.

B. IMMUNOREGULATION OF LYMPHOKINE SECRETION BY T CELL CLONES

Because secretion of lymphokines is a primary means by which T_H cells function, we sought to determine whether lymphokine secretion could be modulated in immunologically relevant ways. Preliminary studies indicated that following exposure to antigen, IL-2-secreting cloned T_H cells (T_H1-type) became temporarily refractory to a restimulation with antigen, secreting little or no lymphokine in response to this second stimulation.[85,86] The antigen-refractory T_H cells recovered responsiveness over a period of several days; however, early in the recovery phase, antigen-stimulation led to secretion of CSF and IFN-γ but IL-2 was not detected.[86] It could not be determined if this discordance reflected differential regulation of these lymphokines. Further studies revealed that exposure to high concentrations of rIL-2, in the absence of antigen or accessory cells, also induced cloned T_H cells to become unresponsive to antigen.[87] This finding suggested that an autocrine mechanism of regulation existed in which IL-2, produced in the initial response to antigen, acted to limit the capacity of T_H clones to secrete lymphokines when subsequently rechallenged with antigen. T_H-dependent T_C clones, which do not to secrete IL-2 and are dependent on IL-2 for growth,[6] were not induced by IL-2 to become unresponsive to antigen-stimulation.[88] Thus, the responsiveness to antigen of T_H-dependent T_C appears not to be influenced by T_H cells. It will be of interest to learn whether T_H2-type clones are similarly down-regulated by IL-2 and whether IL-4, which has T cell growth-promoting activity,[15,89] also down-regulates T_H responses to antigen. Subsequent experiments to determine why IL-2-treated T_H clones were unresponsive to antigen, suggested that exposure of these cells to IL-2 resulted in inhibition of the transmembrane or intracellular signaling processes which link receptor-antigen binding to the activation of lymphokine synthesis.[87] Responsiveness of cloned T_H cells to antigen could be reconstituted by adding a calcium ionophore, implying that calcium-dependent signaling was inhibited.[90] Moreover, receptor-dependent increases in intracellular calcium ion levels were discovered to be almost completely inhibited in cloned T_H cells made unresponsive to antigen by prior exposure to IL-2.[91]

C. T CELL CLONES AS MODEL SYSTEMS FOR STUDYING REGULATION OF LYMPHOKINE GENES

As homogeneous populations of T cells which have a phenotype closely resembling normal T cells, T cell clones are potentially excellent model systems for studying the regulation of lymphokine genes. However, the difficulty in producing cloned T cells in sufficient numbers, the relatively complex conditions necessary for growth in culture, and the potential for variability in responsiveness to stimulation (as detailed above) may limit the usefulness of T cell clones as subjects for studies of the molecular biology and biochemistry of lymphokine gene regulation. T cell clones nonetheless have been used to study certain aspects of the regulation of lymphokine expression.

Characterization of the mechanism of action of cyclosporin A (CsA) is of great interest because of its potent immunosuppressive effects and clinical value.[92] Using a cloned alloreactive murine T_H clone, Prystowsky et al.[41] found that CsA inhibited Con A-stimulated secretion of CSF without significantly inhibiting total protein synthesis. Herold et al.[93] demonstrated that CsA blocked accumulation of IL-2, IL-3, and IFN-γ mRNAs in T_H and T_C clones which has been stimulated with Con A or with a mAb which specifically identified the antigen receptor on the T_C clone.[94] Taken together, these data suggested that CsA acts to inhibit stimulated lymphokine production at a pretranslational level, a finding supported by studies on T cell tumor lines and normal peripheral T cells.[95,96]

In a study of the immunosuppressive effects of glucocorticoids, Culpepper and Lee[97] found that dexamethasone inhibited accumulation of IL-3 mRNA and prevented the appearance of IL-3 activity in the supernatant of a Con A-activated T_H clone. Thy-1 mRNA, which was constitutively present, was unaffected, suggesting that the effects of dexamethasone may be specific to certain inducible genes. Undoubtedly, future studies will investigate the regulation of lymphokine genes in detail. A question which remains unanswered is how lymphokine genes are regulated during differentiation, i.e., why are T cells restricted in the types of lymphokines they can be stimulated to express? T cell clones would appear to be valuable tools for answering this question.

V. CONCLUSIONS

T cell clones have played several different roles in lymphokine studies. As homogeneous and potent sources of lymphokines, T cell clones have provided the starting material for purification of lymphokines and for isolation lymphokine cDNAs. Studies attempting to correlate the types of lymphokines secreted by T cell clones with their cell surface phenotype or effector function have shown T cell clones to be quite heterogeneous. Nevertheless, subsets of clones which secrete distinct sets of lymphokines can be discriminated, suggesting both a division of labor and specialization among T cells. T cell clones also serve as excellent model systems for studying both the regulation T cell responses to antigenic stimulation and the linkage between T cell recognition of antigen and the activation of inducible lymphokine genes.

REFERENCES

1. **Fathman, C. G. and Fitch, F. W.,** Eds., *Isolation, Characterization and Utilization of T Lymphocyte Clones,* Academic Press, New York, 1982.
2. **Fitch, F. W.,** T-cell clones and T-cell receptors, *Microbiol. Rev.,* 50, 50, 1986.
3. **von Boehmer, H. and Haas, W.,** Eds., *T Cell Clones,* Elsevier, Amsterdam, 1985.
4. **Waksman, B. H.,** Overview: biology of the lymphokines, in *Biology of the Lymphokines,* Cohen, S., Pick, E., and Oppenheim, J. J., Eds., Academic Press, New York, 1979, 585.
5. **Webb, D. R. and Goeddel, D. V.,** Eds., *Molecular Cloning and Analysis of Lymphokines,* Academic Press, Orlando, FL, 1987.
6. **Ely, J. M., Prystowsky, M. B., Eisenberg, L., Quintans, J., Goldwasser, E., Glasebrook, A. L., and Fitch, F. W.,** Alloreactive cloned T cell lines. V. Differential kinetics of IL 2, CSF and BCSF release by a cloned T amplifier cell and its variant, *J. Immunol.,* 127, 2345, 1981.
7. **Johnson, J. P., Cianfriglia, M., Glasebrook, A. L., and Nabholz, M.,** Karyotype evolution of cytolytic T cell lines, in *Isolation, Characterization and Utilization of T Lymphocyte Clones,* Fathman, C. G. and Fitch, F. W., Eds., Academic Press, New York, 1982, 183.
8. **Prystowsky, M. B.,** personal communication, 1985.
9. **Prystowsky, M. B., Ely, J. M., Beller, D. I., Eisenberg, L., Goldman, J., Goldman, M., Goldwasser, E., Ihle, J., Quintans, J., Remold, H., Vogel, S. N., and Fitch, F. W.,** Alloreactive cloned T cell lines. VI. Multiple lymphokine activities secreted by helper and cytolytic cloned T lymphocytes, *J. Immunol.,* 129, 2337, 1982.
10. **Oppenheim, J. J. and Cohen, S.,** Eds., *Interleukins, Lymphokines, and Cytokines,* Academic Press, New York, 1983.
11. **Sorg, C. and Schimpl, A.,** Eds., *Cellular and Molecular Biology of Lymphokines,* Academic Press, Orlando, FL, 1985.
12. **Grabstein, K., Eisenman, J., Mochizuki, D., Shanebeck, K., Conlon, P., Hopp, T., March, C., and Gillis, S.,** Purification to homogeneity of B cell stimulating factor: a molecule that stimulates proliferation of multiple lymphokine-dependent cell lines, *J. Exp. Med.,* 163, 1405, 1986.

13. **Hapel, A. J., Warren, H. S., and Hume, D. A.,** Different colony stimulating factors are detected by the interleukin 3 dependent cell lines FDCP1 and 32Dc1-23, *Blood,* 64, 786, 1984.

14. **Prystowsky, M. B., Ihle, J. N., Otten, G., Keller, J., Rich, I., Naujokas, M., Loken, M., Goldwasser, E., and Fitch, F. W.,** Two biologically distinct colony-stimulating factors are secreted by a T lymphocyte clone, in *Normal and Neoplastic Hematopoiesis,* Golde, D. W. and Marks, P. A., Eds., Alan R. Liss, New York, 1983, 369.

15. **Mosmann, T. R., Cherwinski, H., Bond, M. W., Giedlin, M. A., and Coffman, R. L.,** Two types of murine helper T cell clone. I. Definition according to profiles of lymphokine activities and secreted proteins, *J. Immunol.,* 136, 2348, 1986.

16. **Rabin, E. M., Mond, J. J., Ohara, J., and Paul, W. E.,** Interferon-γ inhibits the action of B cell stimulatory factor (BSF)-1 on resting B cells, *J. Immunol.,* 137, 1573, 1986.

17. **Horowitz, J. B., Kaye, J., Conrad, P. J., Katz, M. E., and Janeway, C. A., Jr.,** Autocrine growth inhibition of a cloned line of helper T cells, *Proc. Natl. Acad. Sci. U.S.A.,* 83, 1886, 1986.

18. **Wong, G. H. W., Clark-Lewis, I., Hamilton, J., and Schrader, J. W.,** P cell stimulating factor and glucocorticoids oppose the action of interferon-γ in inducing Ia antigens on T-dependent mast cells (P cells), *J. Immunol.,* 133, 2043, 1984.

19. **Zurawski, G., Benedik, M., Kamb, B. J., Abrams, J. S., Zurawski, S. M., and Lee, F. D.,** Activation of mouse T-helper cells induces abundant preproenkephalin mRNA synthesis, *Science,* 232, 772, 1986.

20. **Okayama, H. and Berg, P.,** A cDNA cloning vector that permits expression of cDNA inserts in mammalian cells, *Mol. Cell. Biol.,* 3, 280, 1983.

21. **Yokota, T., Arai, N., Lee, F., Rennick, D., Mosmann, T., and Arai, K.,** Use of a cDNA expression vector for isolation of mouse interleukin 2 cDNA clones: expression of T-cell growth-factor activity after transfection of monkey cells, *Proc. Natl. Acad. Sci. U.S.A.,* 82, 68, 1985.

22. **Yokota, T., Lee, F., Arai, N., Rennick, D., Zlotnick, A., Mosmann, T., Miyajima, A., Takebe, Y., Kastelein, R., Zurawski, G., and Arai, K.,** Strategies for cloning mouse and human lymphokine genes using a mammalian cDNA expression vector, *Lymphokines,* 13, 1, 1987.

23. **Noma, Y., Sideras, P., Naito, T., Bergstedt-Lindqvist, S., Azuma, C., Severinson, E., Tanabe, T., Kinashi, T., Matsuda, F., Yaoita, Y., and Honjo, T.,** Cloning of cDNA encoding the murine IgGl induction factor by a novel strategy using SP6 promoter, *Nature,* 319, 640, 1986.

24. **Sideras, P., Bergstedt-Lindqvist, S., MacDonald, H. R., and Severinson, E.,** Secretion of IgG₁ induction factor by T cell clones, *Eur. J. Immunol.,* 15, 586, 1985.

25. **Sideras, P., Bergstedt-Lindqvist, S., and Severinson, E.,** Partial characterization of IgG₁-inducing factor, *Eur. J. Immunol.,* 15, 593, 1985.

26. **Kinashi, T., Harada, N., Severinson, E., Tanabe, T., Sideras, P., Konishi, M., Azuma, C., Tominaga, A., Bergstedt-Lindqvist, S., Takahashi, M., Matsuda, F., Yaoita, Y., Takatsu, K., and Honjo, T.,** Cloning of complementary DNA encoding T-cell replacing factor and identity with B-cell growth factor II, *Nature,* 324, 70, 1986.

27. **Herold, K. C., Lancki, D. W., Dunn, D. E., Arai, K., and Fitch, F. W.,** Activation of lymphokine genes during stimulation of cloned T cells, *Eur. J. Immunol.,* 16, 1533, 1986.

28. **Smith, K. A.,** T-cell growth factor, *Immunol. Rev.,* 51, 337, 1980.

29. **Brooks, C. G. and Henney, C. S.,** Interleukin-2 and the regulation of natural killer activity in cultured cell populations, in *Contemporary Topics in Molecular Immunology,* Vol. 10, Gillis, S. and Inman, F. P., Eds., Plenum Press, New York, 1985, 63.

30. **Rosenberg, S. A. and Lotze, M. T.,** Cancer immunotherapy using interleukin-2 and interleukin-2 activated lymphocytes, *Annu. Rev. Immunol.,* 4, 681, 1986.

31. **Lowenthal, J. W., Zubler, R. H., Nabholz, M., and MacDonald, H. R.,** Similarities between interleukin-2 receptor number and affinity on activated B and T lymphocytes, *Nature,* 315, 669, 1985.

32. **Ihle, J. N. and Weinstein, Y.,** Immunological regulation of hematopoietic/lymphoid stem cell differentiation by interleukin 3, *Adv. Immunol.,* 39, 1, 1986.

33. **Yang, Y.-C., Ciarletta, A. B., Temple, P. A., Chung, M. P., Kovacic, S., Witek-Giannotti, J. S., Leary, A. C., Kriz, R., Donahue, R. E., Wong, G. C., and Clark, S. C.,** Human IL-3 (multi-CSF): identification by expression cloning of a novel hematopoietic growth factor related to murine IL-3, *Cell,* 47, 3, 1986.

34. **Lee, F., Yokota, T., Otsuka, T., Meyerson, P., Villaret, D., Coffman, R., Mosmann, T., Rennick, D., Roehm, N., Smith, C., Zlotnik, A., and Arai, K.,** Isolation and characterization of a mouse interleukin cDNA clone that expresses B-cell stimulatory factor 1 activities and T-cell- and mast-cell-stimulating activities, *Proc. Natl. Acad. Sci. U.S.A.,* 83, 2061, 1986.

35. **Yokota, T., Otsuka, T., Mosmann, T., Banchereau, J., DeFrance, T., Blanchard, D., De Vries, J. E., Lee, F., and Arai, K.,** Isolation and characterization of a human interleukin cDNA clone, homologous to mouse B-cell stimulatory factor-1, that expresses B-cell- and T-cell-stimulating activities, *Proc. Natl. Acad. Sci. U.S.A.,* 83, 5894, 1986.

36. **Hirano, T., Yasukawa, K., Harada, H., Taga, T., Watanabe, Y., Matsuda, T., Kashiwamura, S., Nakajima, K., Koyama, D., Iwamatsu, A., Tsunasawa, S., Sakiyama, F., Matsui, H., Takahara, Y., Taniguchi, T., and Kishimoti, T.,** Complementary DNA for a novel human interleukin (BSF-2) that induces B lymphocytes to produce immunoglobulin, *Nature,* 324, 73, 1986.
37. **Howard, M. and Paul, W. E.,** Regulation of B-cell growth and differentiation by soluble factors, *Ann. Rev. Immunol.,* 1, 307, 1983.
38. **Wong, G. H. W. and Schrader, J. W.,** Regulation of H-2, Ia, TL, and Qa antigen expression by interferon γ, *Lymphokines,* 11, 48, 1985.
39. **Schreiber, R. D. and Celada, A.,** Molecular characterization of interferon γ as a macrophage activating factor, *Lymphokines,* 11, 87, 1985.
40. **Lengyel, P.,** Biochemistry of interferons and their actions, *Annu. Rev. Biochem.,* 51, 251, 1986.
41. **Prystowsky, M. B., Otten, G., Pierce, S. K., Shay, J., Olshan, J., and Fitch, F. W.,** Lymphokine production by cloned T lymphocytes, *Lymphokines,* 12, 13, 1985.
42. **Glasebrook, A. L. and Fitch, F. W.,** Alloreactive cloned T cell lines. I. Interactions between clones amplifier and cytolytic T cell lines, *J. Exp. Med.,* 151, 876, 1980.
43. **Widmer, M. B. and Bach, F. H.,** Antigen-driven helper cell independent cloned cytolytic T lymphocytes, *Nature,* 294, 750, 1981.
44. **Glasebrook, A. L., Kelso, A., and MacDonald, H. R.,** Cytolytic T lymphocyte clones that proliferate autonomously to specific alloantigenic stimulation. II. Relationship of the Lyt-2 molecular complex to cytolytic activity, proliferation, and lymphokine secretion, *J. Immunol.,* 130, 1545, 1983.
45. **Kelso, A. and Glasebrook, A. L.,** Secretion of interleukin 2, macrophage-activating factor, interferon, and colony-stimulating factor by alloreactive T lymphocyte clones, *J. Immunol.,* 132, 2924, 1984.
46. **Widmer, M. B., Roopenian, D. C., Biel, L. W., and Bach, F. H.,** Characterization of alloreactive murine T cell clones *in vitro,* in *T Cell Clones,* von Boehmer, H. and Haas, W., Eds., Elsevier, Amsterdam, 1985, 131.
47. **Kelso, A., MacDonald, H. R., Smith, K. A., Cerottini, J.-C., and Brunner, K. T.,** Interleukin 2 enhancement of lymphokine secretion by T lymphocytes: analysis of established clones and primary limiting dilution microcultures, *J. Immunol.,* 132, 2932, 1984.
48. **Andrus, L., Granelli-Piperno, A., and Reich, E.,** Cytotoxic T cells both produce and respond to interleukin 2, *J. Exp. Med.,* 59, 647, 1984.
49. **Ledbetter, J. A., Evans, R. L., Lipinski, M., Cunningham-Rundles, C., Good, R. A., and Herzenberg, L. A.,** Evolutionary conservation of surface molecules that distinguish T lymphocyte helper/inducer and cytotoxic/suppressor subpopulations in mouse and man, *J. Exp. Med.,* 153, 310, 1981.
50. **Meuer, S. C., Hodgdon, J. C., Hussey, R. E., Protentis, J. P., Schlossman, S. F., and Reinherz, E. L.,** Antigen-like effects of monoclonal antibodies directed at receptors on human T cell clones, *J. Exp. Med.,* 158, 988, 1983.
51. **White, R. A. H., Mason, D. W., Williams, A. F., Galfre, G., and Milstein, C.,** T-lymphocyte heterogeneity in the rat: separation of functional subpopulations using a monoclonal antibody, *J. Exp. Med.,* 148, 664, 1978.
52. **Engleman, E. G., Benike, C. J., Glickman, E., and Evans, R. L.,** Antibodies to membrane structures that distinguish suppressor/cytotoxic and helper T lymphocyte sub-populations block the mixed leukocyte reaction in man, *J. Exp. Med.,* 154, 193, 1981.
53. **I.U.I.S.-W.H.O. Nomenclature Subcommittee,** Nomenclature, *J. Immunol.,* 134, 659, 1985.
54. **Spickett, G. P., Brandon, M. R., Mason, D. W., Williams, A. F., and Woollett, G. R.,** MRC OX-22, a monoclonal antibody that labels a new subset of T lymphocytes and reacts with the high molecular weight form of the leukocyte-common antigen, *J. Exp. Med.,* 158, 759, 1983.
55. **Mason, D. and Arthur, R. P.,** T cells that help B cell responses to soluble antigen are distinguishable from those producing interleukin 2 on mitogenic or allogeneic stimulation, *J. Exp. Med.,* 163, 774, 1986.
56. **Morimoto, C., Letvin, N. L., Distaso, J. A., Aldrich, W. R., and Schlossman, S. F.,** The isolation and characterization of the human suppressor inducer T cell subset, *J. Immunol.,* 134, 1508, 1985.
57. **Morimoto, C., Letvin, N. L., Rudd, C. E., Hagan, M., Takeuchi, T., and Schlossman, S. F.,** The role of the 2H4 molecule in the generation of suppressor function of Con A-activated T cells, *J. Immunol.,* 137, 3247, 1986.
58. **Haskins, K., Kappler, J., and Marrack, P.,** The major histocompatibility complex-restricted antigen receptor on T cells, *Annu. Rev. Immunol.,* 2, 51, 1984.
59. **Hecht, T. T., Longo, D. L., and Matis, L. A.,** The relationship between immune interferon production and proliferation in antigen-specific T lymphocytes, *J. Immunol.,* 131, 1049, 1983.
60. **Nau, G. J., Moldwin, R. L., Lancki, D. W., Kim, D.-K., and Fitch, F. W.,** Inhibition of IL-2-driven proliferation of murine T lymphocyte clones by supraoptimal levels of immobilized anti-T cell receptor monoclonal antibody, *J. Immunol.,* 139, 114, 1987.
61. **Sitkovsky, M. V., Pasternack, M. S., Lugo, J. P., Klein, J. R., and Eisen, H. N.,** Isolation and partial characterization of Concanavalin A receptors on cloned cytolytic T lymphocytes, *Proc. Natl. Acad. Sci. U.S.A.,* 81, 1519, 1984.

62. **Weiss, A. and Stobo, J.,** Requirement for the coexpression of T3 and the T cell antigen receptor on a malignant human T cell line, *J. Exp. Med.,* 160, 1284, 1984.
63. **O'Flynn, K., Krensky, A. M., Beverly, P. C. L., Burakoff, S. J., and Linch, D. C.,** Phytohaemagglutinin activation of T cells through the sheep red blood cell receptor, *Nature,* 313, 686, 1985.
64. **Fox, D. A., Schlossman, S. F., and Reinherz, E. L.,** Regulation of the alternative pathway of T cell activation by anti-T3 monoclonal antibody, *J. Immunol.,* 136, 1945, 1986.
65. **Meuer, S. C., Hussey, R. E., Fabbi, M., Fox, D. A., Acuto, O., Fitzgerald, K. A., Hodgdon, J. C., Protentis, J. P., Schlossman, S. F., and Reinherz, E. L.,** An alternative pathway of T cell activation; a functional role for the 50KD T11 sheep erythrocyte receptor protein, *Cell,* 36, 897, 1984.
66. **Hara, T., Fu, S. M., and Hansen, J. A.,** Human T cell activation. II. A new activation pathway used by a major T cell population via a disulfide-bonded dimer of a 44 kilodalton polypeptide (9.3 antigen), *J. Exp. Med.,* 161, 1513, 1985.
67. **Moretta, A., Pantaleo, G., Lopez-Botet, M., and Moretta, L.,** Involvement of T44 molecules in an antigen-independent pathway of T cell activation. Analysis of correlation to the T cell antigen-receptor complex, *J. Exp. Med.,* 162, 823, 1985.
68. **Rock, K. L., Yeh, E. T. H., Gramm, C. F., Haber, S. I., Reiser, H., and Benacerraf, B.,** TAP, a novel T cell-activating protein involved in the stimulation of MHC-restricted T lymphocytes, *J. Exp. Med.,* 163, 315, 1986.
69. **Malek, T. R., Ortega, G., Chan, C., Kroczek, R. A., and Shevach, E. M.,** Role of Ly-6 in lymphocyte activation. II. Induction of T cell activation by monoclonal anti-Ly-6 antibodies, *J. Exp. Med.,* 164, 709, 1986.
70. **Gunter, K. C., Malek, T. R., and Shevach, E. M.,** T cell-activating properties of an anti-Thy-1 monoclonal antibody: possible analogy to OKT3/Leu-4, *J. Exp. Med.,* 159, 716, 1984.
71. **Lancki, D. W., Ma, D. I., Havran, W. L., and Fitch, F. W.,** Cell surface structures involved in T cell activation, *Immunol. Rev.,* 81, 65, 1984.
72. **MacDonald, H. R., Bron, C., Rousseaux, M., Horvath, C., and Cerottini, J.-C.,** Production and characterization of monoclonal anti-Thy-1 antibodies that stimulate lymphokine production by cytolytic T cell clones, *Eur. J. Immunol.,* 15, 495, 1985.
73. **Dustin, M. L., Sanders, M. E., Shaw, S., and Springer, T. A.,** Purified lymphocyte function-associated antigen 3 binds to CD2 and mediates T lymphocyte adhesion, *J. Exp. Med.,* 165, 677, 1987.
74. **Plunkett, M. L., Sanders, M. E., Selvaraj, P., Dustin, M. L., and Springer, T. A.,** Rosetting of activated human T lymphocytes with autologous erythrocytes. Definition of the receptor and ligand molecules as CD2 and lymphocyte function-associated with antigen 3 (LFA-3), *J. Exp. Med.,* 165, 664, 1987.
75. **Benjamin, W. R., Steeg, P. S., and Farrar, J. J.,** Production of immune interferon by an interleukin 2-dependent murine T cell line, *Proc. Natl. Acad. Sci. U.S.A.,* 79, 5379, 1982.
76. **Kasahara, T., Hooks, J. J., Dougherty, S. F., and Oppenheim, J. J.,** Interleukin 2-mediated immune interferon (IFN-γ) production by human T cells and T cell subsets, *J. Immunol.,* 130, 1784, 1983.
77. **Vilcek, J., Henriksen-DeStefano, D., Siegel, D., Klion, A., Robb, R., and Le, J.,** Regulation of IFN-γ production in human peripheral blood cells by exogenous and endogenously produced interleukin 2, *J. Immunol.,* 135, 1851, 1985.
78. **LeFrancois, L., Klein, J. R., Paetkau, V., and Bevan, M. J.,** Antigen-independent activation of memory cytotoxic T cells by interleukin 2, *J. Immunol.,* 132, 1845, 1984.
79. **Havran, W. L., Kim, D.-K., Moldwin, R. L., Lancki, D. W., and Fitch, F. W.,** Interleukin-2 differentially regulates IL-2 receptors on murine cloned cytolytic and helper T cells, *Clin. Immunol. Immunopathol.,* 39, 368, 1986.
80. **Howard, M., Farrar, J., Hilfiker, M., Johnson, B., Takatsu, K., Hamaoka, T., and Paul, W. E.,** Identification of a T-cell derived B cell growth factor distinct from interleukin 2, *J. Exp. Med.,* 155, 914, 1982.
81. **Kelso, A., Metcalf, D., and Gough, N. M.,** Independent regulation of granulocyte-macrophage colony-stimulating factor and multilineage colony-stimulating factor production in T lymphocyte clones, *J. Immunol.,* 136, 1718, 1986.
82. **Kelso, A. and Gough, N.,** Expression of hemopoietic growth factor genes in murine T lymphocytes, *Lymphokines,* 13, 209, 1987.
83. **Ythier, A. A., Abbud-Filho, M., Williams, J. M., Loertscher, R., Schuster, M. W., Nowill, A., Hansen, J. A., Maltezos, D., and Strom, T. B.,** Interleukin-2 dependent release of interleukin 3 activity by T4+ human T-cell clones, *Proc. Natl. Acad. Sci. U.S.A.,* 82, 7020, 1985.
84. **Dunn, D. E., Herold, K. C., Otten, G., Lancki, D. W., Vogel, S. N., Gajewski, T., and Fitch, F. W.,** Interleukin 2 and Concanvalin A stimulate gamma interferon production in a cloned T cell line by distinct pathways, manuscript in preparation, 1987.
85. **Wilde, D. B. and Fitch, F. W.,** Antigen-reactive cloned helper T cells. I. Unresponsiveness to antigenic restimulation develops after stimulation of cloned helper T cells, *J. Immunol.,* 132, 1632, 1984.

86. **Wilde, D. B., Prystowsky, M. B., Ely, J. M., Vogel, S. N., Dialynas, D. P., and Fitch, F. W.,** Antigen-reactive cloned helper T cells. II. Exposure of murine cloned helper T cells to IL 2-containing supernatant induces unresponsiveness to antigenic restimulation and inhibits lymphokine production after antigenic stimulation, *J. Immunol.,* 133, 636, 1984.

87. **Otten, G., Wilde, D. B., Prystowsky, M. B., Olshan, J., Rabin, H., Henderson, L. E., and Fitch, F. W.,** Cloned helper T lymphocytes exposed to interleukin 2 become unresponsive to antigen and to concanavalin A but not to calcium ionophore and phorbol ester, *Eur. J. Immunol.,* 16, 217, 1986.

88. **Fitch, F. W., Otten, G., and Kim, D.-K.,** Two T cell clones respond differently to antigen after exposure to IL-2, *Fed. Proc.,* 44, 1695, 1985.

89. **Fernandez-Botran, R., Krammer, P. H., Diamanstein, T., Uhr, J. W., and Vitetta, E. S.,** B cell-stimulatory factor 1 (BSF-1) promotes growth of helper T cell lines, *J. Exp. Med.,* 155, 914, 1986.

90. **Otten, G., Herold, K. C., and Fitch, F. W.,** Interleukin 2 inhibits antigen-stimulated lymphokine synthesis in helper T cells by inhibiting calcium-dependent signalling, submitted for publication, 1987.

91. **Otten, G.,** unpublished observations, 1987.

92. **Shevach, E.,** The effects of Cyclosporin A on the immune system, *Annu. Rev. Immunol.,* 3, 397, 1985.

93. **Herold, K. C., Lancki, D. W., Moldwin, R. L., and Fitch, F. W.,** Immunosuppressive effects of Cyclosporin A on cloned T cells, *J. Immunol.,* 136, 1315, 1986.

94. **Lancki, D. W., Lorber, M. I., Loken, M. R., and Fitch, F. W.,** A clone-specific monoclonal antibody that inhibits cytolysis of a cytolytic T cell clone, *J. Exp. Med.,* 157, 921, 1983.

95. **Kronke, M., Leonard, W. J., Depper, J. M., Arya, S. K., Wong-Stahl, F., Gallo, R. C., Waldmann, T. A., and Greene, W. C.,** Cyclosporin A inhibits T-cell growth factor gene expression at the level of mRNA transcription, *Proc. Natl. Acad. Sci. U.S.A.,* 81, 5214, 1984.

96. **Wiskocil, R., Weiss, A., Imboden, J., Kamin-Lewis, R., and Stobo, J.,** Activation of human T cell line: a two-stimulus requirement in the pretranslational events involved in the coordinate expression of interleukin 2 and γ-interferon genes, *J. Immunol.,* 134, 1599, 1985.

97. **Culpepper, J. A. and Lee, F.,** Regulation of IL 3 expression by glucocorticoids in cloned murine T lymphosytes, *J. Immunol.,* 135, 3191, 1985.

98. **Tartakovsky, B., Kovacs, E., Takacs, L., and Durum, S. K.,** T cell clone producing an IL 1-like factor after stimulation by antigen-presenting B cells, *J. Immunol.,* 137, 160, 1986.

99. **Acres, R. B., Larsen, A., and Conlon, P. J.,** IL 1 expression in a clone of human T cells, *J. Immunol.,* 138, 2132, 1987.

100. **Yokota, T., Lee, R., Rennick, D., Hall, C., Arai, N., Mosmann, T., Nabel, G., Cantor, H., and Arai, K.,** Isolation and characterization of a mouse cDNA clone that expresses mast-cell growth-factor activity in monkey cells, *Proc. Natl. Acad. Sci. U.S.A.,* 81, 1070, 1984.

101. **Gough, N. M., Gough, J., Metcalf, D., Kelso, A., Grail, D., Nicola, N. A., Burgess, A. W., and Dunn, A. R.,** Molecular cloning of cDNA encoding murine haematopoietic growth regulator, granulocyte-macrophage colony stimulating factor, *Nature,* 309, 763, 1984.

102. **Lee, F., Yokota, T., Otsuka, T., Gemmell, L., Larson, N., Luh, J., Arai, K., and Rennick, D.,** Isolation of cDNA for a human granulocyte-macrophage colony-stimulating factor by functional expression in mammalian cells, *Proc. Natl. Acad. Sci. U.S.A.,* 82, 4360, 1985.

Chapter 4

RECEPTORS ON T AND B LYMPHOCYTES

Robert E. Cone and John J. Marchalonis

TABLE OF CONTENTS

I. INTRODUCTION

Lymphocytes, like all cells, utilize cell membrane receptors to communicate with their environment. Their environment contains other lymphocytes as well as many factors which mediate the lymphocyte's homeostatic activities. Thus, cell-cell interactions (by contact or extracellular products) are requisite to normal lymphocyte function and therefore a viable immune system. Moreover, the singular function of lymphocytes is to respond and sometimes eliminate molecules and/or cells recognized as foreign to the organism. This function, like homeostatic mechanisms, is also mediated via cell membrane receptors. The immediate products of the interaction of receptor molecules and ligand which results in the activation or inactivation of lymphocytes are complex and are only recently being unraveled (see below). The designation of a molecule as a "receptor" has been widely used, and to define a molecule as a receptor the standard criteria of saturability, specificity, and reversibility of ligand binding should be established. Moreover, the binding of ligand to its receptor should affect the activity of the cell.[1] Accordingly, if antibody to a membrane protein activates (or inactivates) the cell the molecule is not necessarily a receptor unless a ligand is identified. On the other hand, the specific binding activity of some molecules (e.g., E or erythrocyte receptor of human T lymphocytes) may be identified but the functional consequences of this binding are not clear. At least the membrane molecules are defined by binding a ligand. A common erroneous use of "receptor" is the designation of cell surface molecules bound by lectins as "lectin receptors". In point of fact, the surface molecule is a "receptee" and not the receptor. The combining site involved is part of the lectin which is detecting a carbohydrate group at the cell surface.

Table 1 lists lymphocyte receptors and the 19 listed receptors are grouped according to Marchalonis and Galbraith[2] into functional categories. The first group (I) of receptors central to lymphocyte function are the antigen binding/specific receptors which mediate recognition of antigen. The second group (II) determines the response of the cell by triggering the cell into division and/or differentiation. Supportive (III) receptors are not necessarily involved in the initial activation of a cell but are involved in modulating or maintaining events initiated by triggering receptors and/or normal homeostatic processes. The fourth (IV) miscellaneous group is really a receptable for receptors with a ligand but no known function. As the functional role of these receptors is defined they would be moved to groups II or III since all antigen binding proteins (I) may have been described.

II. ANTIGEN BINDING/SPECIFIC RECEPTORS

That antigen-specific lymphocyte clones are "selected" by antigen through the aegis of membrane receptors is a fact that took years to develop. Immunoglobuins, the secreted antigen-specific product of B lymphocytes, serve as the B cell receptor for antigen and polypeptides structurally similar to immunoglobulins are T cell receptors for antigen. On the other hand, the diversity of functionally distinct T cell subsets may hold also for the nature and distribution of T cell receptors for antigen. Accordingly, we consider separately antigen receptors of B cells and T cells (Figure 1).

A. B CELLS

That B lymphocytes utilize immunoglobulin molecules as membrane receptors for antigen is derived from the demonstration that (1) B lymphocytes readily bind antigen specifically, (2) B lymphocyte antigen binding and function is inhibited by antibodies to immunoglobulins, (3) immunoglobulins are present in B lymphocyte membranes and molecules which bind antigen specifically have been isolated from the membrane of antigen-specific B cells, and (4) some anti-immunoglobulin antibodies stimulate B cells.[3,4] The antigen specificity for

TABLE 1
Lymphocyte Receptors

I	Antigen binding	Cell	Ref.
	MHC restricted heterodimers α/β, γ/δ	T	20—22, 24
	Antigen-binding molecule	T	32—38, 40—43
	Immunoglobulin, IgM, IgD	B	1—6

II	Triggering	Cell	Ref.
	BCGF	B	50
	BCDF	B	51
	IL-2 low/high	T, (B)	52, 53
	IL-1	T	51
	T3/TCR	T	24, 29, 45

III	Supportive	Cell	Ref.
	Insulin	T	58, 59
	Growth hormone	T	60
	Transferrin	Activated T, B	61, 62
	LDL	T, B	63
	Gc	Activated T, B	56
	α-2HS	T, B	64

IV	Miscellaneous	Cell	Ref.
	Fc, IGg	T, B	69—72
	Fc, IgE, IgA, IgD	T	73—75
	C3	B, activated T	76
	Histamine	T	79
	β-Adrenergic	B, T	78
	Enkephalin	T	68

individual B lymphocytes is derived from V, J, and gene segment rearrangements of immunoglobulin genes.[5] All membrane immunoglobulins of an individual cell have the same V region but may have constant regions (inserted into the membrane) which are both IgM or IgD isotype. The membrane IgM molecule resembles the monomeric subunit of pentameric IgM although the membrane μ heavy chain differs somewhat from the secreted μ chain based on a peptide sequence for membrane insertion. It is not clear why two isotypes (μδ) are expressed in the membrane while both molecules bear the same V region and bind antigen. Membrane IgM is shed rapidly ($T^1/_2$ = 6 h) by large B cells as an intact molecule which does not bear membrane lipids[9-9] while it is turned over slowly by small B cells.[8] Membrane IgD also shows a rapid turnover phase;[9] however, the shed molecule is degraded.[9] Microfilaments regulate the shedding of membrane IgM, whereas microtubules (but not microfilaments) regulate the turnover of membrane IgD.[9] These observations suggest a different cytoskeletal association of these receptors which might bear on their function for the cell. There are differences in the proportion of μ + δ + . μ + δ- and μ − δ − cells in ontogeny with δ + cells representing more mature B cells.[10] Moreover, when B cells are stimulated there are switches in the synthesis of isotypes and some secondary B cells express other isotypes (e.g., IgA, IgE, IgG) as receptors;[11] however, cells expressing isotypes other than μ or are rarc and likely are the result of stimulation of B cells.

When membrane immunoglobulins interact with antigen, the receptors become cross-linked, associate demonstrably with actin,[12] and usually aggregate to form a cap which is internalized and/or released from the cell.[13] The net effect of this phenomenon is a temporary

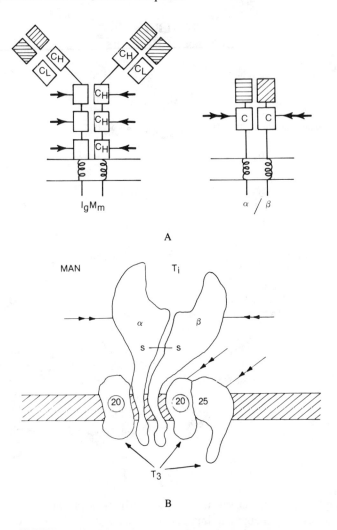

FIGURE 1.   (A) Schematic representation of the domains of receptor immunoglobulin of B cell (IgM) and T cells (α/β heterodimer). Variable (V) regions are denoted by shading. Constant regions (C) are indicated by the letter C within the domain blocks. The arrows indicate the attachment of glycosyl moieties; the transmembrane segments are represented as helices. (B) Diagrammatic representation of the T-cell receptor complex containing the α/β heterodimer as expressed by helper and cytotoxic T cells of man. The α/β heterodimers form disulfide-bonded structures resembling monomeric Fab fragments with long hinge regions, membrane-spanning segments, and cytoplasmic segments. These antigen receptors (Ti) are associated with invariant molecules (termed T3) that are involved in activation. The apparent masses of the molecules of the T3 complex are given as numerals within circles. Double arrows represent glycosyl moieties.

loss of membrane immunoglobulin which is replaced within 12 h. The actual role of capping, endocytosis, etc., of receptor-antigen complex in stimulation of the cell is not known and this event may not be necessary to stimulate the B cell. Based on studies with T cells (see below) there is speculation that during cross-linking membrane immunoglobulins become associated with other membrane proteins which may form a triggering complex.

B. T CELLS

That T lymphocytes recognize antigen specifically has been established for some time;[14]

however, demonstrable antigen binding by T cells and the nature of T cell receptors for antigen has been, until recently, problematic. Some T cells do bind foreign antigen, generally in solid phase[14-18] (e.g., cells, derivatized nylon) and the antigen-binding cells bear Lyt2 antigens.[15] In fact the generation of such cells during an immune respone *in vitro* indicates that the appearance of these cells is highly dose-dependent and parallels the development of suppressor T cells.[15] On the other hand, Lyt1[+] and -2[-] cells have not been demonstrated to bind antigen, yet their function is highly specific.[15] The recognition of foreign (nominal) antigen by helper T cells and cytotoxic T cells is restricted by classes II and I major histocompatibility complex (MHC) antigens, respectively.[19] Whether this recognition involves a neoepitope created by association of an MHC antigen with processed nominal antigen or separate recognition of nominal antigen and self MHC is not known. T cell membrane proteins (receptors, TCR) involved in recognition of antigen and MHC have been identified as heterodimeric (M_r 90,000) molecules comprised of two glycopolypeptide chains (M_r approximately 40,000) distinct in charge.[20-23] The polypeptides initially were designated α and β and a second group, defined as γ/δ, have been described[24] based on demonstration of genes for these polypeptides. Comparisons of gene sequence (and sometimes protein sequence) α, β, and γ molecules show strong homologies to immunoglobulins and immunocompetent cells display variable gene rearrangements indicating further the immunoglobulin nature of these molecules.[25-28] In addition, genes for human MHC-restricted T cell receptors map to chromosomes bearing immunoglobulin heavy chains (α-chain) and light chain (β-chain). That these proteins are receptors is suggested by the finding that antibodies specific for clonal receptors block the function of the clone only or may stimulate the clone;[20-22] however with some exceptions[23] these molecules have not been shown to bind nominal antigen.[29] It could be argued that antigen binding by heterodimeric TCR cannot be demonstrated until the appropriate antigen (antigen and MHC) is used.

Unlike helper and cytotoxic T cells, T cells with the suppressor phenotype bind nominal antigen[15] and are not restricted by MHC antigens in their recognition of antigen. Moreover, TCRβ chain genes are absent from many T cell hybrids with the suppressor phenotype.[30,31] However, suppressor cells and some helper T cells produce soluble polypeptides which bind nominal antigen specifically. These T cell (derived) antigen binding molecules (TABM)[32] are found in the culture fluids of suppressor T cells,[33,34] hybrids,[35,36] and clones[37] and in serum[38-40] and ascites fluid[41] containing some T cell hybrids and are M_r 68,000 to 140,000 and comprised of M_r 22,000 subunits.[32] Membrane forms of TABM have been demonstrated[42,43] which bind specifically the antigen to which the cell shows specificity[42] and anti-TABM antibodies inhibit the ability of an antigen binding T cell hybrid to bind antigen.[42] These data indicate that membrane TABM function as an receptor for antigen. The relationship of these proteins to MHC-restricted TCR is unknown. Preliminary studies indicate that TCR and TABM are basically distinctive, although TABM, immunoglobulins, and TCRβ chain share a peptide sequence in the V region.[44]

III. TRIGGERING RECEPTORS

MHC-restricted T cells are not activated solely by the interaction of the MHC-antigen receptor. This event is coincident with interaction with group membrane (T3) glycoproteins.[24,29,45] In fact, antibodies to T3 will activate T cells and maintain the proliferarion of T clones in the absence of antigen.[24,29,45,46] In humans, the T3 complex is comprised of 28,000 and 22,000 mol wt polypeptides[47] while the mouse MHC/antigen receptor is associated with two glycoproteins, 23,000 T3γ and 21,000 (T3δ) and two nonglycosylated peptides, 26,000 (T3ε) and 16,000.[48] T3 and MHC/antigen receptors can be coprecipitated by antireceptor anti-T3 antibodies if the complex is isolated in mild (digitonin) detergents,[49] indicating physical association between these moieties. Since T3 is associated with the antigen receptor and required for triggering we included it in the *triggering* category.

Once a T or B cell interacts with antigen subsequent events leading to proliferation, then differentiation leads to the expression of receptors which bind ligands that contribute to proliferation and/or differentiation of the cell. B cells express receptors for T cell-derived B cell growth factor (BCGF)[50] and B cell differentiation factor (BCDF),[51] which promotes the progression of proliferating B cells into effector cells. The biochemical nature of these receptors has not yet been defined.

T cells express receptors which bind macrophage (antigen presenting cell) -derived interleukin-1 (IL-1)[51] and helper T cells do not proliferate in response to antigen unless IL-1 delivers a signal to the helper T cell. Similarly, activated T cells express receptors for T cell-derived IL-2.[52,53] This receptor has been defined further by monoclonal antireceptor antibodies (anti-Tac), which bind proteins of 55,000 to 60,000 mol wt. Like receptors for IL-1 and chemotactic F-met-leu-phe[54] of polymorphonuclear leukocytes, receptors of IL-2 can be defined as high or low affinity receptors. Anti-Tac antibodies apparently isolate high and low affinity receptors while only high affinity receptors can be isolated by affinity for IL-2. It may be that high affinity receptors must be engaged to activate the cell;[55] however, it is not certain whether high and low affinity receptors are separate molecules or high affinity receptors are formed by multimerization of low affinity receptors.[53] Resting T cells may not express receptors for IL-2 (high affinity) but when the cells are activated by antigen binding to T3/Ti, receptors for IL-2 are expressed and IL-2 is produced.[53] Thus, IL-2 and its receptors represents an autocrine system of growth control. To summarize, B cells express receptor for two lymphokines (BCGF and BCDF) regulating the proliferation and differentiation of B cells. T cells express receptors for a monokine (IL-1) and a lymphokine (IL-2). Since IL-2 influences B cells some B cells also express IL-2 receptor;[52,53] however, a receptor for a ligand modulating only T cell differentiation has not been identified. Activated T cells do express receptors for the vitamin D metabolite 1,25-(DH) D_3[56] which might be involved in the final phase of differentiation.[57] Presumably as other cytokines are described (e.g., IL-3), receptors for these will also be defined eventually. Other T cell surface molecules have been implicated in triggering the cell because antibodies to these polypeptides activate the cell (T11, Ly6, for example). It is premature, however, to label these proteins as receptors since there is (presently) no ligand.

IV. SUPPORTIVE RECEPTORS

Receptors thus far described function in recognition/triggering in that ultimately the receptor-ligand interaction activates (or inactivates) the cell. Supporitve receptors act as elements that bind a ligand which then influences the activity of the cell. For example, receptors for insulin[58,59] and growth hormone[60] focus these molecules which then influence cellular activity. Like receptors for IL-2, insulin receptors generally are detected *after* activation of the cell. Activated cells (T and B) express binding sites for transferrin[61,62] which binds a variety of divalent metallic cations essential for optimal cell growth. Transferrin receptors are expressed by activated T and B cells, neoplastic cells, and virus-infected cells. Similarly, lymphocytes may express receptors for low density lipoproteins (LDL)[63] which can influence cell membrane lipid composition and α2-HS glycoprotein[64] carrying zinc.[65]

V. MISCELLANEOUS

Lymphocytes express receptors for a host of molecules whose biological influence on the lymphocyte is not clear and therefore fall in this category (temporarily?). In addition, lymphocytes are influenced by molecules, e.g., IFN-γ,[67] and neuropeptides[68] known to function through surface receptors. Most B cells express receptors for the Fc portion of IgG.[69] While some Fc (IgG) receptors are 45,000 to 55,000 mol wt proteins, the heterogeneity in Fc receptors[70-72] suggests that multiple forms may be distributed on different cell lineages. T cell receptors for immunoglobulins are more complex. IgA, IgE, and IgD can induce the proliferation of T cells with receptors for these immunoglobulins,[73-75] and these T cells may be involved in the regulation of the expression of these isotypes. Some B cells and activated T cells express receptors for the third component of complement,[76] but the biological relevance of these receptors is not yet clear.

The specificity of infection of lymphocyte lineages by viruses (e.g., EBV and B cells, HIV, and helper T cells) indicates receptors for these viruses. In humans, T4 is a receptor for HIV.[77] This raises the question whether there is as an endogenous ligand for T4 which HIV mimics. Quite possibly this putative ligand may have immunological significance. Moreover, anti-idiotypic antibodies to antibodies to the ligand might prevent infection with HIV. Finally, lymphocytes express receptors for several pharmacologically active molecules, e.g., β-adrenergic receptors[78] and histamine.[79] Thus, lymphocytes are modulated by a host of homeostatic mechanisms before and/or after they respond to antigen.

VI. RECEPTOR-MEDIATED SIGNAL TRANSDUCTION

Membrane receptor-ligand interactions must be transduced into the cell to signal the genome and/or biosynthetic or secretory mechanisms. This signal occurs through a cascade of second messengers which amplify the initial signal.[80,81]

Although this complex pathway (Figure 2) may vary with a given receptor, we will consider generally this system, since most (perhaps all) receptors are associated with this system. The second messengers are found in membrane phospholipids, the precursor lipid being phosphotidyl inositol (PtdIns). PtdIns is phosphorylated in stages to phosphatidyli-nositol 4,5 biphosphate (PtdIns4,5P$_2$). Receptor-ligand interaction activates a phosphoinos-itidase via the agency of a coupling G protein. The enzyme hydrolyzes Ptd Ins to second messengers inositol 1,4,5 triphosphate (ins 1,4,5 P$_3$) and diaceylglycerol (DAG) Ins 1,4,5P$_3$ may be dephosphorylated to free inositol of (which reenters the pathway by being phos-phorylated to Ptd Ins) phosphorylated to Ins 1,3,4P$_4$, another second messenger. The two second messengers, DAG and Ins 1,4,5P$_3$ may mediate distinct events during activation of the cell. Ins 1,4,5P$_3$ is involved in Ca^{2+}-dependent processes. Internal calcium is mobilized by Ins 1,4,5P$_3$. The calcium and DAG activate protein kinase C which phosphorylates proteins. Subsequent events could be membrane depolarization, secretion, or genomic ac-tivation (or inactivation).[80-82] The activity of the receptors listed in Table 1 have been found to be mediated by phospholipids, and in fact receptor activity can be bypassed by the exogenous addition of agents (such as phorbol esters) which enter the activation pathway.[82] The activation pathway may be general, although some receptors may be associated with one aspect of the pathway. For example, a receptor which activates cyclic nucleotides might activate protein kinase C without activation of the phosphoinositol pathway. Thus, the activity of a given receptor could be selective depending on with what aspect of the signaling system the receptor is associated. Thus, the final outcome of the influence of a ligand on the lymphocyte will depend on the receptor or complexity of the ligand.

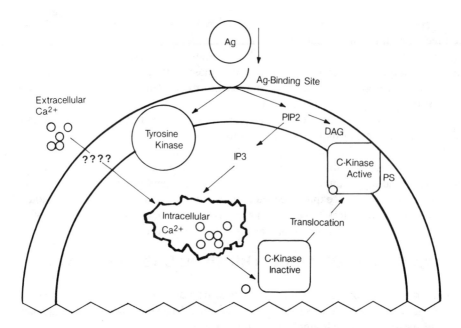

FIGURE 2. Schematic model of major biochemical events apparently common to both T and B cells after stimulation through antigen-binding sites. The stimulus for activation would be antigen or antibody to surface immunoglobulin in the case of the B cells and antigen or antibodies to members of the T3 complex in the T cell case. The binding of ligand initiates hydrolysis of phosphatidylinositol diphosphate (PIP_2), yielding inositol triphosphate (IP_3), which mobilizes Ca^{2+}. The resulting increase in intracellular Ca^{2+}, a phenomenon that may also involve the influx of extracellular ions, contributes to the translocation of C-kinase from the cytosol to the membrane. Interaction of C-kinase with Ca^{2+} (DAG) and phospholipid, such as phosphatidylserine (PS), leads to enzyme activation and the specific phosphorylation of several membrane-associated substrates. Tyrosine kinases may also be activated upon modulation of antigen-binding sites by either antigen or antibody. The potential involvement of phosphodiesterase and relevant controlling mechanisms (G or N proteins and GTP) of phospholipase A, arachidonate, cyclic nucleotides, lymphokines, and interactions with adherent cells are omitted from this diagram in the interest of clarity.

REFERENCES

1. **Marchalonis, J. J. and Cone, R. E.,** *Transplant. Rev.,* 14, 30, 1973.
2. **Marchalonis, J. J. and Galbraith, R.,** Receptors on lymphoid cells: an overview, *Methods Enzymol.,* 150, 377, 1987.
3. **Julius, M. H., Heusser, C. H., and Hautmann, K.-U.,** Induction of resting B cells to DNA synthesis by soluble monoclonal anti-immunoglobulin, *Eur. J. Immunol.,* 14, 753, 1984.
4. **Cambier, J. C., Justement, L. B., Newell, K., Chen, Z. Z., Harris, L. K., Sandoual, V. M., Klemsz, M. J., and Ransom, J. T.,** Transmembrane signals and intracellular "second messengers" in the regulation of quiescent B lymphocyte activation, *Immunol. Rev.,* 95, 37, 1987.
5. **Alt, F. W., Blackwell, T. K., DePinho, R. A., Reth, M. G., and Yancopoulos, G. D.,** *Immunol. Rev.,* 89, 5, 1986.
6. **Rogers, J. and Wall, R.,** Immunoglobulin RNA rearrangements during B lymphocyte differentiation, *Adv. Immunol.,* 35, 39, 1984.
7. **Melchers, F., Cone, R. E., and Von Bochmer, H.,** Immunoglobulin turnover in B lymphocytes sub-populations, *Eur. J. Immunol.,* 5, 382, 1975.
8. **Emerson, S. G. and Cone, R. E.,** I-A^k and H-2K^k antigens are shed as supramolecular particles in association with membrane lipids, *J. Immunol.,* 127, 482, 1981.
9. **Emerson, S. G. and Cone, R. E.,** Regulation of murine B lymphocyte plasma membrane protein turnover and shedding, *J. Cell Physiol.,* 109, 25, 1981.

10. **Parkhouse, R. M. E. and Cooper, M. D.,** A model for the differentiation of B lymphocytes with implications for the biological role of IgD, *Immunol. Rev.,* 37, 105, 1977.

11. **Vitetta, E. S. and Uhr, J. W.,** IgD and B cell differentiation, *Immunol. Rev.,* 37, 50, 1977.

12. **Loor, F.,** Plasma membranes and cell cortex interactions in lymphocyte functions, *Adv. Immunol.,* 30, 1, 1980.

13. **Cone, R. E.,** Dynamic aspects of the lymphocyte surface, in *The Lymphocyte: Structure and Function II,* Marchalonis, J. J., Ed., Marcel Dekker, New York, 1988, 567.

14. **Cone, R. E. and Beaman, K. D.,** T cell antigen binding proteins (immunoproteins) and their cell membrane analogues, in *Antigen-Specific T Cell Receptors and Factors,* Vol. 2, Marchalonis, J. J., Ed., Academic Press, Orlando, FL, 1987, 67.

15. **Eardley, D., Shen, F. W., Cone, R. E., and Gershon, R. K.,** Antigen binding T cells: dose response and kinetics studies on the development of different subsets, *J. Immunol.,* 122, 140, 1979.

16. **Cramer, M.,** Isolated hapten-specific T cell receptor material — final view, in: *Antigen-Specific T Cell Receptors and Factors,* Marchalonis, J. J., Ed., Vol. 2, Academic Press, Orlando, FL, 1987, 33.

17. **Cone, R. E.,** Molecular basis for t lymphocyte recognition of antigen, *Progr. Allergy,* 29, 114, 1981.

18. **Ruddle, N. H., Beezley, B. B., Lewis, G. K., and Goodman, J. W.,** Antigen-specific T cell hybrids. II. T cell hybrids which bind azobenzene arsonate, *Mol. Immunol.,* 17, 925, 1980.

19. **Benacerraf, B.,** Overview of the major histocompatibility complex, *Science,* 212, 1229, 1981.

20. **Haskins, K., Kubo, R.,White, J., Pigeon, M., Kappler, J., and Marrack, P.,** The major histocompatibility complex-restricted antigen receptor on T cells. I. Location with a monoclonal antibody, *J. Exp. Med.,* 157, 1149, 1983.

21. **Reinherz, E. L., Acuto, O., Fabbi, M., Bensussan, A., Milanese, C., Royer, H. D., Meuer, S. C., and Schlossman, S. F.,** Clonotypic surface structure on human T lymphocytes: functional and biochemical analysis of the antigen receptor complex, *Immunol. Rev.,* 81, 95, 1984.

22. **Kaye, J., Porcelli, S., Tite, J., Jones, B., and Janeway, C. A., Jr.,** Both a monoclonal antibody and antisera specific for determinants unique to individual cloned helper T cell lines can substitute for antigen and antigen presenting cells in the activation of T cells, *J. Exp. Med.,* 158, 836, 1983.

23. **Silliciano, R. F., Hemesath, T. J., Pratt, J. C., Dintz, R. Z., Dintzis, H. M., Acuto, O., Shim, H. S., and Reinherz, E. L.,** Direct evidence for the existence of nominal antigen binding sites on T cell surface Ti α-β heterodimers of MHC-restricted T cell clones, *Cell,* 47, 161, 1986.

24. **Pardoll, D. M., Kruisbeek, A. M., Fowlkes, B. J., Coligan, J. E., and Schwartz, R. H.,** The unfolding story of T cell receptor, *FASEB J.,* 1, 103, 1987.

25. **Hedrick, S. M., Cohen, D. I., Nielson, E. A., and Davis, M. M.,** Isolation of cDNA clones encoding T cell-specific membrane associated proteins, *Nature,* 308, 149, 1984.

26. **Yanagi, Y., Yoskikai, Y., Leggett, K., Clark, S. P., Aleksander, I., and Mak, T. W.,** A human T cell specific cDNA clone encodes a protein having extensive homology to immunoglobulin chains, *Nature,* 308, 145, 1984.

27. **Hayday, A. C., Saito, H., Gillies, S.D., Kranz, D. M., Tanigawa, G., Eisea, H. N., and Tonegawa, S.,** Structure, organization and somatic rearrangement of T-cell gamma genes, *Cell,* 40, 259, 1985.

28. **Brenner, M. B., McLean, J., Scheft, H., Riberdy, J., Ang., S.-L., Seidman, J. G., Devlin, P., and Krangel, M. S.,** Two forms of the T-cell receptor protein found on peripheral blood cytotoxic T lymphocytes, *Nature,* 325, 689, 1987.

29. **Kubo, R. T., Kappler, J. W., Haskins, K. and Marrack, P.,** The major histocompatibility complex-restricted T cell antigen receptor, in *Antigen-Specific T Cell Receptors and Factors,* Vol. 1, Marchalonis, J. J., ed., Academic Press, Orlando, FL, 1987, 77.

30. **Medrick, S. M., Germain, R. N., Bevan, M. J., Dorf, M., Engel, I., Fink, P., Gascoign, N., Heber-Katz, E., Kapp, J., Kaufman, Y., Kaye, J., Melchers, F., Pierce, C., Schwartz, K. H., Sorensen, C., Taniguchi, M., and Davis, M. M.,** Rearrangement and transcription of a T cell receptor β-chain gene in different T cell subsets, *Proc. Natl. Acad. Sci. U.S.A.,* 82, 531, 1985.

31. **Mak, T. W. and Yanagi, Y.,** Genes encoding the human T cell antigen receptors, *Immunol. Rev.,* 81, 222, 1984.

32. **Cone, R. E.,** Non-MHC restricted T cell antigen binding proteins, in *Methods in Enzymology: Immunochemical Techniques,* Part K, Vol. 150, DiSabato, G., Ed., Academic Press, Orlando, FL, 1987, 666.

33. **Cone, R. E., Rosenstein, K. W., Janeway, C. A., Iverson, G. M., Murray, J. H., Cantor, H., Fresno, M., Mattingly, J. A., Cramer, M., Krawinkel, U., Wigzell, H., Binz, H., Frischknecht, H., Ptak, W., and Gershon, R. K.,** Affinity-purified, antigen-specific products produced by T cell share epitopes recognized by heterologous antisera raised against several different antigen-specific products from T cells, *Cell Immunol.,* 82, 233, 1983.

34. **Ptak, W., Gershon, R. K., Rosenstein, R. W., Murray, J. H., and Cone, R. E.,** Purification and characterization of TNP-specific immunoregulatory molecules produced by T cells sensitized to picryl-chloride (PCLF), *J. Immunol.,* 131, 2859, 1983.

35. **Healy, G. T., Kapp, J. A., and Webb, D. R.**, Purification and biochemical analysis of antigen-specific suppressor factors obtained from the supernatant or the cytosol of a T cell hybridoma, *J. Immunol.,* 131, 2843, 1983.

36. **Steele, J. K., Stammers, A. T., and Levy, J. G.**, Isolation and characterization of a tumor-specific suppressor factor from a T cell hybridoma, *J. Immunol.,* 134, 2767, 1985.

37. **Fresno, M., McVay-Boudreau, L., Nable, G., and Cantor, H.**, Antigen-specific T lymphocyte clones. II. Purification and biological characterization of an antigen-specific protein synthesized by cloned T cells, *J. Exp. Med.,* 173, 250, 1981.

38. **Iverson, G. M., Eardley, D. P., Janeway, C. A., and Gershon, R. K.**, The use of anti-idiotypic immunoabsorbents to isolate circulating antigen-specific T cell-derived molecules from hyperimmune sera, *Proc. Natl. Acad. Sci. U.S.A.,* 80, 1435, 1981.

39. **Cone, R. E., Gerardi, D. A., Davidoff, J., Petty, J., Kobayashi, K., and Cohen, S.**, Quantitation of T cell antigen binding molecules (TABM) in the sera of non-immunized, immunized and desensitized mice, *J. Immunol.,* 138, 234, 1987.

40. **Pasemen, V. J. and Möller, G.**, ELISA assay for the detection of a dextran binding product secreted by a T cell hybrid Th1, *Scand. J. Immunol.,* 25, 349.

41. **Beaman, K. D. and Cone, R. E.**, Production and purification of monoclonal T lymphocyte antigen binding molecules (TABM), *Biochem. Biophys. Res. Commun.,* 25, 349, 1985.

42. **Cone, R. E., Beaman, K. D., and Ruddle, N. A.**, Isolation of antigen binding molecules from the membrane of an antigen binding, antigen-specific T cell hybrid, *Cell. Immunol.,* 99, 257, 1986.

43. **Callahan, H. J. and Maurer, P. H.**, Preparation of an antigen-binding fragment from a murine T lymphocyte membrane, *Mol. Immunol.,* 17, 897, 1980.

44. **Marchalonis, J. J., Schluter, S. F., Hubbard, R. A., McCabe, C., and Allen, R. C.**, Immunoglobulin epitopes defined by synthetic peptides correlated to joining region sequence: conservation of determinants and dependence upon the presence of an arginyl or a lysyl residue for cross-reaction between light chains and T cell receptor chains, *Mol. Immunol.,* 25(8), 771, 1988.

45. **Alcover, A., Ramarli, D., Richardson, N. E., Chang, H.-C., and Reinherz, E.**, Functional and molecular aspects of human T lymphocyte activation via T3-Ti and T11 pathways, *Immunol. Rev.,* 95, 5, 1987.

46. **Padula, S. G., Pollard, M. K., Lingenheld, E. G., and Clark, R. B.**, Maintenance of antigen specificity by human IL-2 dependent T cell lines. Use of antigen presenting cells and OK T3 antibody in the absence of antigen, *J. Clin. Invest.,* 75, 788, 1985.

47. **Acuto, O., Fabbi, M., Bensussan, A., Milanese, C., Campen, T. J., Royer, H. D., and Reinherz, E. L.**, The human T-cell receptor, *J. Clin. Immunol.,* 5, 141, 1985.

48. **Samuelson, L. E., Hartford, J. B., and Klausner, R. D.**, Identification of the components of the murine T cell antigen receptor complex, *Cell,* 43, 223, 1985.

49. **Tsoukas, C., Landgraf, B., Bentin, J., Lamberti, J. F., Carson, D. A., and Vaughan, J. H.**, Structural and functional characteristics of the CD3 (T3) molecular complex on human thymocytes, *J. Immunol.,* 138, 388, 1987.

50. **Kehrl, J. H., Muraguchi, A., Butler, J. L., Falkoff, R. J. M., and Fauci, A. S.**, Human B cell activation proliferation and differentiation, *Immunol. Rev.,* 78, 75, 1984.

51. **Dower, S. K., Kronhelm, S. R., March, C. J., Conlon, P. J., Hopp, T. P., Gillis, S., and Urdal, D. L.**, Detection and characterization of high affinity plasma membrane receptors for interleukin 1, *J. Exp. Med.,* 162, 501, 1985.

52. **Malek, T. R., Ashwell, J. D., Germain, R. N., Shevae, E. M., and Miller, J.**, The murine interleukin-2 receptor: biochemical structure and regulation of expression, *Immunol. Rev.,* 92, 81, 1986.

53. **Greene, W. C., Depper, J. M., Kronke, M., and Leonard, W. J.**, The human interleukin-2 receptor: analysis of structure and function, *Immunol. Rev.,* 92, 49, 1986.

54. **Mackin, W. M., Huang, C.-K., and Becker, E.**, The formylpeptide chemotactic receptor on rabbit peritoneal neutrophils. I. Evidence for two binding sites with different affinities, *J. Immunol.,* 129, 1608, 1982.

55. **Robb, R. J., Greene, W. C., and Rusk, C. M.**, Low and high affinity cellular receptors for interleukin-2: implications for the level of Tac antigen, *J. Exp. Med.,* 160, 1126, 1984.

56. **Provvedini, D. M., Tsoukas, C. D., Deftos, L. J., and Manolagas, S. C.**, 1,25-Dihydroxyvitamin D_3 receptors in human leukocytes, *Science,* 221, 1181, 1983.

57. **Bhalla, A. K., Amento, E. P., Clemens, T. L., Holick, H. F., and Krane, S. M.**, Specific high affinity receptors for 1,25-dihydroxyvitamin D_3 in human peripheral blood mononuclear cells: presence in monocytes and induction in T lymphocytes following activation, *J. Clin. Endocrinol. Metab.,* 57, 1308, 1983.

58. **Galbraith, R. A., Buse, M. G., and Marchalonis, J. J.**, Insulin binding to cultured B- and T-lymphocytes, *Immunol. Lett.,* 4, 141, 1982.

59. **Helderman, J. H., Reynolds, T. C., and Strom, T. B.**, The insulin receptor as a universal marker of activated lymphocytes, *Eur. J. Immunol.,* 8, 589, 1978.

60. **Barazzone, P., Lesniak, M. A., Gordon, P., Van Obberghen, E., Carpentier, J.-L., and Orci, L.,** Binding, internalization and lysosomal association of ^{125}I-human growth hormone in cultured human lymphocytes: a quantitative morphological and biochemical study, *J. Cell Biol.,* 87, 360, 1980.

61. **Galbraith, R. M., Werner, P., Arnaud, P., and Galbraith, G. M. P.,** Transferrin binding to peripheral blood lymphocytes activated by phytohemagglutinin involves a specific receptor. Ligand interaction, *J. Clin. Invest.,* 66, 1135, 1980.

62. **Trowbridge, I. S. and Lopez, F.,** Monoclonal antibody to transferrin receptor blocks transferrin binding and inhibits human tumor cell growth *in vitro, Proc. Natl. Acad. Sci. U.S.A.,* 79, 1175, 1982.

63. **Bilheimer, D.W., Ho, Y. K., Brown, M. S., Anderson, R. G. W., and Goldstein, J. L.,** Genetics of the low density lipoprotein receptor. Diminished receptor activity in lymphocytes from heterozygotes with familian hypercholesterolemia, *J. Clin. Invest.,* 61, 678, 1978.

64. **Lewis, J. G., Crosier, P. S., and Andre, C. M.,** α_2HS glycoprotein binds to lymphocytes transformed by Epstein-Barr virus, *FEBS Lett.,* 138, 37, 1982.

67. **Aiyer, R. A., Serrano, L. E., and Jones, P. P.,** Interferon-γ binds to high and low affinity receptor components on murine macrophages, *J. Immunol.,* 136, 3329, 1986.

68. **Heijnen, C. J., Croiset, G., Zijzstra, J., and Ballieux, R. E.,** Modulation of lymphocyte function by endorphins, *Ann. N.Y. Acad. Sci.,* 496, 161, 1987.

69. **Dickler, H.,** Lymphocyte receptors for immunoglobulin, *Adv. Immunol.,* 24, 167, 1976.

70. **Cone, R. E., Chi, D. S., Grebenau, M. D., and Thorbecke, G. J.,** Characteristics of avian lymphocyte surface proteins which bind membrane and circulating immunoglobulins, *Mol. Immunol.,* 18, 597, 1981.

71. **Cooper, S. M. and Sambray, Y.,** Isolation of a murine leukemia Fc receptor by selective release induced by surface redistribution, *J. Immunol.,* 117, 511, 1976.

72. **Rask, L., Klareskoy, L., Ostberg, L., and Peterson, P. A.,** Isolation and properties of a murine spleen cells Fc receptor, *Nature,* 257, 231, 1975.

73. **Spiegelberg, H. L.,** Structure and function of Fc receptors for IgE on lymphocytes, monocytes and macrophages, *Adv. Immunol.,* 35, 61, 1984.

74. **Coico, R.F., Xue, D., Wallace, B., Pernis, B., and Thorbecke, G. J.,** T cells with receptors for IgD, *Nature,* 316, 744, 1985.

75. **Daeron, M., Neuport-Sautes, Y., Junji, J., and Fridman, W. H.,** Receptors for immunoglobulin isotypes (FcR) on murine T cells. II. Multiple FcR induction on hybridoma T cell clones, *Eur. J. Immunol.,* 15, 668, 1985.

76. **Ross, G. D. and Medof, M. E.,** Membrane complement receptors specific for bound fragments of C3, *Adv. Immunol.,* 37, 217, 1985.

77. **Dalgleish, A. G., Beverley, P. C. L., Clapham, R., Crawford, D. H., Greaves, M. F., and Weiss, R. P.,** The CD4 (T4) antigen is an essential component of the receptor for the AIDS retrovirus, *Nature,* 312, 763, 1984.

78. **Aarons, R. D., Nies, A. S., Gal, J., Hegstrand, L. R., and Molinoff, P. B.,** Elevation of β-adrenergic receptor density in human lymphocytes after propranolol administration, *J. Clin. Invest.,* 65, 949, 1980.

79. **Takahashi, K., Tavassoli, M., and Jacobsen, D. W.,** Receptor binding and internalization of immobilized transcobalamin II by mouse leukemia cells, *Nature,* 288, 713, 1980.

80. **Petrini, M., Galbraith, R. M., Werner, P. A. M., Emerson, D. L., and Arnaud, P.,** Gc (vitamin D binding protein) binds to cytoplasm of all human lymphocytes and is expressed on B-cell membranes, *Clin. Immunol. Immunopathol.,* 31, 282, 1984.

81. **Berridge, M. J.,** Inositol triphosphate and diacyglycerol: two interacting second messengers, *Ann. Rev. Biochem.,* 56, 159, 1987.

82. **Sklar, L. A.,** Ligand-receptor dynamics and signal amplification in the neutrophil, *Adv. Immunol.,* 39, 95, 1986.

83. **Cambier, J. C., Justement, L. B., Newell, M. K., Chen, Z. Z., Harris, L. K., Sandoval, V. M., Klemsz, M. J., and Ranson, J. T.,** Transmembrane signals and intracellular "second messengers" in the regulation of quiescent B-lymphocyte activation, *Immunol. Rev.,* 95, 37, 1987.

Chapter 5

INTRACELLULAR AND EXTRACELLULAR FACTORS PROMOTING LYMPHOCYTE ACTIVATION AND PROLIFERATION

Kerin L. Fresa, Meera R. Hameed, and Stanley Cohen

TABLE OF CONTENTS

I. INTRODUCTION

A. THE IMMUNE RESPONSE

The immune system is composed of a complex, interdigitated network of cells and soluble factors. The function of the immune system is primarily to maintain homeostasis by providing resistance against "nonself" invaders, such as pathogenic microorganisms, toxins, and perhaps neoplastic cells. The induction of an immune response depends on three critical processes: *proliferation* of appropriate subpopulations of lymphoid and associated cells, *differentiation* to various specialized states and phenotypes, and *activation* of functional capabilities.

The cells involved in the generation of an immune response toward a particular agent include macrophages, which secrete various monokines as well as process and present antigen to other cells; B lymphocytes, which upon appropriate stimulation, differentiate to become antibody-secreting plasma cells or memory cells; and T helper or suppressor lymphocytes, which both interact directly with other cells and secrete soluble lymphokines that either facilitate or diminish the proliferation, differentiation, and activation of a large number of cell types, including the cells of the immune system themselves.

This chapter focuses largely on lymphocyte proliferation, but overviews some of the early intracellular events following the triggering of these cells in comparison to other cell types in order to identify similar mechanisms occurring in the activation of diverse cellular processes. Chapters 6 and 7 discuss these topics as they specifically relate to B and T cell activation in greater detail. In this chapter, we deal primarily with later events in the process of transduction, with specific attention to the chemical signals that appear to directly trigger DNA replication.

B. LYMPHOKINES AND CYTOKINES

The lymphokine concept was discussed in great detail in Chapter 2. Here, we review briefly general aspects of lymphokines and cytokines. The history of lymphokines probably dates back to 1926 when Zinsser and Tamiya[1] found permeability factors in supernatants of tuberculin-sensitized guinea pig cells exposed to tuberculoprotein; however, the first of the factors that we conventionally recognize as a lymphokine, migration inhibition factor (MIF), was first described in 1966 by Bloom and Bennett[2] and by David.[3] MIF is one of a family of inflammatory lymphokines that are involved in the effector arm of the immune response, and that function by influencing inflammatory responses. More recently, it was recognized that there are also lymphokines which play critical roles in the afferent component of immune responses, the best-known example of which is interleukin-2 (IL-2). The bulk of the initial molecular biological characterization of lymphokines has focused on these lymphokines.

It is now apparent that many diverse cell types produce soluble factors that are functionally and chemically similar to the known monokines and lymphokines. The first such factors to be described were substances produced by virally infected nonlymphoid cells, which were chemotactic for neutrophils and macrophages.[3-6] The term "cytokines" was coined by us to describe this entire family of mediators.[7] Thus, lymphokines and monokines represent subsets of cytokines. One of the best examples of a cytokine is interleukin-1 (IL-1), which has been shown to be produced by a variety of cell types in addition to macrophages.[8]

In general, cytokines appear to act by triggering appropriate cellular receptors; however, at least one factor, leukocyte migration inhibition factor, has intrinsic enzymatic (esterase) activity.[9,10] The cytokines are rapidly-acting factors with half-lives usually measured in minutes. Because of their effects on cells, however, their "physiologic" half-life, namely the period of time during which their effects may be observed, is often substantially longer. Now that large amounts of pure mediators may be produced by recombinant techniques, it has become possible to study the effects of these substances at the intracellular level. We will first describe intracellular signaling mechanisms involved in cellular activation and proliferation in several cell types, and then address the lymphocyte directly, with comparisons to neutrophil activation in order to underscore the generality of some of the cellular processes involved. We then describe the role of an important cellular intermediate, ADR, in the final stages of IL-2-induced activation for proliferation. The chapter concludes with a discussion of some abnormal responses involving this factor, its regulator, and its intracellular target that occur during aging and neoplastic disease.

II. INTRACELLULAR SIGNALING MECHANISMS

A. HISTORICAL EVIDENCE THAT NUCLEAR ACTIVITY IS CONTROLLED BY CYTOPLASMIC FACTORS

The lymphokines and cytokines described in the previous sections are secreted into the extracellular milieu. These factors exert their effects on lymphoid cell differentiation, activation for effector function, and proliferation through binding to specific receptors at the cell surface. Perhaps the best studied and characterized factors are those that promote cell division; however, even in this case, the mechanisms by which these signals are relayed to the nucleus, where DNA replication and transcription occur, remain poorly understood.

Early studies, performed in nonlymphoid cells, indicated that nuclear activity is controlled by factors and events that occur outside the nucleus. For example, it was observed that the individual nuclei within binucleate and multinucleate cells often progress from G_1 into S phase of the cell cycle synchronously, suggesting that this activity was regulated by extranuclear factors.[11] The role of cytoplasmic factors and events in the control of nuclear DNA synthesis was demonstrated by Graham et al.,[12,13] who showed that nuclei from normally quiescent cells such as adult frog brain cells or liver cells can be induced to undergo DNA synthesis when injected into the cytoplasm of metabolically active frog eggs. Similar results were obtained in studies by Harris and his associates.[14,15] Using Sendai virus-mediated cell fusion techniques, they demonstrated that nuclear DNA synthesis in differentiated cells could be induced following fusion of these cells with continuously proliferating HeLa or Ehrlich ascites cells. However, since heterokaryons formed by the simple fusion of the parental cells contained nuclei and cytoplasm from both parents, it was difficult to determine the origin of factors that were controlling DNA synthesis in the heterokaryon. To overcome this difficulty, nucleated erythrocytes were employed as a source of quiescent, differentiated cells for Sendai-virus-mediated fusion, because the nuclei of these cells were completely dormant.[15] Furthermore, since the virus was hemolytic at the concentrations required to induce cell fusion, the erythrocytes effectively contained little to no cytoplasm at the time of fusion. Thus, the heterokaryons that were generated in these fusions were composed of both nuclei and cytoplasm from the HeLa cell parent and nuclei alone from the erythrocyte ghost. When the dormant nuclei were introduced into the HeLa cytoplasm by cell fusion, these nuclei underwent substantial enlargement and commenced DNA and RNA synthesis. These results suggest that nuclear DNA synthesis may be regulated by factors present in the cytoplasm.

Studies performed by Das[16] support the role of cytoplasmic intermediates in the control of nuclear DNA synthesis. She demonstrated that stimulation of quiescent 3T3 cells with epidermal growth factor (EGF) resulted in the appearance of extractable cytoplasmic factors that were capable of inducing DNA synthesis in isolated, quiescent frog nuclei. In contrast, cytoplasmic extracts from quiescent, contact-inhibited 3T3 cells were unable to induce DNA synthesis, suggesting that this factor was only present in actively dividing cells. The ability to induce DNA synthesis in isolated nuclei appeared to be mediated by nondialyzable protein(s) that were susceptible to heat and trypsin digestion. These factors appeared to be distinct from internalized EGF or its receptor. These results suggest that actively dividing cells may contain cytoplasmic factors that are capable of inducing DNA synthesis in isolated nuclei and also suggest that growth factors, after binding at the cell surface, may induce one or a series of cytoplasmic factors that relay the "message" to the nucleus to begin DNA synthesis.

B. PHOSPHATIDYLINOSITOL HYDROLYSIS AND OTHER INTRACELLULAR SECOND MESSENGER SYSTEMS

The results described in the previous section indicate that nuclear activity is controlled by cytoplasmic factors; however, the nature of these factors has remained poorly understood. In recent years, much information has accumulated concerning the initial intracellular biochemical events that occur following interaction of extracellular modulator molecules such as hormones, growth factors, neurotransmitters, and cytokines, with specific receptors at the cell surface. These events include rearrangement and endocytosis of membrane receptors with internalization of the bound ligands, autophosphorylation of receptors, phosphorylation of other cellular proteins, ionic fluxes, alterations in intracellular enzyme activities and in cyclic nucleotide and intracellular lipid metabolism, and changes in intracellular pH and in the cytoskeleton.[17-19] These intracellular events appear to be involved in the regulation of cellular metabolism, secretion, and DNA synthesis and thus appear to serve as "second messengers" that transmit signals provided by the bound growth factor or hormone at the cell surface to the interior of the cell.

The best described second messenger or signal transduction system utilized cyclic adenosine monophosphate (cAMP) and has been reviewed extensively elsewhere.[20-22] Briefly, binding of certain hormones to specific cell surface receptors activates adenylate cyclase, through transducing proteins, called G proteins, which bind guanosine phosphates. This process leads to a rise in the intracellular concentration of cAMP and the subsequent activation of cAMP-dependent protein kinases. These protein kinases then phosphorylate various cellular proteins, resulting in either activation or inhibition of cellular enzyme systems, such as those involved in glycogen metabolism.

Many hormones and growth factors, upon binding to their specific receptors cause an increase in the intracellular concentration of Ca^{2+}.[23] The rise in intracellular Ca^{2+} appears to occur through the breakdown of cellular phosphoinositides, which are ubiquitous components of eukaryotic cell membranes. These phosphoinositides include phosphatidylinositol (PI), which comprises about 7% of the cellular phospholipids, and its phosphorylated derivatives, phosphatidyl-inositol-4 phosphate (PIP), which comprises about 1% of cellular phospholipids, and phosphatidyl-inositol-4,5 diphosphate (PIP_2), which comprises about 0.4% of cellular phospholipids.[24,25] The phosphoinositides are in equilibrium with each other through the actions of kinases and phosphatases.[24,26,27] These phosphoinositides are metabolized following the interaction of certain growth factors, hormones, and neurotransmitters with their specific receptors at the cell surface. Breakdown of these phospholipids by a receptor-associated phospholipase C yields a diglyceride and one of the inositol phosphates (IP).[24] The IPs are rapidly degraded to inositol, which are consumed in the resynthesis of PI.[24] Diglycerides are either hydrolyzed via lipases to monoglycerides, then to free arachidonate and glycerol; or are phosphorylated by diglyceride kinase to form phosphatidic acid (PA). PA is then converted back into PI.[24]

Diacylglycerol (DAG) and inositol triphosphate (IP_3) are metabolites of hydrolysis of PIP_2 by activated phospholipase C.[24] IP_3 functions as a signal to mobilize Ca^{2+} from an intracellular pool, resulting in increased cytoplasmic concentrations of Ca^{2+}.[27,28] DAG functions to increase the affinity of protein kinase C (PKC) for Ca^{2+} and activates this enzyme.[29] PKC has a broad substrate specificity, phosphorylating serine and threonine residues of many endogenous proteins, and may be involved in the phosphorylation events that are associated with cellular activation. IP_3 is rapidly degraded to inositol and is used in the resynthesis of

PI.[24] DAG is rapidly converted to phosphatidic and arachidonic acids, which are also consumed in the resynthesis of PI.[24] Thus, it appears that the interaction of growth factors, hormones, and neurotransmitters with specific receptors at the cell surface results in the activation of intracellular signaling mechanisms, which appear to transmit that signal to the cell nucleus.

C. INTRACELLULAR SIGNALING MECHANISMS IN NEUTROPHIL ACTIVATION

Although this chapter and the entire volume deal mainly with the lymphoid system, it is instructive to begin by examining another cell type that functions in host defense before reviewing lymphocyte activation in detail. Of the various cells that participate in effector mechanisms of defense, perhaps the best studied is the neutrophil. In the lymphocyte, multiple activating events often occur simultaneously, For example, a given cell may receive signals for proliferation, activation, and differentiation, and as many of the signal transduction reactions may overlap, the analysis of critical pathways is often difficult. As the mature neutrophil is an end-stage cell that does not proliferate, it is relatively easy to study activation of specific functions.

The mature neutrophil has a lobulated nucleus, trilaminar structured plasma membrane which extends pseudopods toward a chemical gradient, microfilaments (actin and myosin), specific granules and azurophilic granules, and lacks nucleoli. It does not undergo cell division. The activation of these cells leads to chemotaxis, respiratory burst, aggregation, and granule release, which in turn result in inactivation or destruction of invading microorganisms, The biochemical events of this cellular activation appear to involve inositol phospholipid metaboilism, increased intracellular Ca^{2+} levels, and PKC activation, not unlike that seen in the activation of other cells such as T lymphocytes.

The response of neutrophils to chemotactic stimuli is important in host defense mechanisms. Signal transduction for chemotaxis is initiated when chemoattractant binds to specific receptors on the cell surface. Chemoattractant receptors on leukocytes trigger a number of cellular responses including cytoskeletal reorganization, changes in cell shape, directed motility, lysozymal enzyme secretion, and activation of respiratory burst. The receptors for these chemoattractants, which include the N-formylated peptides, C5a and leukotriene B4, have been characterized. The most widely studied chemoattractant receptor is that for the N-formylated peptide, formyl-methionyl-leucine-phenylalanine (fMet-Leu-Phe).[32,33] There appear to be two receptors for this peptide on the neutrophil surface,[34,35] one with high affinity and one with low affinity, which are interconvertible. These receptors are linked to G proteins.[20]

Following binding of chemoattractant to receptors on the neutrophil cell surface, PIP_2 is hydrolyzed to DAG and IP_3,[36-40] probably through the action of phospholipase C. Indeed, leukocyte plasma membranes have been shown to contain phospholipase C activity with apparent specificity for polyphosphoinositides.[41] The involvement of G proteins in this process was demonstrated by Smith et al.[42] They showed that stimulation of PIP_2 hydrolysis in leukocyte plasma membranes by chemoattractants required GTP and this action was mediated by phospholipase C. Further evidence of the same is shown by the ability of guanine nucleotides to modulate receptor affinity and of bacterial toxins to attenuate PI metabolism and leukocyte function. Stimulation of guanine nucleotides require the presence of low concentrations of Ca^{2+}, similar to that in resting cytosol.[43] In the absence of GTP, supraphysiological concentrations of Ca^{2+} (>100 nM) are required for PIP_2 hydrolysis in PMN membranes.[41-43] Pertussis toxin and cholera toxin prevent chemoattractant-induced stimulation of PMNs by interacting with a G protein, thus blocking phospholipase C activation. Both the toxins inhibited high affinity fMet-Leu-Phe binding, suggesting that the same G protein is a substrate for both; however, the specificities of G proteins involved in phospholipase C binding have yet to be investigated.

As mentioned previously, chemoattractants induce the rapid and transient formation of IP$_3$,[36-40,44,45] causing an increase in intracellular Ca^{2+} levels.[37,45] The increase in cytosolic Ca^{2+} is biphasic.[45,47] The first phase is dependent on intracellular Ca^{2+} stores,[37,45] as the chemoattractant-induced increase in cytosolic Ca^{1+} is only partially reduced by chelation of extracellular Ca^{2+}.[45] In contrast, the second phase depends on extracellular Ca^{2+} and is slower than the initial response.[48]

Stimulation of PMNs with chemoattractants also results in increased DAG levels,[33] partially as a result of PIP$_2$ hydrolysis. However, chemoattractant-induced changes in phosphoinositide metabolism exhibit minimal enhancement by cytochalasin-B,[38,49] suggesting that the majority of DAG is from sources other than phosphoinositides. Studies show that exogenous phospholipase C (which leads to activation of respiration and a minimal secretion of specific granules) activates DAG and stimulates PKC through a mechanism independent of inositol phospholipids and changes in cytosolic Ca^{2+} concentration. It appears that DAG seems to be primarily derived from phosphatidyl choline and ethanolamine.[50] Addition of active phorbol esters to PMNs or to monocytes resulted in the redistribution of PKC from cytosol to cells' particulate fraction,[51,53] and also stimulated superoxide production at the same potency,[51] suggesting that activation of PKC is involved in neutrophil activation. It appears that PKC activation and translocation are necessary for activation of NADPH oxidase activity in plasma membrane preparations.[54,55]

In conclusion, neutrophil activation involves a common pathway through inositol phospholipids, Ca^{2+} mobilization, and PKC activation which leads to specialized cell function in the form of cell division or granule release and phagocytosis. These ultimately play a major role in the host's defense mechanism.

D. INTRACELLULAR SIGNALING MECHANISMS IN LYMPHOCYTE ACTIVATION FOR PROLIFERATION

Since the events described in the previous sections appear to be common pathways for signal transduction following interaction of a wide variety of substances with specific receptors at the cell surface, it seems very likely that these same mechanisms would be involved in activation of lymphocytes by antigen or mitogen, or in the induction of proliferation by specific growth factors such as IL-2. The intracellular biochemical events that occur during T and B cell activation will be considered in the following sections.

1. Signal Transduction in T Cell Activation and Proliferation

The generation of a T cell-dependent immune response against a specific antigen appears to occur in two phases. Resting T cells are at G$_0$ in the cell cycle. Following the interaction of specific populations of resting T cells with appropriately processed antigen, these cells progress to G$_1$ of the cell cycle, during which time the cells become responsive to the proliferative signals provided by IL-2 through the expression of specific IL-2 receptors (IL-2R) at the cell surface. Concurrently, appropriate subsets of lymphocytes produce IL-2 on stimulation with IL-1. Binding of IL-2 to these receptors results in progression through the cell cycle and proliferation of those cells. Thus, these events lead to the selective expansion of T cells with effector function directed against a specific antigen. Conversely, the interaction of mitogen with T cell populations results in the polyclonal activation of these cells with production of lymphokines, induction of cell surface IL-2R, and polyclonal proliferation.

a. Antigen- and Mitogen-Induced Changes in Intracellular Signaling Mechanisms

Several investigators have examined signal transduction mechanisms in T cells stimulated with antigen or mitogen, in an effort to understand the intracellular signaling mechanisms that occur during T cell activation. Addition of relevant antigen, in the presence of autologous antigen-presenting cells (APC), to resting populations of antigen-specific T cell clones has been shown to result in significant increases in IP_3,[56] suggesting that PI hydrolysis occurs following interaction of antigen or mitogen with appropriate receptors at the cell surface. Furthermore, addition of antigen, in the presence of APC, has also been shown to increase intracellular Ca^{2+} levels in T cell clones specific for tetanus toxoid and keyhold limpet hemocyanin.[57] These results suggest that stimulation of resting T cells with antigen results in the activation of phospholipase C and the hydrolysis of PIP_2 with the formation of IP_3 and DAG. These results also implicate PKC in the intracellular pathways leading to T cell activation. These hypotheses are substantiated by the results of Kozumbo et al.,[58] who examined the intracellular biochemical changes that were associated with lymphokine production in cloned murine cytotoxic T lymphocytes (CTL) following stimulation with antigen or mitogen. They found that stimulation of CTL clones with antigen or mitogen resulted in increased PI hydrolysis. Specifically, they observed increased intracellular concentrations of PI and PA, decreased intracellular concentrations of PIP_2, and increased production of IPs and DAG in CTL clones that were stimulated with antigen or mitogen. These changes occurred within minutes of addition of antigen or mitogen and were maintained for approximately 6 to 8 h. The duration of these changes approximated the time required for optimum production of macrophage-activating factor (MAF). Addition of irrelevant antigen failed to induce either MAF production or changes in PI hydrolysis. These results provide further evidence that activation of lymphocytes with either mitogen or antigen, as measured by lymphokine production, is associated with increased PI turnover with production of IPs and DAG.

Recent studies have identified the T cell receptor for antigen as a noncovalently bound molecular complex consisting of a disulfide-linked heterodimer containing variable amino acid sequences, termed the Ti molecule, and invariable glycoproteins, called CD_3.[59,60] Monoclonal antibodies (mAb) generated against either T3 or Ti have been utilized to mimic the effects of antigen or mitogen in T cell activation.[61,62] Because the T3 molecule is invariable and present on all mature T cells, binding of mAb to the T3 antigen can be utilized for polyclonal activation of T cells, whereas mAb to individual Ti molecules can be utilized in the activation of specific antigen-reactive T cell clones. These agents can be used to mimic the effects of antigen or mitogen binding, respectively, on intracellular signal transduction pathways. Binding of mAb to the T cell receptor complex appears to activate T cells via increases in intracellular Ca^{2+} levels, activation of PI hydrolysis pathways, and resultant translocation and activation of PKC.[62-65] In the presence of the phorbol ester, phorbol myristate acetate (PMA), mAb to either T3 or Ti has been shown to induce T cell activation, as measured by IL-2 production in the human T cell line, Jurkat.[62-67] Production of IL-2 following stimulation is associated with prompt, sustained increases in intracellular Ca^{2+} levels, as measured by the Ca^{2+}-sensitive fluor, quin-2. Furthermore, stimulation of Jurkat cells with mAb to the T3-antigen receptor complex leads to the appearance of new intracellular phosphoproteins, suggesting that activation of protein kinases, possibly Ca^{2+}-dependent PKC, is involved in the process of T cell activation. As reported by Imboden and Stobo,[65] the rise in intracellular Ca^{2+} by these agents initially appeared to be the result of release of Ca^{2+} from intracellular stores. However, in the absence of extracellular Ca^{2+}, the CD3/Ti-mediated increase in intracellular Ca^{2+} was shown to be of only several minutes duration, compared to increases of greater than 30 min in the presence of extracellular Ca^{2+}, suggesting that the sustained rise in intracellular Ca^{2+} was due to a subsequent influx of extracellular Ca^{2+}, possibly through opening of Ca^{2+} channels. Binding of mAb against T3 or Ti also resulted in an increase in intracellular inositol phosphates, including IP_3, presumably through the hydrolysis of PIP_2, providing further evidence that T cell activation following ligand binding to the T cell receptor complex involves activation of PKC.[29]

Indeed, it has been demonstrated that the addition of mAb to CD3/Ti results in an increased translocation of PKC activity from the cytosol to the membrane via DAG, the other product of PI hydrolysis.[66,67] Since translocation of PKC is generally thought to reflect receptor-mediated activation of PKC via hydrolysis of PIs, including PIP_2, these results suggest that T cell activation by ligand binding to the T cell receptor complex is mediated through the production of DAG and IP_3, which function to raise intracellular Ca^{2+} levels and activate PKC.

b. Signal Transduction in IL-2-Induced T Cell Proliferation

Induction of proliferation in antigen- or mitogen-activated T cells appears to be mediated through binding of IL-2 to high-affinity receptors that are expressed on the activated T cell membrane. Several investigators have studied intracellular signal transduction mechanisms in T cell populations that had been activated by antigen or mitogen and subsequently stimulated with IL-2 in an effort to further elucidate the signal transduction pathways that are involved in T cell proliferation. Gaulton and Eardley[68] have demonstrated that the addition of IL-2 to Concanavalin A (Con-A) or PHA-activated murine splenic T lymphocytes or IL-2-dependent T cell lines results in the rapid phosphorylation of a variety of membrane-associated proteins, including the IL-2 receptor itself. The phosphorylation of the IL-2R was evident within 1 min after addition of IL-2 and peaked approximately 15 min after IL-2 addition. In order to determine which protein kinases regulate protein phosphorylation associated with IL-2 stimulation, they examined protein phosphorylation in lymphocytes that were treated with cAMP and cyclic guanosine monophosphate (cGMP) agonists. Based on the results of these studies, they suggested that IL-2-induced protein phosphorylation was perhaps regulated in part by protein kinase A, and perhaps in part by PKC. This hypothesis is supported by the work of Farrar and Anderson,[69] who studied the intracellular mechanisms by which the IL-2-receptor interaction induces cellular proliferation. Specifically, they examined PKC activity in the plasma membrane and cytoplasmic fractions of cloned murine IL-2-dependent T cells at various times after addition of IL-2. Within 3 min after addition of IL-2, a fourfold increase in plasma membrane-associated PKC activity was observed, with a concomitant decrease in cytoplasmic PKC. Peak plasma membrane-associated PKC activity was observed 10 min after IL-2 stimulation, when cytoplasmic PKC activity was lowest. Plasma membrane-associated PKC activity declined by 20 min after stimulation, and was at baseline levels by 60 min. In order to determine if there was a direct correlation between association of PKC with the plasma membrane and proliferation, proliferation was assessed in response to increasing concentrations of IL-2. Farrar and Anderson observed a clear correlation between the degree of proliferation and the level of plasma membrane-associated PKC activity. It is interesting to note, however, that Kozumbo et al.[58] failed to detect PI hydrolysis, as measured by the production of IPs and DAG, in mitogen- or antigen-activated cells that were stimulated with IL-2. Similarly, Mills et al.[70] were unable to detect hydrolysis of PIP_2 in human T lymphocytes that were stimulated with IL-2. These results appear to contradict those of Farrar and Anderson,[69] who postulated that IL-2 transmits its proliferative signal to the nucleus via PI hydrolysis and activation of PKC. It is possible that the binding of IL-2 to its receptor at the cell surface leads to the translocation and activation of PKC, but through a mechanism distinct from PI hydrolysis. It should also be kept in mind that activation of lymphocytes by antigen or mitogen to secrete lymphokines, including IL-2, with concomitant expression of IL-2R at the cell surface, may be intrinsically tied to proliferation of these cells. Thus, activation of PKC by PIP_2 hydrolysis may be indirectly involved in the intracellular signaling mechanisms for cell proliferation.

c. Effect of Phorbol Esters and Ca^{2+} Ionophores on Intracellular Signaling Mechanisms in T Cells

Recent studies, in a variety of cell types, indicate a remarkable synergy between Ca^{2+} ionophores and phorbol esters, such as PMA, in cellular activation.[27,63,71] Ca^{2+} ionophores function to raise the intracellular concentration of Ca^{2+} and phorbol esters have been demonstrated to activate PKC by significantly increasing the affinity of this enzyme for required co-factors Ca^{2+} and phospholipid.[72] Thus, these agents are useful in determining the role of PKC and increased Ca^{2+} levels in T cell activation and proliferation. The combination of PMA and Ca^{2+} ionophore has been shown to induce lymphokine production and subsequent proliferation in T cell populations,[63,71] providing additional support for the role of PKC and increased intracellular Ca^{2+} levels in T cell activation processes. Treatment with Ca^{2+} ionophore alone or PMA alone appear to be insufficient to activate T cells, suggesting that the rise in intracellular Ca^{2+} alone is insufficient to activate T cells. A notable exception is the ability to induce IL-2R expression following treatment with PMA alone;[37] however, the combination of Ca^{2+} ionophore and phorbol ester cannot induce proliferation of IL-2-dependent T cell lines in the absence of that lymphokine, suggesting that while phorbol ester and Ca^{2+} ionophore can activate T cells for the production of lymphokines, including IL-2, and can render T cells responsive to proliferative signals through the induction of IL-2 receptors, these agents cannot override the requirement for IL-2 in T cell proliferation. The implication of these studies is that the initial phase of T cell activation, as measured by lymphokine production and IL-2R expression, is dependent on a rise in intracellular Ca^{2+} levels and activation of PKC. However, the second, IL-2-dependent proliferative stage cannot be mimicked by phorbol esters and Ca^{2+} ionophore. These results may have two interpretations: (1) other signal transduction mechanisms in addition to increased intracellular Ca^{2+} levels and activation of PKC are required for T cell proliferation or (2) increased intracellular Ca^{2+} levels and activation of PKC are not involved in the intracellular signaling mechanisms for T cell proliferation.

2. Intracellular Changes Accompanying B Cell Activation

As appears to be the case with T lymphocytes that are stimulated with antigen or mitogen, stimulation of B lymphocytes with anti-immunoglobulin appears to lead to receptor (surface immunoglobulin) cross-linking with PI hydrolysis and PKC activation.[73-76] Recent reports have also described the appearance of novel cytoplasmic proteins that may be involved in signal transduction to the nucleus in B lymphocytes stimulated with anti-immunoglobulin. Following binding of anti-immunoglobulin to the B lymphocyte cell membrane, a membrane-bound, trypsin-like serine protease is activated.[77] This serine protease appears to split precursor proteins in the cytoplasm into active cytoplasmic factors that were capable of inducing nonhistone protein-specific protein kinase activity in the nucleus.

Similar cytoplasmic factors have been detected in lymphocytes from the lipopolysaccharide (LPS)-responsive C3H/HeN strain of mice following stimulation with that endotoxin.[78] Microinjection of cytoplasmic extracts from LPS-stimulated C3H/HeN lymphocytes into B lymphocytes of nonresponder C3H/HeJ origin resulted in the ability of C3H/HeJ lymphocytes to proliferate in response to stimulation with LPS. These data suggest that the ability to respond to LPS stimulation was associated with a cytoplasmic mediator which is induced in responder strains of mice following stimulation with LPS. Furthermore, transfer of this factor into lymphocytes from nonresponder strains of mice confers the ability to proliferate in response to stimulation with LPS. Gel filtration of the cytoplasmic extracts from LPS-stimulated C3H/HeN lymphocytes indicated that the factor responsible for this activity had a molecular weight of 100 kDa. These results all suggest that the intracytoplasmic factors that directly influence nuclear function may be accessible to experimental manipulation.

E. ACTIVELY DIVIDING LYMPHOCYTES CONTAIN A CYTOPLASMIC ACTIVATOR OF DNA SYNTHESIS

Since most of the pathways described in the previous sections reflect early cell membrane-related events involved in signaling for activation and proliferation, we thought it of interest to study instead the subsequent steps that are more directly and immediately involved in nuclear activation. In order to do so, we began by examining the ability of cytoplasmic extracts from actively dividing lymphocytes and lymphoid cell lines to induce DNA synthesis in isolated nuclei.[79] For these studies, cytoplasmic extracts were prepared from spontaneously proliferating human T cell lymphoblastoid cells (MOLT-4), murine plasmacytoma cells (P3X63Ag8.653), human B lymphoma cells (RPMI 8392), and from mitogen-stimulated normal human lymphocytes. Because previous embryological investigations making use of similar assays found a lack of species specificity, we assayed these extracts for their ability to induce DNA synthesis in isolated, quiescent frog spleen cell nuclei. This reaction was carried out in a cocktail containing 2'-deoxyadenosine 5'-triphosphate, 2'-deoxyguanosine 5'-triphosphate 2'-deoxycytidine 5'-triphosphate, adenosine 5'-triphosphate (ATP), phosphoenolpyruvate, pyruvate kinase, and ^{3}H-thymidine triphosphate (^{3}H-TTP). Several lines of evidence indicated that this assay measures DNA synthesis and not DNA repair. First, the presence of all four deoxyribonucleotides and ATP were required for ^{3}H-TTP incorporation. Second, under essentially identical experimental conditions, Jazwinski et al.[80] were able to document replicative "forks" and "eyes" in the DNA of stimulated nuclei by electron microscopy.

Cytoplasmic extracts from spontaneously proliferating lymphoid cell lines and from mitogen-stimulated lymphocytes induced high levels of DNA synthesis in isolated nuclei from adult frog spleen cells, as measured by ^{3}H-TTP incorporation into trichloroacetic acid (TCA)-precipitable material.[79] Maximal levels of ^{3}H-TTP incorporation was observed after 90 min of incubation. Furthermore, a sigmoidal dose-response curve could be elicited with increasing concentrations of extract. This pattern of response differs from that of several extracellular inducers of DNA synthesis, such as antigens, mitogens, or growth hormones which typically show a bell-shaped dose-response curve, with inhibition at higher inducer concentrations. Minimal DNA synthesis was observed in nuclei incubated without extract or in nuclei incubated with cytoplasmic extracts from nonproliferating cells, including nonstimulated normal human lymphocytes. Cytoplasmic extracts incubated alone also failed to incorporate ^{3}H-TTP. These results suggest that continuously proliferating lymphoblastoid cells and proliferating normal lymphocytes contain a cytoplasmic factor that may be involved in induction of nuclear DNA synthesis. We have termed the factor that is present in the cytoplasms of actively dividing cells that can induce DNA synthesis in isolated nuclei the activator of DNA replication (ADR).

ADR activity could also be detected in cytoplasmic extracts from IL-2 responsive lymphocyte populations that had been stimulated with that factor.[81] In both dose-response and kinetic studies, the ADR response paralleled the proliferative response, suggesting that ADR is also involved in IL-2-dependent T cell growth. However, since the IL-2-responsive T cell blasts that were used in this study had been stimulated with PHA, it was important to determine that ADR was stimulated as a result of IL-2 treatment, and that the ADR activity that we had observed under these conditions was not residual activity stimulated by PHA. Since dexamethasone inhibits PHA-induced proliferation in a dose-dependent manner, presumably by blocking IL-2 production, we examined the ability of lymphocytes treated with dexamethasone to produce ADR. Addition of dexamethasone to lymphocytes stimulated with PHA resulted in a significant decrease in ADR activity in these cells. This decrease in ADR activity could be reversed if exogenous IL-2 was added to the cultures. These results suggest that induction of ADR is not an early event in T cell activation by PHA, but rather appears to be a later event resulting either directly or indirectly from binding of IL-2 to specific receptors on activated T cells.

III. CHARACTERIZATION OF ADR

A. PHYSICAL PROPERTIES OF ADR

Cytoplasmic extracts from actively dividing lymphoid cells that were treated with trypsin failed to induce DNA synthesis in isolated nuclei,[79] suggesting that the factor(s) responsible for induction of DNA synthesis was a protein. Furthermore, ADR was found to be stable at 4°C for 24 h, and could still be detected after freeze-thawing.[79] ADR activity could also be retained following lyophilization and reconstitution of the cytoplasmic extracts.[79] However, ADR could be inactivated by incubating at 60°C for 20 min.[87] Dialysis studies indicated that ADR had a molecular weight larger than 3500.[79] Thus, ADR appeared to be a relatively stable protein with a molecular weight larger than 3.5 kDa.

In order to more closely approximate the size of the protein, cytoplasmic extracts containing ADR activity were subjected to Amicon ultrafiltration. For these studies, cytoplasmic extracts of 8392 cells were serially filtered through XM50 and XM100A membranes. The fractions that were retained by the membranes and the filtrates were collected and assayed for ADR activity. Only the fraction that was retained by the XM100A membrane possessed ADR activity, suggesting that ADR had a molecular weight greater than 100,000.[79] Similar results were obtained using MOLT-4 cytoplasmic extracts as a source of ADR. The XM100A retentate could then be enriched for ADR activity by ammonium sulfate precipitation. ADR activity precipitated under 30 to 50% ammonium sulfate saturation. Using these methodologies, we were able to preserve 100% of the ADR activity in preparations from which the protein had been reduced by 73%.[79]

B. ADR IS AN INTRACELLULAR MEDIATOR

In order to determine if ADR was secreted by lymphocytes like a conventional lymphokine, supernatants from 8392 cells were collected and dialyzed against extraction buffer.[79] The dialysate was then either diluted or concentrated, so that concentrations ranging from 0.1X to 10X of the original starting concentration were tested for ADR activity. No ADR activity could be detected at any of the concentrations tested.[79] The lack of activity in these preparations was not due to loss of the factor through dialysis as we had previously shown that ADR activity was not dialyzable.[79]

While initial experiments showed that ADR could induce DNA synthesis in isolated nuclei, it was also of interest to determine if ADR had any effect on intact cells. For these experiments, intact frog spleen cells were incubated with cytoplasmic extracts of 8392 cells. These extracts, even when concentrated fivefold, failed to induce DNA synthesis in intact frog spleen cells.[79] Since intact frog spleen cells were capable of proliferation after stimulation with Con-A, the inability of intact frog spleen cells to respond to ADR could not be attributed to an inability of these cells to divide. It was also possible that despite a lack of species-specificity in the effect of ADR on isolated nuclei, a species-specific membrane attachment step may be necessary when intact cells are used as an indicator of ADR activity. Therefore, cytoplasmic extracts of murine origin were tested for ADR activity using intact murine lymphocytes as indicator cells. No induction of DNA synthesis was observed under these conditions. Thus, it appears that ADR is neither secreted from cells nor has it any effect on intact cells.[79] It appears therefore, that ADR is entirely an intracellular mediator.

C. BIOCHEMICAL CHARACTERISTICS OF ADR

For a variety of reasons, we suspected that ADR might be a protease. In a preliminary study, cytoplasmic extracts of MOLT-4 cells were tested for protease activity by the ability to degrade fibrin, in the presence and absence of an exogenous source of plasminogen.[82] Even in the absence of plasminogen, significant degradation of fibrin was observed following 21 h of co-incubation; however, a marked, time-dependent enhancement of proteolysis was observed following addition of plasminogen. Plasminogen alone was proteolytically inactive. Extract fractions with maximal ADR activity had maximal protease activity, raising the possibility that ADR itself is a protease. Since ADR has not been purified to homogeneity, we explored this possibility with the aid of protease inhibitors. Isolated frog spleen nuclei were incubated with increasing concentrations of MOLT-4 derived-ADR preparations in the presence and absence of protease inhibitors.[82] Addition of aprotinin to wells containing ADR and isolated nuclei resulted in a significant inhibition of ADR activity. Aprotinin could also inhibit ADR activity derived from IL-2 activated, normal human lymphoblasts. Other protease inhibitors, specifically N-α-tosyllysine chloromethyl ketone and leupeptin, were also able to block ADR activity. Aminobenzamidine also blocked ADR activity, although higher concentrations of the inhibitor were required. Interestingly, addition of soybean trypsin inhibitor, at comparable concentrations, had no effect on ADR activity. The ability of protease inhibitors to block ADR activity was due to an effect on component(s) of the extract and not a direct effect on the nuclei, as nuclei that were preincubated with concentrations of aprotinin that were inhibitory for ADR activity, were still able to synthesize DNA upon removal of the aprotinin and stimulation with ADR-containing extracts.

These results suggest either that the ADR-nuclear interaction is protease-dependent or that ADR itself is a protease. We therefore performed experiments utilizing aprotinin. For these studies, aprotinin, and as a control, soybean trypsin inhibitor (SBTI), were conjugated to agarose beads, Cytoplasmic extracts of MOLT-4 cells were then incubated with aprotinin-agarose, SBTI-agarose, or unconjugated agarose beads. The majority of ADR activity could be removed from cytoplasmic extracts of MOLT-4 cells by aprotinin-agarose. The beads could then be collected, packed into a column, and the ADR activity could be eluted from the beads in the presence of $0.4\ M$ NaCl/$0.05\ M$ sodium acetate, pH 5.0. The recovery of ADR from the columns provides strong evidence that ADR itself is a protease. As controls, adsorption of MOLT-4 cytoplasmic extracts with either plain or SBTI-conjugated agarose had no effect on ADR activity. As expected, no ADR activity could be eluted from control columns containing unconjugated agarose beads. Preliminary biochemical characterization of the aprotinin-agarose eluate by sodium dodecyl sulfate/polyacrylamide gel electrophoresis (SDS/PAGE) revealed a band with an approximate molecular weight of 100,000 which possessed proteolytic activity. These results are consistent with earlier studies which showed that ADR activity in MOLT-4 extracts was associated with a fraction having a molecular weight of greater than 100 kDa.

D. QUIESCENT CELLS CONTAIN AN INHIBITOR OF ADR ACTIVITY

For these studies, cytoplasmic extracts were prepared from MOLT-4 cells or PBL that were cultured in the presence or absence of PHA.[83] Consistent with previous studies,[79] the MOLT-4 extract and the extracts prepared from PHA-stimulated lymphocytes (positive extracts) induced high levels of DNA synthesis in isolated frog nuclei. Conversely, extracts prepared from nonstimulated lymphocytes (negative extracts) failed to induce detectable DNA synthesis in isolated frog nuclei. However, nuclear DNA synthesis in wells containing both positive and negative extracts was only 10 to 50% of that in wells containing only the positive extract alone. This suppression was maximal after 90 min of co-culture and was also observed when isolated nuclei were obtained from human PBL, instead of frog spleen cells.

We postulated that the ability of the negative extract to suppress induction of DNA synthesis by ADR was due to the presence of an inhibitor of ADR activity. The inhibitory activity was abolished if the negative extracts were treated with trypsin prior to assay, suggesting that the inhibitor was a protein. This inhibitory factor was found to be stable at 4°C for 24 h and was still detectable following freeze-thawing. Furthermore, the majority of the inhibitory activity was retained following heating to 56°C for 20 min. These results suggest that the inhibitor of ADR activity present in cytoplasmic extracts of quiescent lymphocytes was a relatively heat-stable protein.

To determine the approximate molecular weight of this factor, negative extracts were subjected to Amicon ultrafiltration. The inhibitory activity was retained by a XM50 membrane, suggesting that the inhibitory factor was ≥ 50 kDa. Those components of the extract that were <50 kDa were unable to inhibit ADR-induced DNA synthesis in isolated nuclei.

Since the inhibitory factor was isolated from resting PBL that had been cultured *in vitro* for 3 d, we wished to determine if this factor could also be recovered from freshly isolated PBL or if this factor appeared only after *in vitro* cultivation. For these experiments, cytoplasmic extracts were prepared from freshly isolated PBL and from unstimulated PBL after various times of culture. Cytoplasmic extracts of freshly isolated PBL were unable to inhibit the effects of ADR on isolated nuclei; however, inhibitory activity appeared within 2 to 6 h of *in vitro* culture and was maximal after 18 h of culture. Failure to detect inhibitory activity in freshly isolated PBL may be due to the fact that these cells were not truly quiescent, as suggested by the observation that freshly isolated PBLs were able to incorporate low but significant levels of ^{3}H-TdR.

To rule out the possibility that macrophages were either producing the inhibitory factor or were producing a factor that induced lymphocytes to produce the factor, extracts were prepared from unfractionated PBL and macrophage-depleted PBL that were cultured overnight.[83] These extracts were tested for their ability to suppress ADR-induced nuclear DNA synthesis. Extracts prepared from unfractionated PBL and from macrophage-depleted PBL were equally able to inhibit ADR activity, suggesting that the inhibitory factor was neither produced by macrophages, nor was production of the inhibitory factor influenced by macrophages or their products.

IV. DEFECTS IN INTRACELLULAR SIGNALING MECHANISMS IN NEOPLASIA AND AGING

A. DEFECTS IN INTRACELLULAR SIGNALING CONTROL MECHANISMS IN NEOPLASTIC CELLS

The inhibitor of ADR activity was demonstrated by the ability of cytoplasmic extracts from resting cells to inhibit induction of DNA synthesis by ADR in quiescent nuclei; however, it remained to be determined if the inhibitor of ADR activity could suppress ongoing DNA synthesis in activated nuclei.[84] For these experiments, nuclei were prepared from resting lymphocytes (quiescent nuclei) and from lymphocytes that had been treated with PHA (activated nuclei). These nuclei were then incubated with cytoplasmic extracts from resting PBL, which contain the inhibitor of ADR. Addition of the resting extract to nuclei that were actively synthesizing DNA resulted in a marked decrease in DNA synthesis. These results demonstrate that the inhibitor of ADR activity is not only capable of suppressing induction of DNA synthesis in resting nuclei, but can also inhibit ongoing DNA synthesis in activated nuclei.

We postulated that continuous DNA replication in neoplastic cells was associated with a relative insusceptibility of the nucleus of the neoplastic cell to respond to the inhibitory signal. We isolated nuclei from several neoplastic, continuously dividing cell lines, including MOLT-4 cells, RPMI 8392 cells, and BW 5147 cells, and incubated them in the presence or absence of cytoplasmic extracts from resting PBL as a source of the inhibitor of ADR activity. As a control, activated nuclei from mitogen-stimulated PBL were also incubated in the presence or absence of the inhibitor of ADR activity. As shown in previous experiments, cytoplasmic extracts from resting cells were capable of inhibiting DNA replication in nuclei from mitogen-activated PBL; however, these extracts were incapable of suppressing DNA replication in nuclei from neoplastic cells. These results suggest that nuclei from neoplastic cells are relatively insensitive to the suppressive effects of the inhibitor of ADR activity.

B. DEFECTS IN INTRACELLULAR SIGNALING IN LYMPHOCYTES FROM AGED INDIVIDUALS

T lymphocytes from aged individuals have been demonstrated to be less responsive to mitogenic stimulation, as measured by ³H-TdR incorporation, than lymphocytes from young control individuals.[85-88] Several possible mechanisms for this phenomenon have been suggested. It has been postulated that decreased ³H-TdR incorporation in aged lymphocytes is partially due to an increased susceptibility to cell cycle arrest that is induced by the radioisotope and partially due to a decreased susceptibility to the mitogenic signal.[89,90] It has also been postulated that decreased susceptibility to mitogenic stimulation in lymphocytes from aged individuals is due to defective IL-2 production or to a relative inability of these cells to respond to the proliferative signal of IL-2. Addition of exogenous IL-2 to cultures of lymphocytes from aged individuals resulted in only a partial restoration of the proliferative response to mitogen, suggesting that while these lymphocytes may be deficient in their ability to produce IL-2, defects in the ability to respond to IL-2 may also be involved.[91-95] Indirect evidence suggests that lymphocytes from aged individuals may also have a decreased number of and/or affinity for IL-2 receptors at the cell surface.[94,96] Thus, although defects in both the ability to produce and respond to IL-2 are associated with the relative inability of lymphocytes from aged individuals to respond to mitogenic stimulation, the precise intracellular basis for this phenomenon remains undefined.

Several investigators (including ourselves) have shown that decreased proliferative responses observed in lymphocytes from aged individuals is associated with defects in intracellular signaling mechanisms. Proust et al.[97] have studied PKC activity and translocation, PI hydrolysis, and cytoplasmic Ca^{2+} levels in lymphocytes from aged individuals, in order to determine if changes in these intracellular signaling mechanisms were associated with decreased proliferative responses. They found comparable basal levels of PKC in lymphocytes from young and aged individuals; however, following Con-A stimulation of these cells, PKC activity in lymphocytes from aged individuals was only half of that observed in lymphocytes from young control donors simulated in the same manner. In contrast, they were unable to detect differences in PI hydrolysis, as measured by the generation of IP_3, or in free cytoplasmic Ca^{2+} levels in Con-A-stimulated lymphocytes from aged individuals, when compared to Con-A-stimulated young lymphocytes. These results suggest that some intracytoplasmic second messengers may be deficient in lymphocytes from aged individuals and may partially account for the decreased proliferative responses observed in lymphocytes from aged individuals.

We wished to determine if changes in the ability to produce or respond to ADR was also associated with proliferative defects in aged lymphocytes. For these studies, cytoplasmic extracts were prepared from PHA-stimulated PBL from aged (66 to 72 years) and young adult (22 to 30 years) human donors.[98] Cytoplasmic extracts from PHA-stimulated lymphocytes from aged donors were as active in the induction of DNA synthesis in isolated frog nuclei as were extracts from young donors, even though the PHA-induced proliferative capacity of lymphocytes from some, but not all, aged donors was significantly less than that of lymphocytes from young donors. A dose-response analysis was performed to exclude the possibility that we were working at supraoptimal concentrations of ADR and were failing to detect quantitative differences in ADR production in young and old lymphocytes. No quantitative differences in ADR production were found between the groups. As expected, cytoplasmic extracts from unstimulated lymphocytes from both young and aged donors failed to induce significant DNA synthesis in isolated frog nuclei. These results suggest that the decreased proliferative capacity of lymphocytes from aged donors was not associated with an inability to produce ADR.

We then investigated the possibility that decreased proliferation in response to stimulation with mitogen in lymphocytes from aged individuals was associated with a decreased nuclear responsiveness to the proliferative signal provided by ADR. To test this hypothesis, nuclei isolated from resting lymphocytes of aged individuals with either intact or defective mitogen responsiveness were assayed for DNA synthesis in response to an exogenous source of ADR. Control nuclei preparations were derived from resting lymphocytes. Nuclei derived from young lymphocytes and from lymphocytes from aged individuals with intact PHA responsiveness were comparable in their ability to synthesize DNA in response to stimulation with an exogenous source of ADR; however, nuclei derived from lymphocytes of aged individuals with defective proliferative responses to PHA showed a relative inability to synthesize DNA in response to stimulation with ADR.[99] Thus, there was a clear correlation between the response of intact cells to PHA stimulation and the response of isolated nuclei from these cells to ADR. These results suggest that the decreased proliferative capacity observed in lymphocytes from some aged individuals was associated with an inability of the nuclei of these cells to respond to ADR.

V. DISCUSSION

In recent years, our understanding of signal transduction following interaction of hormones and growth factors with their receptors at the cell surface has increased greatly. The immune system provides an excellent model for such study, as lymphoid cells are easily isolated and characterized with respect to surface markers, function, and requirements for both activation and proliferation. The growth factors specific for lymphocytes and the receptors for these factors have also been identified and characterized. T cells, upon interaction with specific antigen or mitogen, become activated, produce lymphokines (including IL-2), and begin to express IL-2R at the cell surface. Binding of IL-2 and other lymphokines to specific receptors on the activated T cell surface, in turn, supports further activation and proliferation of lymphocytes. The intracellular changes that are involved in transmitting these signals for activation and proliferation to the nucleus, where DNA replication and transcription occur, share many similarities to those occurring in nonlymphoid cells following binding of growth factors at the cell surface. These changes include endocytosis of membrane receptors with internalization of the bound ligand, ion fluxes, changes in the cellular cytoskeleton, receptor autophosphorylation, phosphorylation of other cellular proteins through activation of protein kinases, alterations in other enzymatic activities, and changes in phospholipid and cyclic nucleotide metabolism. Hydrolysis of PIP_2, with production of IP_3 and DAG and activation of PKC, appears to represent a common, early event in lymphocyte activation for production of lymphokines and their cell surface receptors. The signal for proliferation provided by binding of IL-2 to its receptor appears to be more complex, but may involve activation of PKC or other protein kinases. The ultimate signal that actually triggers the nucleus to begin DNA synthesis in preparation for cell division is even less well understood. By the nature of its defining assay (an effect on isolated nuclei), ADR would appear to be a good candidate as the mediator of that final triggering event; however, the mechanism by which ADR actually initiates, either directly or indirectly, DNA synthesis is unknown. Possibilities include activation of enzymes involved in DNA replication, alteration of the nuclear membrane to facilitate macromolecular transport or assembly, or proteolytic cleavage of intranuclear regulatory proteins. In addition, the events that link IL-2 binding to activation of ADR activity are also unknown. Both of these issues are currently under investigation. Furthermore, production of ADR-like factors in nonlymphoid cells is also being studied in order to determine if ADR is a common intracellular mediator in regulation of DNA synthesis, regardless of cell type. The studies of Das[16] support this contention. Since perturbations in the production of, and nuclear sensitivity to, ADR and/or its inhibitor, occur in the process of aging and in neoplastic disease, a more complete understanding of this system may provide valuable information about the mechanisms of aberrant proliferative responses in those conditions.

ACKNOWLEDGMENT

Portions of the work described here were supported by NIH Grant CA-39723.

REFERENCES

1. **Zinsser, H. and Tamiya, T,** An experimental analysis of bacterial allergy, *J. Exp. Med.,* 44, 753, 1926.
2. **Bloom, B. R. and Bennett, B.,** Mechanisms of a reaction *in vitro* associated with delayed-type hypersensitivity, *Science,* 153, 80, 1966.
3. **David, J. R.,** Delayed hypersensitivity *in vitro:* its mediation by cell free substances formed by lymphoid cell-antigen interaction, *Proc. Natl. Acad. Sci. U.S.A.,* 56, 73, 1966.
4. **Ward, P., Cohen, S., and Flanagan, T. D.,** Leukotactic factors elaborated by virus-infected tissues, *J. Exp. Med.,* 135, 1095, 1972.
5. **Flanagan, T. D., Yoshida, T., and Cohen, S.,** Production of macrophage migration inhibition factors by virus infected cell cultures, *Infect. Immunol.,* 8, 145, 1973.
6. **Yoshida, T., Flanagan, T. D., Genco, R. J., and Cohen, S.,** Virus-induced migration inhibitory activity in experimental mumps infection, *Clin. Immunol. Immunopathol.,* 2, 472, 1974.
7. **Cohen, S., Ward, P. A., and Bigazzi, P. E.,** Cell cooperation in cell mediated immunity, in *Mechanisms of Cell-Mediated Immunity,* McCluskey, R. J. and Cohen, S., Eds., John Wiley & Sons, New York, 1974, 331.
8. **Dinarello, C. A.,** Interleukin 1, *Rev. Infect. Dis.,* 6, 51, 1984.
9. **Rocklin, R. E. and Rosenthal, A. S.,** Evidence that human leukocyte inhibitory factor (LIF) is an esterase, *J. Immunol.,* 119, 249, 1977.
10. **Bendtzen, K.,** Human leukocyte migration inhibition factor (LIF). I. Effect of synthetic and naturally occurring esterase and protease inhibitors, *Scand. J. Immunol.,* 6, 126, 1977.
11. **Gonzales-Fernandez, A., Gimenez-Martin, G., Diez, J. L., de la Torre, C., and Lopez-Saez, J. F.,** Interphase development and beginning of mitosis in the different nuclei of polynucleate homokaryotic cells, *Chromosoma,* 36, 100, 1971.
12. **Graham, C. F.,** The regulation of DNA synthesis and mitosis in multinucleate frog eggs, *J. Cell Sci.,* 1, 363, 1966.
13. **Graham, C. F., Arms, K., and Gurdon, J. B.,** The induction of DNA synthesis by frog egg cytoplasm, *Devel. Biol.,* 14, 349, 1966.
14. **Harris, H., Watkins, J. F., Ford, C. E., and Schoefl, G. I.,** Artificial heterokaryons of animal cells from different species, *J. Cell Sci.,* 1, 1, 1966.
15. **Johnson, R. T. and Harris, H.,** DNA synthesis and mitosis in fused cells. II. HeLa-chick erythrocyte heterokaryons, *J. Cell Sci.,* 5, 625, 1969.
16. **Das, M.,** Mitogenic hormone-induced intracellular message: assay and partial characterization of an activator of DNA replication induced by epidermal growth factor, *Proc. Natl. Acad. Sci. U.S.A.,* 77, 112, 1980.
17. **Rosen, O. M.,** After insulin binds, *Science,* 237, 1452, 1987.
18. **Moolenaar, W. H.,** Effects of growth factors on intracellular pH regulation, *Ann. Rev. Physiol.,* 48, 363, 1986.
19. **Cohen, P.,** The role of protein phosphorylation in neural and hormonal control of cellular activity, *Science,* 296, 613, 1982.
20. **Gilman, A. G.,** G proteins and dual control of adenylate cyclase, *Cell,* 36, 577, 1984.
21. **Pastan, I.,** Cyclic AMP, *Sci. Am.,* 227, 97, 1970.
22. **Sutherland, E. W.,** Studies on the mechanism of hormone action, *Science,* 177, 401, 1972.
23. **Racker, E.,** Fluxes of Ca^{2+} and concepts, *Fed. Proc.,* 39, 2422, 1980.
24. **Majerus, P. W., Neufeld, E. J., and Wilson, D. B.,** Production of phosphoinositide-derived messengers, *Cell,* 37, 701, 1984.
25. **Nishizuka, Y.,** Turnover of inositol phospholipids and signal transduction, *Science,* 225, 1365, 1984.
26. **Berridge, M. J.,** Inositol triphosphate and diacylglycerol as second messengers, *Biochem. J.,* 220, 345, 1984.

27. **Berridge, M. J. and Irvine, R. F.,** Inositol triphosphate, a novel second messenger in cellular signal transduction, *Nature,* 312, 315, 1984.

28. **Streb, H., Irvine, R. F., Berridge, M. J., and Schultz, I.,** Release of Ca^{2+} from a nonmitochondrial store in pancreatic cells by inositol-1,4,5-triphosphate, *Nature,* 306, 67, 1983.

29. **Kishimoto, A., Takai, Y., Mori, T., Kikkawa, U., and Nishizuka, Y.,** Activation of calcium and phospholipid dependent protein kinase by diacylglycerol, its possible relationship to phosphatidylinositol turnover, *J. Biol. Chem.,* 255, 2273, 1980.

30. **Uhing, R. J., Dillon, S. B., Polakis, P. G., Truett, A. P., and Snyderman, R.,** Chemoattractant receptors and signal transduction processes, in *Cellular and Molecular Aspects of Inflammation. Smith Kline and French Laboratories Research Symposium V,* Post, G. and Crooke, S. T., Eds., Plenum Press, New York, 1988, 355.

31. **Korchak, H. M., Vienne, K., Rutherford, L. E., and Weissman, G.,** Neutrophil stimulation: receptor, membrane, and metabolic events, *Fed. Proc.,* 43, 2749, 1984.

32. **Freer, R. J., Day, A. R., Radding, J. A., Schiffman, E., Answanikumar, S., Showell, H. J., and Becker, E. L.,** Further studies on the structural requirements for synthetic peptide chemoattractants, *Biochemistry,* 19, 2404, 1980.

33. **Showell, H. J., Zigmond, S. H., Schiffman, E., Aswanikumar, S., Corcoran, B., and Becker, E. L.,** The structure-activity relations of synthetic peptides as chemotactic factors and inducers of lysosomal enzyme secretion for neutrophils, *J. Exp. Med.,* 143, 1154, 1976.

34. **Mackin, W. M., Huang, C. K., and Becker, E. L.,** The formyl peptide chemotactic receptor on rabbit peritoneal neutrophils, *J. Immunol.,* 129, 1608, 1982.

35. **Koo, C., Lefkowitz, R. J., and Snyderman, R.,** Guanine nucleotides modulate the binding affinity of the oligopeptide chemoattractant receptor on human polymorphonuclear leucocytes, *J. Clin. Invest.,* 72, 748, 1983.

36. **Dougherty, R. W., Godfrey, P. P., Hoyle, P. C., Putney, J. W., Jr., and Freer, R. J.,** Secretogogue induced phosphoinositide metabolism in human leukocytes, *Biochem. J.,* 222, 307, 1984.

37. **Bradford, P. G. and Rubin, R. P.,** Quantitative differences in inositol 1,4,5-triphosphate in chemoattractant-stimulated neutrophils, *J.Biol. Chem.,* 261, 15644, 1986.

38. **Bradford, P. G. and Rubin, R. P.,** Characterization of formyl-methionyl-leucyl-phenylalanine stimulation of inositol triphosphate accumulation in rabbit neutrophils, *Mol. Pharmacol.,* 27, 74, 1985.

39. **Burgess, G. M., McKenney, J. S., Irvine, R. F., and Putney, J. W., Jr.,** Inositol 1,4,5 triphosphate and inositol 1,3,4 triphosphate formation in calcium mobilizing hormone activating cells, *Biochem. J.,* 232, 237, 1985.

40. **Lew, P. D., Monod, A., Krause, K. H., Waldvogel, F. A., Biden, T. J., and Schlegel, W.,** The role of cytosolic calcium in the generation of inositol 1,4,5 triphosphate and inositol 1,3,4 triphosphate in HL-60 cells: differential effects of chemotactic peptide receptor stimulation at distinct calcium levels, *J. Biol. Chem.,* 261, 13121, 1986.

41. **Cockroft, S., Baldwin, J. M., and Allan, D.,** The calcium activated polyphosphoinositide phosphodiesterase of human and rabbit neutrophil membranes, *Biochem. J.,* 221, 477, 1984.

42. **Smith, C. D., Lane, B. C., Kusaka, I., Verghese, M. W., and Snyderman, R.,** Chemoattractant-receptor induced hydrolysis of phosphatidyl inositol 4,5-biphosphate in human polymorphonuclear leucocyte membranes: requirement of a guanine regulatory protein, *J. Biol. Chem.,* 260, 5875, 1985.

43. **Smith, C. D., Cox, C. C., and Snyderman, R.,** Receptor-coupled activation of phosphoinositide-specific phospholipase C by an G protein, *Science,* 232, 97, 1986.

44. **Andersson, T., Dahlgren, C., Pozzan, T., Stendahl, O., and Lew, D. P.,** Characterization of fMet-Leu-Phe receptor mediated Ca^{++} influx across the plasma membrane of human neutrophils, *Mol. Pharmacol.,* 30, 437, 1986.

45. **Lew, P. D., Wollheim, C. B., Waldvogel, F. A., and Pozzan, T.,** Modulation of cytosolic free calcium by changes in intracellular calcium buffering capacity: correlation with exocytosis and oxygen production in human neutrophils, *Mol. Pharmacol. J. Cell. Biol.,* 99, 1212, 1984.

46. **Prentki, M., Wollheim, C. G., and Lew, P. D.,** Ca^{++} homeostasis in permeabilized human neutrophils: characterization of Ca^{++} sequestering pools and the action of inositol 1,4,5 triphosphate, *J. Biol. Chem.,* 259, 13777, 1984.

47. **Andersson, T., Dahlgren, C., Pozzan, T., Stendahl, O., and Lew, D. P.,** Characterization of fMet-Leu-Phe receptor mediated Ca^{2+} influx across the plasma membrane of human neutrophils, *Mol. Pharmacol.,* 30, 447, 1986.

48. **Korchak, H. M., Rutherford, L. E., and Weissman, G.,** Stimulus response coupling in the human neutrophils. I. Kinetic analysis of changes in calcium permeability, *J. Biol. Chem.,* 259, 4070, 1984.

49. **Serhan, C. N., Broekman, M. J., Korchak, H. M., Smolen, J. E., Marcus, A. J., and Weissman, G.,** Changes in phosphatidylinositol and phosphatidic acid in stimulated human neutrophils: relationship to calcium mobilization, aggregation and superoxide radical generation, *Biochem. Biophys. Acta,* 762, 420, 1983.

50. **Grzeskowiak, M., Della Bianca, V., De Togni, P., Papini, E., and Rossi, F.,** Independence with respect to Ca^{++} changes of the neutrophil respiratory and secretory response to exogenous phospholipase C and possible involvement of diacylglycerol and protein kinase C, *Biochem. Biophys. Acta,* 844, 81, 1985.
51. **Myers, M. A., McPhail, L. C., and Snyderman, R.,** Redistribution of protein kinase C activity in human monocytes: correlation with activation of the respiratory burst, *J. Immunol.,* 135, 3411, 1985.
52. **Wolfson, M., McPhail, L. C., Narsallah, V. N., and Snyderman, R.,** Phorbol myristate acetate mediates redistribution of protein kinase C in human neutrophils: potential role in the activation of the respiratory burst system, *J. Immunol.,* 135, 2057, 1985.
53. **Gennaro, R., Floro, C., and Romeo, D.,** Coactivation of protein kinase C and NADPH oxidase in the plasma membrane of neutrophil cytoplasts, *Biochem. Biophys. Res. Commun.,* 134, 305, 1986.
54. **Cox, C. C., Dougherty, R. W., Ganong, B. R., Bell, R. M., Niedel, J. E., and Snyderman, R.,** Differential stimulation of the respiratory burst and lysozymal enzyme secretion in human polymorphonuclear leucocytes by synthetic diacylglycerols, *J. Immunol.,* 136, 4611, 1986.
55. **Melloni, E., Pontremoli, S., Salamino, F., Sparatore, B., Michetti, M., Sacco, O., and Horeker, B. L.,** ATP induces the release of a neutral serine proteinase and enhances the production of superoxide anion in membranes from phorbol ester activated neutrophils, *J. Biol. Chem.,* 261, 1986.
56. **Imboden, J., Weyand, C., and Goronzy, J.,** Antigen recognition by a human T cell clone leads to increases in inositol triphosphate, *J. Immunol.,* 138, 1322, 1987.
57. **Nisbet-Brown, E., Lee, J. W. W., Cheung, R. K., and Gelfand, E. W.,** Antigen-dependent increases in cytosolic free calcium in specific human T lymphocyte clones, *Nature,* 316, 545, 1985.
58. **Kozumbo, W. J., Harris, D. T., Gromkowski, S., Cerottini, J.-C., and Cerutti, P. A.,** Molecular mechanisms involved in T cell activation. II. The phosphatidylinositol signal transducing mechanism mediates antigen-induced lymphokine production but not interleukin 2 induced proliferation in cloned cytotoxic T lymphocytes, *J. Immunol.,* 130, 606, 1997.
59. **Meuer, S., Acuto, O., Hercend, T., Schlossman, S., and Reinherz, E.,** The human T cell receptor, *Annu. Rev. Immunol.,* 2, 23, 1984.
60. **Brenner, M. B., Trowbridge, I. S., and Strominger, J. L.,** Cross-linking of human T cell receptor proteins: association between the T cell idiotype subunit and the T3 glycoprotein heavy subunit, *Cell,* 40, 183, 1985.
61. **Meuer, S. C., Hodgdon, J. C., Hussey, R. E., Protentis, J. P., Schlossman, S. F., and Reinherz, E. L.,** Antigen-like effects of monoclonal antibodies directed at receptors on T cell clones, *J. Exp. Med.,* 158, 988, 1983.
62. **Weiss, A., Wiskocil, R., and Stobo, J.,** The role of T3 surface molecules in the activation of human T cells: a two-stimulus requirement for IL-2 production reflects events occurring at a pre-translational level, *J. Immunol.,* 133, 1, 1984.
63. **Weiss, A., Imboden, J., Shoback, D., and Stobo, J.,** The role of T3 surface molecules in human T cell activation: T3-dependent activation results in an increase in cytoplasmic free calcium, *Proc. Natl. Acad. Sci. U.S.A.,* 81, 4169, 1984.
64. **Imboden, J., Weiss, A., and Stobo, J.,** The antigen receptor on a human T cell line initiates activation by increasing cytoplasmic free calcium, *J. Immunol.,* 1, 34, 663, 1985.
65. **Imboden, J. B. and Stobo, J. D.,** Transmembrane signalling by the T cell antigen receptor. Perturbation of the T3-antigen receptor complex generates inositol phosphates and releases calcium ions from intracellular stores, *J. Exp. Med.,* 161, 446, 1985.
66. **Ledbetter, J. A., June, C. A., Martin, P. J., Spooner, C. E. Hansen, J. A., and Meier, K. E.,** Valency of CD3 binding and internalization of the CD3 cell-surface complex control T cell responses to second signals: distinction between effects on protein kinase C, cytoplasmic free calcium and proliferation, *J. Immunol.,* 136, 3945, 1986.
67. **Farrar, W. L. and Riuscetti, F. W.,** Association of protein kinase C activation with IL-2 receptor expression, *J. Immunol.,* 136, 1266, 1986.
68. **Gaulton, G. N. and Eardley, D. D.,** Interleukin 2-dependent phosphorylation of interleukin 2 receptors and other T cell membrane proteins, *J. Immunol.,* 136, 2470, 1986.
69. **Farrar, W. L. and Anderson, W. B.,** Interleukin 2 stimulates association of protein kinase C with plasma membrane, *Nature,* 315, 233, 1985.
70. **Mills, G. B., Stewart, D. J., Mellors, A., and Gelfand, E. W.,** Interleukin 2 does not induce phosphatidylinositol hydrolysis in activated T cells, *J. Immunol.,* 136, 3019, 1986.
71. **Truneh, A., Albert, F., Golstein, P., and Schmitt-Verhulst, A.,** Early steps of lymphocyte activation bypassed by synergy between calcium ionophores and phorbol ester, *Nature,* 313, 318, 1985.
72. **Depper, J., Leonard, W., Kronke, M., Noguchi, P., Cunningham, R., Waldmann, T., and Greene, W.,** Regulation of IL-2 receptor expression: effects of phorbol esters, phospholipase C and reexpsoure to lectin or antigen, *J. Immunol.,* 133, 3054, 1984.
73. **Coggeshall, K. M. and Cambier, J. C.,** B cell activation. VIII. Membrane immunoglobulins transduce signals via activation of phosphatidylinositol hydrolysis, *J. Immunol.,* 133, 3382, 1984.

74. **Coggeshall, K. M. and Cambier, J. C.,** B cell activation. VI. Effects of exogenous diglyceride and modulators of phospholipid metabolism suggest a central role for diacylglycerol generation in transmembrane signalling by mIg, *J. Immunol.,* 134, 101, 1985.

75. **Muraguchi, A., Kehrl, J. H., Butler, J. L., and Fauci, A. S.,** Sequential requirements for cell cycle progression of resting human B cells after activation with anti-Ig, *J. Immunol.,* 132, 176, 1984.

76. **Maino, V. C., Hayman, M. J., and Crumpton, M. J.,** Relationship between enhanced turnover of phosphatidylinositol and lymphocyte activation by mitogens, *Biochem. J.,* 146, 247, 1975.

77. **Kishimoto, T., Kikutani, H., Nishizawa, Y., Sakaguchi, N., and Yamamura, Y.,** Involvement of anti-Ig-activated serine protease in the generation of cytoplasmic factor(s) that are responsible for the transmission of Ig-receptor-mediated signals, *J. Immunol.,* 123, 1504, 1979.

78. **Eda, Y., Ohara, J., and Watanabe, T.,** Restoration of LPS responsiveness of C3H/HeJ mouse lymphocytes by microinjection of cytoplasmic factor(s) from LPS-stimulated normal lymphocytes, *J. Immunol.,* 131, 1294, 1983.

79. **Gutowski, J. K. and Cohen, S.,** Induction of DNA synthesis in isolated nuclei by cytoplasmic factors from spontaneously proliferating and mitogen-activated lymphoid cells, *Cell. Immunol.,* 75, 300, 1983.

80. **Jazwinski, S. M., Wang, J. L., and Edelman, G. M.,** Initiation of replication in chromosomal DNA induced by extracts of proliferating cells, *Proc. Natl. Acad. Sci. U.S.A.,* 73, 2231, 1976.

81. **Gutowski, J. K., Mukherji, B., and Cohen, S.,** The role of cytoplasmic intermediates in IL-2-induced T cell growth, *J. Immunol.,* 133, 3068, 1984.

82. **Wong, R. L., Gutowski, J. K., Katz, M., Goldfarb, R. H., and Cohen, S.,** Induction of DNA synthesis in isolated nuclei by cytoplasmic factors: inhibition by protease inhibitors, *Proc. Natl. Acad. Sci. U.S.A.,* 84, 241, 1987.

83. **Gutowski, J. K., West, A., and Cohen, S.,** The regulation of DNA synthesis in quiescent lymphocytes by cytoplasmic inhibitors, *Proc. Natl. Acad. Sci. U.S.A.,* 82, 5160, 1985.

84. **Gutowski, J. K. and Cohen, S.,** Suppression of DNA synthesis in normal, but not neoplastic, nuclei by cytoplasmic extracts from resting cells, *Cell. Immunol.,* 106, 174, 1987.

85. **Weksler, M. and Hutteroth, T. H.,** Impaired lymphocyte function in aged humans, *J. Clin. Invest.,* 53, 99, 1974.

86. **Hori, Y., Perkins, E. H., and Halsall, M. K.,** Decline in phytohemagglutinin responsiveness of spleen cells from aging mice, *Proc. Soc. Exp. Biol. Med.,* 144, 48, 1973.

87. **Foad, B. S. I., Yamaguchi, Y., and Litwin, A.,** Phytomitogen responses of peripheral blood lymphocytes in young and older subjects, *Clin. Exp. Immunol.,* 17, 657, 2974.

88. **Joncourt, F., Bettens, F., Krisktensen, F., and DeWeck, A. L.,** Age-related changes in mitogen responsiveness in different lymphoid organs from outbred NRMI mice, *Immunobiology,* 158, 439, 1981.

89. **Staiano-Coico, L., Darzynkiewicz, Z., Hefton, J. M., Dutkowski, R., Darlington, G., and Weksler, M. E.,** Increased sensitivity of lymphocytes from people over 65 to cell cycle arrest and chromosomal damage, *Science,* 219, 1335, 1983.

90. **Hefton, J. M., Darlington, G. J., Casazza, B. A., and Weksler, M. E.,** Immunologic studies of aging. V. Impaired proliferation of PHA responsive human lymphocytes in culture, *J. Immunol.,* 125, 1007, 1980.

91. **Gillis, S., Kozak, R., Durante, M., and Weksler, M. E.,** Immunological studies of aging: decreased production of and response to T cell growth factor by lymphocytes from aged humans, *J. Clin. Invest.,* 67, 927, 1981.

92. **Thomas, M. L. and Weigle, W. O.,** Lymphokines and aging. Interleukin 2 production and activity in aged animals, *J. Immunol.,* 127, 2101, 1981.

93. **Miller, R. A. and Stutman, O.,** Decline in aging mice of the anti-2,4,6-trinitrophenol cytotoxic T cell response attributable in loss of Lyt-2⁻, interleukin 2 producing helper cell function, *Eur. J. Immunol.,* 11, 751, 1981.

94. **Gilman, S. C., Rosenberg, J. S., and Feldman, J. D.,** T lymphocytes from young and aged rats. II. functional defects and the role of interleukin 2, *J. Immunol.,* 128, 644, 1982.

95. **Cheung, H. T., Wu, W. T., Pahlavani, M., and Richardson, A.,** Effect of age on interleukin 2 messenger RNA level, *Fed. Proc.,* 44, 573, 1985.

96. **Chang, M.-P., Makinodan, T., Peterson, W. J., and Strehler, B. L.,** Role of T cells and adherent cells in age-related decline in murine interleukin 2 production, *J. Immunol.,* 129, 2426, 1982.

97. **Proust, J. J., Filburn, C. R., Harrison, S. A., Buchholz, M. A., and Nordin, A. A.,** Age-related defect in signal transduction during lectin activation of murine T lymphocytes, *J. Immunol.,* 139, 1472, 1987.

98. **Gutowski, J. K., Innes, J., Weksler, M. E., and Cohen, S.,** Induction of DNA synthesis in isolated nuclei by cytoplasmic factors. II. Normal generation of cytoplasmic stimulatory factors by lymphocytes from aged humans with depressed proliferative responses, *J. Immunol.,* 132, 559, 1984.

99. **Gutowski, J. K., Innes, J. B., Weksler, M. E., and Cohen, S.,** Impaired nuclear responsiveness to cytoplasmic signals in lymphocytes from elderly humans with depressed proliferative responses, *J. Clin. Invest.,* 78, 40, 1986.

Chapter 6

TRANSMEMBRANE SIGNALING IN B CELL ACTIVATION

Louis B. Justement and John C. Cambier

TABLE OF CONTENTS

I. INTRODUCTION

B cell physiology is regulated by a large number of ligands which bind to distinct cell surface receptors. The complexity of this regulation is illustrated by the fact that resting B cells are responsive to multiple ligands, and that these specific ligands can exert different effects on the cell depending on its physiologic state. Delineation of the signal transduction mechanisms employed by receptors for these ligands is an important step toward understanding how B cell immune function is controlled via the concerted effects of multiple regulatory species. In view of this, our laboratory and other laboratories have focused on the study of receptor-mediated signal transduction in quiescent B cells. To date, little or nothing is known about transmembrane signaling mechanisms operative in B cell blasts or memory cells. Therefore, the focus of this review is on events associated with the activation and inactivation of resting B lymphocytes.

In the absence of external stimuli, mature peripheral B lymphocytes exist in a quiescent state characterized by a basal level of metabolic activity devoted to housekeeping functions. Left unperturbed, these cells do not progress through the cell cycle and therefore are considered to be in G_0. G_0 B lymphocytes are capable of interacting with a number of ligands which affect their biology. In the parlance of cellular immunology, such effects have come to be known collectively as "activation". Thus, thymus dependent and independent antigens (Ag), antibodies directed against immunoglobulin (anti-Ig) which act as antigen surrogates,[2,3] interleukin 4 (IL-4, formerly B cell stimulatory factor-1, BSF-1),[4] B cell activation factor (BCAF),[5-6] and mitogens such as lipopolysaccharide (LPS)[7] are all capable of inducing B cell activation as manifest by their ability to stimulate hyperexpression of class II MHC molecules (Ia) by resting B cells. Increased expression of Ia presumably promotes the generation of B cell immune responses based solely on the fact that a quantitative increase in expression of these molecules enhances the ability of B cells to interact productively with antigen specific, MHC-restricted helper T cells, resulting ultimately in antibody formation. These activation agents also prepare the B cell for subsequent interaction with additional ligands such as interleukin-1 (IL-1),[8] interleukin-2 (IL-2),[9-10] and interleukin-5 (IL-5, formerly B cell growth factor II) which are necessary for proliferation and differentiation into antibody-secreting cells.

Three additional ligands, the Fc portion of IgG, interferon gamma (IFN-γ), and antibody directed against Ia (anti-Ia) have been shown to exert an effect on resting B cells. Fc receptor ligation has been shown to antagonize anti-Ig induced proliferation of B cells.[12] IFN γ inhibits soluble anti-Ig or IL-4 induced Ia expression, as well as anti-Ig induced proliferation when incubated with resting cells,[13-14] but is a differentiation-inducing factor for activated B cells.[15] Finally, anti-Ia antibodies antagonize LPS and anti-Ig induced B cell proliferation,[16-17] but appear to promote differentiation when added to B cells which have previously been activated.[18] The fact that both IFN-γ and Ia-binding ligands exert a positive effect on the stage of B cell differentiation is interesting in view of their antagonistic effects on early events associated with B cell activation and proliferation. Essentially, these two ligands appear to divert proliferating cells toward differentiation, presumably by initiating intracellular events which antagonize biochemical processes necessary for activation and proliferation.

Toward an understanding of the mode of action of the regulators discussed above, a number of laboratories have begun to dissect the mechanistic link between receptor-ligand complex formation and resultant changes in lymphocyte biology. Of more specific interest is the molecular basis of transmembrane signal transduction by receptors for specific immunoregulators and how relevant second messenger cascades interact to regulate the ultimate biologic response. In the succeeding paragraphs, we discuss the extant literature regarding transmembrane signal transduction mechanisms operative in B cell signaling.

II. AN OVERVIEW OF THE MECHANISMS OF TRANSMEMBRANE SIGNALING

One of the most productive areas of recent study in cell biology, and one which is extremely relevant to an understanding of lymphocyte function, concerns the delineation of mechanisms by which a cell responds to regulatory molecules via plasma membrane receptors. It has become clear that changes in the physiology of a cell, elicited by ligand binding, are controlled by the intracellular generation of specific second messenger molecules which in turn regulate the activity of protein kinases. Thus, in most instances, the receptor transmits the information imparted to it through the binding of a ligand by initiating a cascade of events which culminate in covalent modification of existing enzymes and other proteins, via phosphorylation, thus altering their function. Currently, four distinct second messenger-dependent protein kinase systems have been identified in nonlymphoid tissues: the cyclic AMP (cAMP) and cyclic GMP (cGMP)-dependent,[19] the Ca^{2+}/phospholipid-dependent,[20] and the Ca^{2+}/calmodulin-dependent[21] kinases. Additionally, several receptors have been found to possess intrinsic protein kinase activity which is activated upon ligand binding.[22] Cells may employ these kinases singly or in combination to regulate the function of specific signal transducing enzymes, thus modifying their physiologic state.

Perhaps the best-defined signal transduction system involves binding of catecholamines to the β- and α_2-adrenergic receptors leading to modulation of intracellular levels of the second messenger cAMP. The receptors operative in this system are associated with guanine-nucleotide-binding regulatory molecules termed N_s and N_i respectively. These guanosine-triphosphate (GTP)-binding proteins regulate the activity of the catalytic subunit of adenylate cyclase, thus promoting or inhibiting the conversion of ATP into cAMP.[23-24] Binding of ligand to the β-adrenergic receptor activates the N_s regulatory protein which is a heterotrimer comprised of an α_s subunit with an M_r of 43 kDa, a β subunit of 35 kDa, and a γ subunit of 5 kDa.[25] Activation of the N_s regulatory protein is associated with binding of GTP which causes dissociation of the α_s subunit, bound to GTP, from the βγ complex, and the complex as a whole from the receptor. The α_s-GTP subunit then binds to the inactive adenylate cyclase catalytic subunit resulting in its activation. The active α_s-GTP-adenylate cyclase complex is inactivated by the GTPase activity associated with the α_s subunit of N_s. Once GTP has been converted into guanosine diphosphate (GDP), the α_s subunit recombines with βγ. Activation of the α_2-adrenergic receptor results in dissociation of the α_i subunit of N_i (41 kDa) from the βγ heterodimer which is identical to that found in association with α_s. Activation of N_i results in inhibition of adenylate cyclase-mediated cAMP production either by binding of α_i to adenylate cyclase or by reassociation of free βγ with the α_s subunit.[26] Under conditions where adenylate cyclase is activated, the resultant increase in cAMP has been shown to activate cAMP-dependent protein kinase.[19] A somewhat similar signaling mechanism has been identified for the generation of cGMP which involves components that are analogous to those of the β- and α_2-adrenergic receptors.[27-28]

Studies of the α_1-adrenergic receptor system have elucidated much of the mechanism operative in signal transduction by the vast variety of receptors whose ligation is associated with the generation of diacylglyceride and Ca^{2+} second messengers (Figure 1). Initial observations by Hokin and Hokin[29] defined hormone-mediated effects on phosphoinositide metabolism. Since those initial observations, extensive work has confirmed that α_1-adrenergic receptors are coupled to the generation of multiple intracellular second messengers via activation of hydrolysis of phosphoinositides associated with the plasma membrane.[30] Specifically, ligand binding activates a phospholipase C (PLC) which hydrolyses mono- and polyphosphoinositides including phosphatidylinositol 4,5-bisphosphate (PtdInsP2) yielding diacylglycerol (DAG) and inositol 1,4,5-trisphosphate (InsP3). Work by Streb et al.[31] first demonstrated that InsP3 mediates the release of Ca^{2+} stored in the endoplasmic reticulum.

Nishizuka and co-workers[26] characterized a protein kinase designated protein kinase C (PKC) which is regulated by Ca^{2+} and diacylglycerol. Later studies in a variety of systems demonstrated that this kinase is translocated from the cytosol to the plasma membrane in response to increased levels of DAG and Ca^{2+}.[32] Translocation is associated with activation of this enzyme and new phosphorylation of proteins.[33] In addition, increased intracellular levels of Ca^{2+} can mediate activation of Ca^{2+}/calmodulin-dependent protein kinase by binding to and activating calmodulin which in turn regulates protein kinase activation.[20]

Recent studies conducted, most notably with the insulin receptor, have demonstrated that in certain instances, ligand-receptor interactions can lead to protein kinase activation without the generation of conventional second messengers.[34] In the case of the insulin receptor, protein kinase activity is an intrinsic part of the receptor itself. Ligand binding activates a tyrosine-specific protein kinase resulting in autophosphorylation of the receptor, either increasing or decreasing its kinase activity, which presumably regulates the phosphorylation of other substrates.[34-35] These protein kinases differ from conventional enzymes in that they phosphorylate substrates only on tyrosine residues as opposed to serine and threonine.

The above discussion provides an indication of the various signal transduction mechanisms utilized to transmit information from cell surface receptors to the interior of a cell. Many of these mechanisms appear to be operative in regulation of B lymphocyte activation, proliferation, and differentiation as is discussed below.

III. B CELL ACTIVATION VIA MEMBRANE IMMUNOGLOBULIN

A. MEMBRANE IMMUNOGLOBULIN-MEDIATED SIGNALING VIA AN α_1-ADRENERGIC-LIKE MECHANISM

Studies conducted in several laboratories over the past decade and a half have provided the basis for our current concept of signal transduction by B cell surface IgM, IgD, and IgG. Maino et al.[36] demonstrated in 1975 that cross-linking of membrane immunoglobulin (mIg) by anti-Ig resulted in increased incorporation of $^{32}PO_4$ into phosphatidylinositol (PtdIns) by approximately fourfold within minutes of stimulation. Based on this finding it was proposed that increased metabolism of PtdIns is an early event associated with mIg-mediated signaling. Subsequently, Braun et al.[37] observed that anti-Ig stimulation of B cells leads to mobilization of 20 to 30% of exchangeable Ca^{2+} within 2 min. This response, like PtdIns hydrolysis, was dependent on receptor cross-linking as indicated by the fact that Fab fragments of anti-Ig did not induce the Ca^{2+} mobilization response. Monroe and Cambier[38] subsequently demonstrated that F(ab')$_2$ fragments of anti-Ig were able to induce B lymphocytes to undergo membrane depolarization within 5 min, with the maximal response occurring after 1 h. These observations suggested the existence of a cascade of events culminating in membrane depolarization, an event previously shown to be an early and essential event for activation and entry of nonlymphoid cells into the cell cycle.[39-40] Monroe and Cambier[41] also found that nonspecific depolarization of B cells by K^+ was sufficient to cause hyper-Ia expression, suggesting that membrane depolarization was causally related to anti-Ig-mediated induction of Ia gene expression. Also important were the observations that membrane depolarization is induced by the phorbol diester analogs phorbol-12-myristate-13-acetate (PMA) and 4 β-phorbol-12,13-didecanoate (4 β-PDD), but not 4 α-phorbol-12,13-didecanoate (4 α-PDD). Of the analogs tested, PMA and 4 β-PDD are known to mimic the effects of DAG by activating PKC, while 4 α-PDD does not. These findings suggested that DAG is generated during mIg-mediated signaling and induces membrane depolarization and subsequent Ia expression via activation of PKC. These early studies provided evidence that at least two second messengers, DAG and Ca^{2+} are involved in mIg-mediated activation of

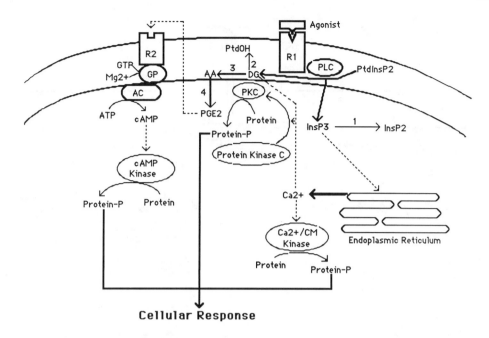

FIGURE 1.   Activation of intracellular second messenger systems and associated protein kinases via ligand binding to the α_1-adrenergic receptor. R1 = α-adrenergic receptor; PLC = phospholipase C; PtdInsP2 = phosphatidylinositol 4,5-bisphosphate; InsP3 = inositol 1,4,5-trisphospha e; InsP2 = inositol 1,4-bis-phosphate; CM = calmodulin; DG = diacylglyceride; PtdOH = phosphatidic acid; AA = arachidonic acid; PGE$_2$ = prostaglandin E$_2$; R2 = prostaglandin receptor; GP = GTP-binding regulatory protein; and AC = adenylate cyclase. 1 = inositol-trisphosphatase; 2 = diacylglycerol kinase; 3 = phospholipase A2; and 4 = cyclooxygenase.

B cells (Figure 2). These findings were analogous to those made concurrently in studies of α_1-adrenergic receptor-mediated signaling in other somatic cell systems.[43]

B. MEMBRANE IMMUNOGLOBULIN-MEDIATED PHOSPHOLIPID HYDROLYSIS

Based on the findings of Monroe and Cambier[38] and Lindsten et al.,[44] who demonstrated the ability of PMA and 4 β-PDD to induce membrane depolarization and hyperexpression of Ia, Coggeshall and Cambier[45] proposed that DAG may be an important second messenger in B cell activation. Based on this hypothesis, DAG or activators of DAG production should mediate membrane depolarization and hyperexpression of Ia in B cells. Similarly, inhibitors of DAG generation should block these events. It was found that exposure of B cells to DAG or induction of DAG synthesis by treatment with exogenous PLC was sufficient to cause membrane depolarization and increased expression of Ia.[45] As expected, anti-Ig (but not PMA) stimulation of membrane depolarization and Ia expression were inhibited by raising the intracellular concentration of cAMP, which blocks PtdIns metabolism in B cells.[45]

More direct evidence that treatment of B cells with anti-Ig results in PtdIns hydrolysis yielding DAG was subsequently provided by Coggeshall and Cambier[46] and Bijsterbosch et al.[47] In these studies, stimulation of B cells with anti-Ig resulted in an increased incorporation of $^{32}PO_4$ into phosphatidic acid (PtdOH), the phosphorylated product of DAG. The kinetics of the response were rapid with maximal stimulation observed after 10 min. A somewhat delayed increase in $^{32}PO_4$ incorporation into PtdIns but not phosphatidylcholine was observed suggesting that anti-Ig treatment specifically alters the metabolism of lipids in the PtdIns cycle with PLC-mediated hydrolysis of phosphoinositides being the earliest step. Raising

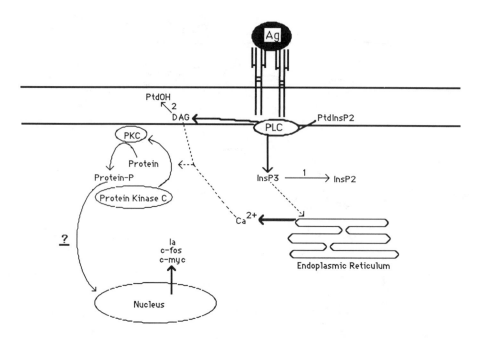

FIGURE 2.   Membrane immunoglobulin-mediated signal transduction. Crosslinking of mIg results in the activation of phospholipase C which hydrolyzes PtdInsP2 to form DAG and InsP3. InsP3 induces mobilization of Ca^{2+} from the endoplasmic reticulum which acts synergistically with DAG to induce PKC translocation and activation. Activation of PKC leads to phosphorylation of a number of endogenous substrates which, via a poorly defined mechanism, induce the transcription of genes encoding Ia, c-fos and c-myc.

the intracellular concentration of cAMP was found to block incorporation of $^{32}PO_4$ into PtdOH and PtdIns, under conditions that were identical to those which block depolarization and increased expression of Ia. The later work of Bijsterbosch et al.[47] supports the above findings. In these experiments, B cells were labeled with ^3H-arachidonic acid and the formation of ^3H-1,2-diacylglycerol was measured following stimulation with various ligands. Treatment with anti-Ig induced a 2-fold increase in the amount of labeled 1,2-diacylglycerol which reached a maximum at 10 min and remained elevated for up to 30 min. Kriz et al.[48] observed a 2-fold increase in the incorporation of $^{32}PO_4$ into PtdOH and PtdIns following treatment of B cells with immobilized anti-Ig. Incorporation of $^{32}PO_4$ was maximal at 2 h, and remained elevated at 3 h. Data concerning $^{32}PO_4$ incorporation prior to 2 h after the addition of Sepharose-bound anti-Ig were not presented, therefore, it is not known whether the kinetics of the PtdIns hydrolytic response are similar following stimulation of B cells with immobilized or soluble anti-Ig.

The source of DAG produced during PtdIns hydrolysis was addressed by Ransom et al.[49] and Bijsterbosch et al.[47] B cells incubated with ^3H-inositol to label PtdIns, PtdInsP, and PtdInsP2 pools were analyzed to determine the release of inositol 1-phosphate (InsP), inositol 1,4-bisphosphate (InsP2), and InsP3 following stimulation with anti-Ig. Bijsterbosch et al.[47] reported a rapid increase (within 10 s) in the level of InsP3, InsP2, and InsP following mIg cross-linking. Inositol trisphosphate exhibited the greatest relative increase compared to InsP2 and InsP. By 1 min, InsP3 levels peaked and then declined. The levels of InsP2 and InsP increased more slowly than InsP3 and remained elevated for a longer period of time. The sequential accumulation of InsP3 followed by InsP2 and InsP is consistent with the finding from other systems that InsP3 is dephosphorylated in a stepwise manner to yield inositol.[43] Thus, it is not possible to distinguish whether anti-Ig induces hydrolysis of only PtdInsP2 or of PtdIns and PtdInsP as well.

The results of Ransom et al.[49] were consistent with those above, in that anti-Ig stimulation resulted in a significant release of InsP3, InsP2, and InsP. The kinetics of this response were slower and more prolonged than those in the study of Bijsterbosch et al.,[47] however. This discrepancy is attributable to differences in the concentration of anti-Ig used to stimulate the response. Thus, it is apparent from these studies that mIg cross-linking results in the activation of PLC which hydrolyzes PtdInsP2 to produce DAG and InsP3, both of which have been demonstrated to affect subsequent cell physiologic events important for activation of the B cell.

While studies using intact cell systems have determined that binding of ligand to mIg results in phospholipid hydrolysis, there is currently no information regarding the mechanism by which mIg activates PLC. Cambier and Harris[50] have recently developed cell-free systems, in which mIg coupling to PtdIns hydrolysis can be demonstrated, to aid in the elucidation of the molecular basis of this phenomenon. A modification of the procedure described by Smith et al.[51] was used in which PtdInsP2, PtdInsP, and PtdOH were labeled by incubation of B cell membranes with ^{32}P-ATP in the presence of magnesium. Incubation of the ^{32}P-labeled membranes with anti-Ig resulted in the rapid hydrolysis of PtdInsP2, which was easily detectable within 40 s, reached a maximum at 2 min, and gradually declined thereafter. Hydrolysis was dependent on the concentration of ligand and occurred following addition of anti-Ig but not anti-IA or anti-H2K antibodies to the reaction mixture. In contrast to other systems in which PLC-mediated hydrolysis of phosphoinositides appears to be dependent on Ca^{2+},[52] no Ca^{2+} requirement was observed in this system, although hydrolysis of PtdInsP2 could be induced in the absence of ligand by elevation of the Ca^{2+} concentration above 2 μM. Further studies revealed that anti-Ig induced very little hydrolysis of PtdInsP2 in the absence of cytosolic protein. It was proposed that cytosol is the source of the phospholipase responsible for inositol lipid hydrolysis following binding of ligand with mIg.[50]

Although Harris and Cambier were able to document hydrolysis of inositol lipids, it is not possible to quantitate the products of the hydrolysis using the ^{32}PO$_4$ labeling system. This is due to the presence of ^{32}P-ATP metabolites which obscure ^{32}P-inositol phosphates. In order to examine the inositol phosphate products formed as a result of PtdInsP2 hydrolysis, and thus determine the specificity of the operative phospholipase, an alternative system was utilized. B cell membranes were labeled with exogenous ^{3}H-PtdInsP2 in sodium cholate based on the technique of Jackowski et al.[53] Addition of anti-Ig to membranes labeled in this manner stimulated release of InsP within 30 s.[54] In contrast to studies carried out in whole cells, anti-Ig stimulated small but detectable changes in InsP2 and no accumulation, in fact a loss, of detectable InsP3. The discrepancy between the results obtained for whole cell vs. cell free hydrolysis of PtdInsP2 appears to be due to the activation of a very active InsP3/InsP2 phosphatase following mIg cross-linking in isolated membranes.[55] Therefore, ^{3}H-InsP3 formed by hydrolysis of ^{3}H-PtdInsP2 is rapidly dephosphorylated to ^{3}H-InsP which is detected. Further studies revealed that this phosphatase is inhibited by ATP at concentrations greater than 1 mM. Thus, in the presence of ATP anti-Ig induction of InsP3 release is detectable. Finally, experiments in which ^{3}H-PtdIns was incorporated into B cell membranes instead of ^{3}H-PtdInsP2 revealed that anti-Ig induces hydrolysis of PtdIns by a PLC, releasing ^{3}H-InsP. Thus, anti-Ig stimulation of isolated B cell membranes leads to hydrolysis of PtdIns and PtdInsP2 by a phospholipase C enzyme(s) and also leads to activation of an InsP3/InsP2 phosphatase.

A number of recent studies in nonlymphoid cell systems have addressed the possibility that GTP-binding proteins are involved in receptor coupling to phosphoinositide hydrolysis. These studies have demonstrated the involvement of GTP or its analogs in the control of α_1-adrenergic receptor function.[56] Studies using isolated plasma membranes from neutrophils[57] and blowfly salivary gland[58] have also shown that GTP modulates the degree of hydrolysis of PtdInsP2 observed in the presence of fMet-Leu-Phe and 5-hydroxytryptamine, respectively, suggesting a role for GTP-binding proteins in the coupling of these receptors to PLC. In the B cell, GTP-γ_s (100 μM) was found to induce a 2-fold increase in PtdInsP2 hydrolysis in isolated membranes, indicating that B cell membranes possess a GTP activatable PLC.[55] However, the anti-Ig-stimulated hydrolysis of PtdInsP2 did not exhibit a dependence on GTP or GTP-γ_s.[54-55] Finally, GDPβ_s, an inhibitor of GTP-dependent protein function, did not specifically inhibit anti-Ig-mediated activation of PLC or the InsP3/InsP2 phosphatase.[54-55] These results indicate that mIg-mediated activation of PLC in B cell membranes differs mechanistically from PLC activation by FMLP in neutrophil membranes by virtue of the fact that it occurs via a GTP-binding protein independent mechanism. It is interesting and perhaps important in this context that mIg must be cross-linked by ligand to induce inositol lipid hydrolysis, while FMLP and α_1-receptors do not. This requirement for receptor cross-linking may in some way reflect the proposed mechanistic difference in receptor coupling to phosphoinositide hydrolysis.

C. MEMBRANE IMMUNOGLOBULIN-DEPENDENT MOBILIZATION OF Ca^{2+}

Findings from a number of systems suggest a role for Ca^{2+} in mIg-mediated signaling. As discussed, Braun et al.[37] were the first to demonstrate anti-Ig induction of Ca^{2+} mobilization in B cells. Subsequently, Klaus et al.[56] and Ransom and Cambier[57] demonstrated that the Ca^{2+} ionophores A23187 and ionomycin could replace anti-Ig and stimulate B cell activation as measured by an increase in the expression of surface Ia. Calcium ionophore treatment also accelerated the onset of DNA synthesis in cells stimulated with anti-Ig.[56] In contrast to anti-Ig, the ionophores did not stimulate PtdIns breakdown or RNA synthesis.[56] Based on these findings, Klaus and co-workers concluded that Ca^{2+} ionophores induce B cells to leave G_0 but not to enter the G_1 phase of the cell cycle. Subsequent studies by Klaus et al.[58] revealed that like certain anti-Ig antibodies, the combination of PMA and Ca^{2+} ionophore is mitogenic for normal B cells. These findings suggest that under appropriate conditions the two second messengers which are formed following receptor-mediated hydrolysis of phosphoinositides (Ca^{2+} and DAG) are sufficient to drive B cell proliferation. In agreement with these findings is the work of Monroe and Kass,[59] which documented the ability of Ca^{2+} ionophores and PMA to synergize, causing B cells to exit from G_0 and enter into the cell cycle as indicated by increased RNA synthesis. Under no condition did PMA and the Ca^{2+} ionophore stimulate Ig production, suggesting that additional signals are essential to drive B cell differentiation. Finally, recent studies have demonstrated that Ca^{2+} ionophores and PMA, like anti-Ig, synergize with IL-4 to promote B cell proliferation,[4] indicating that IL-4 receptor ligation may mediate the generation of a qualitatively distinct growth signal necessary for entry into the cell cycle. This possibility is consistent with observations that IL-4 does not stimulate Ca^{2+} mobilization, phosphoinositide hydrolyisis, or PKC translocation in B cells (see below).

With the development of Ca^{2+}-sensitive fluorescent dyes, it has become possible to measure changes in the level of intracellular free Ca^{2+} in cells responding to ligand. Pozzan et al.[60] were the first to examine the effect of anti-Ig reagents on Ca^{2+} mobilization in B cells using the Ca^{2+}-sensitive fluorescent indicator quin-2. Binding of anti-Ig was found to 100 nM to greater than 500 nM. Ransom et al.[61] and Bijsterbosch et al.[47] also used quin-2 to show that anti-Ig treatment of B cells results in Ca^{2+} mobilization. A synchronous initial increase in intracellular free Ca^{2+} was observed by Ransom and co-workers[61] in all small splenic B cells stimulated with anti-Ig. This is consistent with the ability of anti-Ig to induce virtually all small B cells to increase expression of Ia.[62] The Ca^{2+} response to anti-Ig in both studies was rapid, with mobilization being maximal within 3 min. Calcium levels then returned toward baseline, maintaining a mean Ca^{2+} concentration of 250 nM for several hours afterward (>24). The intracellular concentration of free Ca^{2+} was reported by Ransom et al.[61] to reach a level of approximately 1 μM from a resting concentration of 150 nM.

Bijsterbosch et al.[47] reported values for basal and stimulated intracellular free Ca^{2+} concentrations similar to those of Pozzan et al.[60] Partain et al.[63] carried out experiments in which dinitrophenyl-specific B cells were stimulated with DNP-Ficoll and Ca^{2+} mobilization measured based on quin-2 fluorescence. Antigen stimulation of B cells resulted in an increase in intracellular free Ca^{2+} from 100 nM to approximately 450 nM within 10 min.

Studies to determine the source of Ca^{2+} mobilized in response to anti-Ig and to identify the mediator of that mobilization were carried out by Ransom et al.[49] These studies were inspired in part by the studies of Streb et al.,[31] who demonstrated that InsP3, a hydrolytic product of PtdInsP2, mediated the release of Ca^{2+} from intracellular organelles of pancreatic cells. Neither InsP1 nor InsP were found to induce Ca^{2+} release, ruling out nonspecific effects of inositol phosphates on the system. Experiments carried out by Burgess et al.[64] were similar to those above except that saponin permeabilized hepatocytes were used. These studies led Ransom et al.[49] to examine the ability of InsP3 to mobilize $^{45}Ca^{2+}$ which had been preaccumulated in the endoplasmic reticulum of B cells in the presence of Mg^{2+}-ATP and sodium azide resulted in sequestration of Ca^{2+}. Loading of B cells with $^{45}Ca^{2+}$ in the presence of Mg^{2+}-ATP and sodium azide resulted in sequestration of Ca $^{2+}$ in the endoplasmic reticulum via an ATP-dependent pumping mechanism. Addition of 1.0 μM InsP3 to $^{45}Ca^{2+}$ loaded B cells caused a rapid release of approximately 70% of the Ca^{2+} from the endoplasmic pool. These findings are consistent with those in other systems, which suggest that receptor-ligand coupling leads to InsP3 formation and subsequent mobilization of internal stores of Ca^{2+}.

Recent studies by Bijsterbosch et al.[65] indicate that a significant proportion of Ca^{2+} mobilized following mIg cross-linking is derived from extracellular stores. Specifically, depletion of extracellular Ca^{2+} using EGTA causes a significant reduction in the Ca^{2+} mobilization response. Studies by Ransom and Cambier[67] indicate that approximately 80% of the Ca^{2+} mobilized in response to anti-Ig comes from outside the cell. This Ca^{2+} influx as well as internal Ca^{2+} release is blocked by neomycin under conditions which inhibit phosphoinositide hydrolysis, suggesting that phosphoinositide hydrolysis is necessary for mobilization of Ca^{2+} from both sources.

D. MEMBRANE IMMUNOGLOBULIN-MEDIATED TRANSLOCATION AND ACTIVATION OF PROTEIN KINASE C

Ogawa et al.[68] and Ku et al.[69] were the first to identify and characterize PKC from human peripheral lymphocytes. A role for PKC in B cell activation is suggested by the fact that cross-linking of mIg stimulates a rapid increase in the hydrolysis of phosphoinositides, releasing DAG and InsP3.[70] The observation that PKC activators PMA and DAG mimic the effects of mIg cross-linking by inducing membrane depolarization and hyper-Ia expression[42] provides further support for this hypothesis. Chen et al.[71] and Nel et al.[72] have demonstrated PKC translocation in B cells in response to anti-Ig stimulation, providing direct evidence of a role for this enzyme in B cell activation. Translocation of PKC from the cytosol to the Triton soluble membrane fraction was rapid (maximal translocation occurred within 2 and 4 min, respectively). In the study reported by Chen et al.,[71] translocation of 80 to 90% of the cytosolic enzyme occurred following treatment of cells with anti-IgM or anti-IgD, but not anti-H2K antibody. Translocation of PKC to the Triton soluble membrane fraction was transient as determined by a decrease in the level of PKC activity within a period of 10 to 15 min. Chen et al.[71] determined that this decrease in activity was accompanied by an increase in PKC activity within the Triton insoluble fraction of the cell. It has subsequently been determined that this secondary translocation represents movement of PKC into the nuclear compartment of the B cell.[73] Further, it was observed that F(ab')$_2$ fragments of anti-Ig do not cause translocation of PKC to the nuclear compartment, which suggests that the Fc portion of anti-Ig is involved, probably through binding to the Fc receptor. Stimulation of B cells with the tumor promoter PMA was found to cause translocation of PKC to the plasma membrane where it was reported by Nel et al.[72] to remain for as long as 60 min. The prolonged association of PKC with the plasma membrane following PMA, but not anti-Ig stimulation, may be due to the fact that PMA is metabolized much more slowly than DAG.

Studies of PtdIns hydrolysis in platelets have revealed that cAMP has an inhibitory effect on the formation of the hydrolytic products DAG and InsP.[74-75] As a result, the accumulation of DAG following ligand stimulation is blocked by cAMP, in turn affecting the activation of PKC. Coggeshall and Cambier[46] have demonstrated that cAMP and theophylline block anti-Ig induction of PtdIns hydrolysis in the B cell. Thus, the ability of dibutyryl cAMP and theophylline to block PKC translocation in response to anti-Ig further supports the findings from other systems that PKC translocation is dependent on receptor-mediated phosphoinositide hydrolysis.[71]

Association of PKC with phosphatidylserine, Ca^{2+}, and DAG (or PMA) on the inner face of the plasma membrane apparently leads to enzyme activation.[33] In a number of tissues, new protein phosphorylation events have been documented following ligand-receptor interaction or PMA stimulation. Perhaps the most notable example is PMA or thrombin-induced phosphorylation of a 40-kDa substrate in platelets, now thought to be lipomodulin.[32] Several studies in the B cell have examined ligand-induced activation of PKC and subsequent protein phosphorylation by monitoring the incorporation of $^{32}PO_4$ into endogenous proteins associated with either the cytosol or plasma membrane following stimulation with PMA or anti-Ig. Nel et al.[72] observed that cytosolic proteins with molecular weights of 94, 66, 60, 56, 50, 43, 38, 35, 28 to 30, 20 to 23, and 15 to 18 kDa, and a membrane-associated protein of 29 kDa were substrates of PKC. Hornbeck and Paul[76] also observed several substrates which were phosphorylated following stimulation of B cells with anti-Ig or PMA. The six most prominent phosphoproteins with M_r values of 47, 55, 62, 68, and 65 to 70 kDa were associated with the plasma membrane. Of these six, four were found to be associated with the cytoskeleton, suggesting that the phosphorylation of cytoskeletal proteins may be an important event early in B cell activation. It was observed that prolonged pretreatment of B cells with PMA (14 h) blocked subsequent anti-Ig induced phosphorylation, presumably by depleting intracellular PKC, indicating that anti-Ig induced protein phosphorylation is mediated by PKC.

Recent work by Newell et al.[77] has demonstrated that stimulation of resting B cells with either PMA or anti-Ig results in phosphorylation of members of an mIg-associated protein complex. This complex is resolved by sodium dodecyl sulfate/polyacrylamide gel electrophoresis (SDS-PAGE) under nonreducing conditions into a doublet with mol wt of 240 and 250 kDa. When separated under reducing conditions four subunits with M_r of 24, 51, 76, and 83 kDa are observed. Phosphorylation of these proteins is detectable within 3 min following the addition of either PMA or anti-Ig (monoclonal anti-δ or anti-μ). Based on affinity chromatography and two-dimensional gel electrophoresis (nonreducing/reducing), these proteins were found to be associated noncovalently with mIg, but not Ia or class I molecules. None of the components of this complex were labeled following exposure of intact cells to ^{125}I-lactoperoxidase, suggesting that none have significant extracellular domains.

It was observed that these phosphoproteins could not be isolated by detergent extraction following stimulation of cells with polyclonal antibodies which induce rapid capping of mIg. It has been reported that cross-linking of mIg by anti-Ig reagents results in the association of mIg with cytoskeletal elements.[78] Thus, in situations where ligand binding induces the association of mIg with cytoskeletal elements, the phosphoprotein complex may, by virtue of its association with mIg, be sequestered in the detergent insoluble fraction which contains cytoskeletal components. The identity and function of these phosphoproteins remain obscure at this time; however, it is possible that phosphorylation of these proteins is associated with uncoupling of mIg from subsequent cell physiologic events (see below).

Experiments by Nel et al.[79] have examined the phosphorylation of endogenous B cell substrates on tyrosine residues following complexing of mIg. Treatment of B lymphocytes with anti-Ig caused an increase in the phosphorylation of two proteins associated with the Triton insoluble fraction. The molecular weights of these tyrosine-kinase substrates were 56 and 60 kDa, which agree with the molecular weights reported for tyrosine kinase substrates in the B cell by Earp et al.[81-82] and Harrison et al.[80] Additional work by Nel et al.[83] revealed that in normal B cells tyrosine phosphorylation of substrates with M_r of 75, 66, 43, and 28 kDa in the Triton soluble material, and 56 and 61 kDa in the Triton insoluble material, occurred following stimulation with PMA. A quantitative increase in the phosphorylation of these proteins was observed over a period of 2 to 48 h. These results provide evidence implicating activation of a tyrosine kinase[5] during mIg-mediated B cell activation. Furthermore, they suggest that activation of PKC following mIg cross-linking may in turn activate a tyrosine kinase(s).

E. UNCOUPLING OF THE MEMBRANE IMMUNOGLOBULIN RECEPTOR FROM ITS SIGNAL TRANSDUCTION CASCADE (MEMBRANE IMMUNOGLOBULIN DESENSITIZATION)

Recent studies by Mizuguchi et al.[84] have revealed that mIg is uncoupled from its associated signal transduction cascade by pretreatment of B cells with varied concentrations of PMA. Preincubation of resting B cells for as short a period as 4 min was sufficient to block anti-IgM induction of phosphoinositide metabolism, mobilization of intracellular Ca^{2+}, and DNA synthesis. The inhibitory effect of PMA on anti-Ig-induced events was not due to diminished expression of mIg. Thus, it is apparent that PMA inhibits the response of resting B cells by interrupting signal transmission at a point distal to mIg. Additional studies by Mizuguchi et al.[85] have further characterized the PMA-induced desensitization of mIg to ligand stimulation. In these studies, dioctanoylglycerol (DOG) was found to mimic the effects of PMA. Additionally, the inhibitory action of both PMA and DOG was reversed by the addition of H-7, an inhibitor of PKC. These findings suggested that activation of PKC results in the phosphorylation of a key protein(s) which results in uncoupling of mIg from subsequent signal transduction processes. Interestingly, the induction of phosphoinositide hydrolysis in B cells by NaF was also subject to inhibition by PMA. This finding indicates that PKC phosphorylates a protein which is common to the anti-Ig and NaF signaling pathways.

Cambier et al.[86] have carried out similar experiments using reciprocal combinations of isotype specific antibodies, i.e, anti-IgD to prestimulate followed by treatment with anti-IgM or vice versa. In these studies, pretreatment of resting B cells with anti-IgD was found to significantly reduce the ability of the cells to mobilize Ca^{2+} and translocate PKC in response to subsequent stimulation with anti-IgM. Similarly, if cells were prestimulated with anti-IgM, they responded poorly to anti-IgD. In agreement with the results of Mizuguchi et al.,[84] prestimulation of B cells with anti-IgM was not observed to decrease the expression of membrane IgD or vice versa. Therefore, desensitization is not explained by modulation of mIg from the surface of the cell. Additional experiments indicated that prestimulation of cells with concentrations of IgD which saturate 1 to 10% of the available surface mIgD results in desensitization of the remaining receptors. These results suggest that ligand binding to mIg blocks induction of Ca^{2+} mobilization in response to subsequent stimulation with anti-Ig.

PMA has been found to mediate disruption of signal transduction in several nonlymphoid systems. In certain instances, receptor desensitization is due to phosphorylation of the receptor itself resulting in a lowered affinity for ligand.[23,25,87] In the case of the B cell antigen receptor, it is unlikely that such a mechanism is responsible for desensitization in view of the fact that the cytoplasmic tails of mIgM and mIgD do not possess phosphate acceptor sites.[88] Furthermore, it is highly unlikely that PLC activity is regulated directly by mIg since mIgM and mIgD have cytoplasmic tails which are three amino acids in length. Thus, it is possible that PKC activation following mIg cross-linking leads to the phosphorylation of a molecule(s) which is responsible for coupling mIg to phosphoinositide hydrolysis. Phosphorylation may render this transducer inoperative. The identity of this molecule is unknown, however, we view the mIg-associated phosphoprotein complex identified by Newell et al.[77] as a likely candidate.

IV. B CELL ACTIVATION VIA BSF-1/IL-4

A. ACTIONS OF B CELL STIMULATORY FACTOR-1

B cell stimulatory factor-1 is a 20-kDa protein produced by certain activated T cells.[4] It was first identified in supernatants of the PMA stimulated EL-4 thymoma cell line, and was found to act as a costimulant with anti-Ig causing resting B cells to enter S phase.[89] More recently, BSF-1 has been shown to be co-mitogenic with antigen.[90]

Studies in several laboratories have shown that BSF-1 affects resting B cells, inducing an increase in expression of Ia and proto-oncogenes including c-fos and c-myc. Roehm et al.[91] and Noelle et al.[92-93] observed a significant increase in the expression of class II MHC molecules on resting B cells following treatment with BSF-1. The increase in Ia expression was detectable within 6 to 8 h and reached a maximum level by 24 h. Stimulation with BSF-1 resulted in increased expression of Ia by virtually every B cell, indicating that all resting B cells are capable of responding to this lymphokine.

Klemsz et al.[94] carried out experiments in which the kinetics of the increase in Ia expression induced by anti-Ig and BSF-1 were compared. Treatment of resting B cells with anti-Ig was found to induce a rapid increase in surface Ia expression within 2 h. This increase was insensitive to cyclohexamide or actinomycin D, suggesting that this phase of the response was independent of gene transcription and translation. A second phase of anti-Ig-induced Ia expression (from 2 to 24 h) was inhibitable by cyclohexamide and actinomycin D. In contrast, BSF-1 stimulation of Ia expression was totally dependent on new gene transcription and translation. While anti-Ig induced a significant increase in Ia within 2 h, BSF-1 treatment did not significantly increase the amount of Ia expressed on the surface of B cells until 3 to 4 h after its addition. Both anti-Ig and BSF-1 were found to induce the accumulation of mRNA coding for Ia, although with different kinetics. Maximal levels of mRNA encoding Ia were observed within 2 h following treatment with anti-Ig, whereas BSF-1 induction of Ia-mRNA did not reach a peak until 7 h. These results suggest that transcription and translation of the genes encoding Ia may be regulated differently following stimulation by anti-Ig and BSF-1. In contrast, the expression of mRNA for the proto-oncogenes c-fos and c-myc appear to be regulated in a similar manner by anti-Ig and BSF-1.[95] Maximal expression of mRNA for c-fos and c-myc is observed by 30 and 60 min, respectively, following treatment with anti-Ig or BSF-1. Results from nuclear run-on assays suggest that the induction of transcription of mRNA encoding Ia and c-fos by these two stimuli can be accounted for, in part, by new gene transcription. The increase in levels of mRNA encoding c-myc, however, is controlled at least in part by posttranslational events. Based on these observations, it is apparent that BSF-1 and anti-Ig regulate the expression of certain genes by distinct mechanisms, while others are under the control of similar or common regulatory pathways.

Recently, two laboratories have isolated and characterized cDNA clones that express BSF-1 activity. Noma et al.[96] successfully cloned cDNA encoding the murine IgG1 induction factor. Upon further characterization of the biological activities of this recombinant lymphokine, it was found that the IgG1 induction factor also functions in the anti-Ig costimulator assay and induces an increase in the expression of Ia by resting B cells. Lee et al.[97] cloned a cDNA coding for a lymphokine with BSF-1 activity and provided evidence that this factor also enhances IgG1 and IgE production. Supernatants from COS monkey cells transfected with this cDNA also exhibited T cell and mast cell growth factor activity, providing direct evidence that BSF-1 can regulate more than one type of hematopoietic cell.[4,97] In view of the fact that BSF-1 has been cloned and appears to have multiple effects on the B cell in addition to regulating other cells types, it has been proposed that the designation interleukin-4 (IL-4) be used when referring to this lymphokine.[4]

B. BSF-1 RECEPTOR-MEDIATED TRANSMEMBRANE SIGNALING

BSF-1 has been shown to regulate events associated with activation, proliferation, and differentiation of B cells.[4] This might suggest the need for a versatile signal transduction system to mediate distinct responses to BSF-1 depending on the cell's state of activation. This versatility could be provided by coupling BSF-1 receptors to distinct second messengers and their associated protein kinase depending on the cell's physiologic state. Alternatively, a single second messenger and its target protein kinase may be coupled to distinct signal cascades which control the transcription and translation of genes important during different stages of B cell biology. Another level of control may be provided by quantitative differences in the amount of second messenger generated as a result of BSF-1-receptor interaction. Finally, other cofactors (lymphokines, etc.) may impinge on the BSF-1 receptor-associated signal transduction cascade. Gaining an insight into the signal transduction mechanism(s) utilized by the BSF-1 receptor is particularly important in view of the pluripotent regulatory influences that this lymphokine exerts on the B cell and other cells of the hematopoietic lineage.

Nothing is known about the mechanism of BSF-1-mediated signaling in any cell except B cells. We know a great deal regarding which second messengers the BSF-1 receptor does not utilize to transduce a signal across the plasma membrane. The difficulty experienced so far in identifying the transmembrane signal transduction pathway associated with the BSF-1 receptor may in part be due to the low numbers of receptors present on resting B cells. Park et al.[98] and Ohara and Paul[99] have carried out binding studies using ^{125}I-labeled BSF-1 to determine the number and affinity of BSF-1 receptors on the B cell. Park and co-workers reported that resting B cells express 65 receptors on their surface while Ohara and Paul measured approximately 300. The latter is in agreement with the work of Howard[100] and collaborators who found approximately 300 to 400 receptors per resting cell. Interestingly, stimulation of resting cells with anti-Ig or LPS has been shown to up-regulate the number of BSF-1 receptors to approximately 1500 per cell within 24 h.[4] BSF-1 modulates the number of BSF-1 receptors that are expressed by B cells in a similar fashion.[4] Only one class of BSF-1 receptor has been identified on the B cell, and it exhibits a high affinity for BSF-1 with an equilibrium binding constant of 2 to 3 $\times$ 10^{10} M^{-1}.[99] Studies using ^{125}I-labeled BSF-1 and heterobifunctional cross-linkers have resulted in the isolation of BSF-1 binding proteins with mol wt of 60,000 kDa as reported by Ohara and Paul[99] and 75,000 kDa in the study carried out by Park et al.[98] Further characterization of these proteins is necessary to determine whether they are identical and are in fact the BSF-1 receptor.

Based on the observation that BSF-1, like anti-Ig, induces Ia expression on resting B cells, studies have been carried out to determine whether BSF-1 and anti-Ig share a common signal transduction pathway which controls the transcription and translation of genes coding for Ia molecules. Mizuguchi et al.[101] and Justement et al.[102] demonstrated that the early effects of BSF-1 on resting B cells are independent of phospholipid hydrolysis and mobilization of Ca^{2+}. BSF-1 induction of Ia expression was also found to be independent of extracellular Ca^{2+}. Chelation of extracellular Ca^{2+} with 1 mM EGTA did not affect the response observed in BSF-1-treated cultures, whereas increased Ia expression in response to anti-Ig was completely inhibited.[101] Studies by O'Garra et al.[103] also support the hypothesis that BSF-1 induction of Ia expression is mediated by a signal transduction cascade distinct from that used by mIg. It was found that cyclosporine inhibits the induction of Ia on B cells following stimulation with anti-Ig, but not with BSF-1. One possible explanation for the differential susceptibility of BSF-1 and anti-Ig to inhibition by cyclosporine may be due to the ability of cyclosporine to inhibit activation of normal lymphocytes by agents that mobilize Ca^{2+}.[104] Therefore, the fact that BSF-1-dependent activation of B cells is resistant to cyclosporine suggests that the effects of BSF-1 are independent of Ca^{2+}.

Additional findings made by Justement et al.[102] indicate that BSF-1 does not induce translocation of PKC from the cytosol to the plasma membrane. This is not unexpected in view of the fact that no detectable phospholipid second messengers are generated and no significant amount of Ca^{2+} is mobilized following treatment with BSF-1. Furthermore, membrane depolarization, an event associated with anti-Ig-mediated induction of Ia, does not occur in response to BSF-1. Membrane depolarization has been shown to be dependent on the activation of PKC,[62] therefore, the inability of BSF-1 to induce membrane depolarization provides additional evidence indicating that PKC is not activated. Thus, it is clear that signals are delivered through the BSF-1 receptor via a transduction pathway which is distinct from that associated with mIg.

Preliminary studies have been carried out in our laboratory which suggest that BSF-1 does not activate a cAMP-dependent signal transduction cascade. Resting B lymphocytes treated with BSF-1 do not exhibit an increase in intracellular concentrations of cAMP as measured by radioimmunoassay.[105] BSF-1 does not appear to stimulate adenylate cyclase activity either, and may in fact inhibit the activity of this enzyme.[106] Additionally, cAMP does not induce increased expression of Ia on resting B cells and actually inhibits Ia induction when cells are cocultured with BSF-1. Studies by Chen and Cambier[107] have shown that dibromo- and 8-butyryl analogs of cAMP induce a rapid and transient shift of PKC activity from the cytosol to the nucleus of B cells. The fact that BSF-1 does not induce PKC translocation to the nucleus again indicates that it does not induce an increase in the intracellular concentration of cAMP. Additional studies with the cyclic nucleotide cGMP have failed to demonstrate any effect of this agent on the expression of Ia, providing preliminary evidence which suggests that BSF-1 does not stimulate an increase in Ia via a cGMP-dependent mechanism.[108]

If in fact BSF-1 does not stimulate the production of phospholipid, cAMP, or cGMP second messengers, and does not depend on Ca^{2+} mobilization or influx for signal transduction, then it is possible that the receptor for BSF-1 has a tyrosine-specific protein kinase associated with it which is activated by the binding of ligand. Several growth factor receptors have been identified which possess tyrosine kinase activity that is activated following ligand binding resulting in autophosphorylation of the receptor.[22] Studies on resting B cells using a cell-free system have identified certain membrane-associated proteins which are phosphorylated in response to binding of BSF-1.[70,102] Incubation of plasma membranes from B cells with ^{32}P-ATP and BSF-1, but not anti-Ig, LPS, INFγ, or IL-2, results in an increase in the phosphorylation of 3 proteins with M_r of 103, 44, and 36 kDa (Figure 3). These proteins are single polypeptide chains as determined by two-dimensional gel electrophoresis. Analysis by nonequilibrium pH gel electrophoresis has revealed that these phosphoproteins resolve between a pI of 8.0 to 8.5. Phosphorylation of the 103, 44, and 36 kDa proteins takes place rapidly (within 1 min) and can be observed at 4°C, a characteristic of tyrosine kinase-mediated substrate phosphorylation. The protein kinase that is activated following BSF-1 stimulation requires the divalent cation Mn^{2+} or Mg^{2+}, but not Ca^{2+} as a cofactor. Addition of Ca^{2+} to the reaction mixture actually inhibits all phosphorylation at concentrations greater than 5 mM. The divalent cation requirements of the protein kinase activated by BSF-1 are similar to those identified for receptor-associated tyrosine kinases.[22]

103

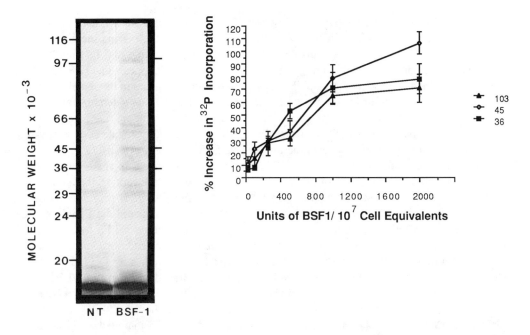

FIGURE 3. BSF-1 stimulation of protein phosphorylation in isolated B cell plasma membranes. (A) Isolated membranes were incubated with or without BSF-1 (1000 U/10^7 cells) in the presence of ^{32}P-ATP. BSF-1 dependent phosphorylation of membrane-associated proteins was visualized after SDS-PAGE on 10% acrylamide gels by autoradiography. (B) Dose dependence of BSF-1 induced phosphorylation of the 103, 44, and 36 kDa proteins.

The finding that BSF-1 can induce the phosphorylation of membrane-associated proteins in a cell-free system suggests that it directly activates a membrane-associated protein kinase. While this observation is potentially important in terms of understanding BSF-1 mediated transmembrane signaling, it remains to be determined whether this enzyme is a tyrosine-specific kinase. Finally, whole cell phosphorylation studies have not yet revealed the 103, 44, and 36 kDa membrane-associated phosphoproteins in BSF-1 treated cells.[109] This raises the question of whether these phosphoproteins are physiologically relevant. It seems more likely that in the whole cell, the phosphorylation of these proteins is simply masked by high background levels of phosphorylation which are not encountered in the cell-free system. In any event, further study is required to determine the relevance of these phosphoproteins in BSF-1 mediated signal transduction.

V. LPS-MEDIATED B CELL ACTIVATION

The mitogen LPS is known to modulate several aspects of B cell biology. Treatment of resting B cells with LPS results in increased expression of Ia, entry into the cell cycle, proliferation, and ultimately production of immunoglobulin.[110] Neither anti-Ig nor BSF-1 have been shown to drive resting B cells to secrete antibody, indicating that LPS affects the B cell via a signal transduction system which is either qualitatively or quantitatively distinct from the signaling pathways employed by either anti-Ig or BSF-1.

Bijsterbosch et al.[47] determined that LPS does not induce phospholipid hydrolysis based on measurements of inositol phosphate and diacylglycerol formation. Accordingly, it was observed that LPS treatment does not stimulate mobilization of intracellular Ca^{2+}. The finding that LPS is resistant to the effects of cyclosporine, similar to BSF-1, provides further evidence in favor of the hypothesis that LPS-induced activation of the B cell, is qualitatively different from mIg-mediated activation. However, Chen et al.[71] have shown that LPS stimulates translocation of PKC from the cytosolic compartment to the plasma membrane of resting B cells. This response is equivalent to that observed following anti-Ig stimulation with regard to its kinetics and efficiency. Based on these findings, it appears that LPS mimics the ability of PMA to directly activate PKC by providing a binding site in the membrane.[111] In support of this possibility is the work of Wightman and Raetz[112] who demonstrated that a lipid A precursor from LPS directly activates PKC isolated from the murine macrophage cell line RAW 264.7. Thus, LPS activates PKC which presumably regulates a series of distal events that are common to both the anti-Ig and LPS pathways of activation.

While LPS and anti-Ig both activate PKC, and as a result, appear to share a common signal transduction mechanism from this point, a question arises concerning the ability of LPS but not anti-Ig to induce antibody production. The ability of LPS to induce B cell differentiation to date has not been attributed to a qualitative difference in the signal that is transmitted to the cell via PKC activation. This suggests that binding of LPS to the B cell may affect multiple intracellular processes through the activation of additional second messenger generating systems which drive the differentiative step. Studies by DeFranco et al. have identified a second pathway for LPS-dependent signal transduction in the WEHI-231 murine B lymphoma cell line. Growth of the WEHI-231 cell line is arrested by treatment with anti-Ig. LPS is one of three polyclonal B cell activators which have the ability to protect these cells from the effects of anti-Ig.[114] It was determined that LPS inhibits both basal and prostaglandin E_{2-} or isoproterenol-stimulated adenylate cyclase activity in saponin permeabilized WEHI-231 cells.[113] A similar response observed in the P388D1 macrophage cell line was inhibited by pretreatment of cells with pertussis toxin, suggesting that the ability of LPS to inhibit adenylate cyclase is dependent on a pertussis toxin-sensitive molecule. This result implies that LPS acts through the N_i signaling component described for the α_2-adrenergic receptor. LPS was also shown to activate the N_i protein, or a similar regulatory molecule, based on *in vitro* ADP-ribosylation experiments using pertussis toxin.[115] Finally, pretreatment of WEHI-231 cells with pertussis toxin was found to block the ability of LPS to reverse anti-Ig-mediated growth inhibition of WEHI-231 cells. These studies provide functional evidence indicating that LPS acts on the WEHI-231 cell line by activating an N_i-like protein which in turn decreases adenylate cyclase activity in the cells. (Whether such a dual pathway is induced by LPS in normal resting B cells remains to be seen.) Thus, available evidence suggests that LPS-mediated signals are transduced via PKC and N_i activation.

VI. ANTAGONISM OF B CELL ACTIVATION BY IA-BINDING LIGANDS AND INTERFERON-γ

Two distinct ligands have been identified which exhibit the ability to block activation of resting B cells. These are antibodies directed against Ia and the T cell-derived lymphokine IFN-γ.

Several studies have demonstrated that surface Ia on B cells may, in addition to its role as a restricting element, act as a receptor which delivers a signal to the cell. Niederhuber et al.[116] first showed that antiserum directed against Ia was able to block the mitogenic effect of LPS. Later experiments confirmed this, demonstrating that monoclonal antibodies with specificity for IA or IE which blocked LPS induced B cell proliferation.[16] Forsgren et al.[117] subsequently extended these observations to show that anti-Ia acts directly on the B cell and therefore does not mediate its effect through the inhibition of accessory cell function. It was also determined based on kinetic studies that anti-Ia was inhibitory for only the first 16 h of culture, after which B cells could no longer be inhibited. This implies that the activation phase is the most sensitive to the inhibitory effects of anti-Ia.

Anti-Ia treatment has also been shown to block induction of Ia expression on resting B cells by LPS and BSF-1.[118] These studies were carried out using anti-IA to block, and fluoresceinated anti-IE to measure increased Ia expression, or vice versa. Pretreatment of cells for 30 min to 6 h, with anti-Ia followed by either LPS or BSF-1 for an additional 24 h, resulted in significant inhibition of Ia expression (approximately 90% after a 6-h pre-treatment). PMA-mediated hyper-Ia expression was also inhibited by pretreatment with anti-Ia which again suggests that inhibition of B cell activation occurs via depletion of the cytosolic pool of PKC. The ability of anti-Ia to block BSF-1 mediated increases in Ia expression is important because it suggests that there may be a common point in the signal transduction pathway activated by anti-Ig or LPS and that activated by BSF-1 which is subject to inhibition by anti-Ia. Based on these studies, it can be concluded that ligand binding to Ia on the surface of a resting B cell delivers a down-regulatory signal which affects early events associated with activation.

The molecular mechanism by which cross-linking of Ia leads to inhibition of B cell activation is not well documented; however, it has been shown that binding of anti-Ia to B cells does not induce detectable changes in phosphoinositide metabolism or intracellular free Ca^{2+} levels.[119] In our laboratory, we have observed that monoclonal antibodies directed against Ia have the ability to modulate early events associated with B cell activation. Chen et al.[120] demonstrated that anti-Ia treatment induces translocation of PKC from the cytosolic compartment to the nucleus. This response was documented based upon enzymatic activity, phorbol binding, western blot analysis, and immunohistochemistry. The kinetics of this translocation are similar to those observed following stimulation with anti-Ig. Translocation is detected within 2 min of stimulation, is transient, and requires cross-linking of Ia. Anti-IgD-induced translocation of PKC to the plasma membrane is inhibited following treatment of B cells with anti-Ia for 2 to 4 min. Therefore, it can be concluded that treatment with anti-Ia results in a depletion of PKC from the cytosolic pool which would normally be utilized following anti-Ig stimulation. Therefore, depletion of PKC from the cytoplasm may in turn effectively attenuate the response of the B cell to anti-Ig or LPS, resulting in inhibition of activation. Finally, an important role for PKC translocated to the nucleus in response to cross-linking of Ia, may be the phosphorylation of several nuclear substrates.[121]

Activation of a distinct second messenger-dependent signaling pathway, following Ia cross-linking, has been suggested by several studies which document the fact that analogs of cAMP exert suppressive effects on B cell activation which are similar to those seen following cross-linking of surface Ia.[118] The ability of cAMP analogs to cause a blockade in the activation of B cells provides circumstantial evidence implicating cAMP as the potential second messenger involved in signal transduction following cross-linking of Ia. Cambier et al.[122] have examined this possibility further and have shown that treatment of resting B cells with anti-Ia results in an accumulation of intracellular cAMP which is detectable within 1 min and reaches maximum (a 3-fold increase) after 10 min. This observation and the fact that analogs of cAMP induce translocation of PKC to the nucleus[107] suggests that cross-linking of Ia may lead to the activation of adenylate cyclase. The resultant increase in intracellular cAMP, acting through cAMP-dependent protein kinase, could potentially mediate the inhibition of several events such as phosphoinositide hydrolysis and PKC translocation to the plasma membrane, in addition to more distal events necessary for activation, effectively blocking the response of the B cell to anti-Ig, LPS, or BSF-1 (Figure 4).[70]

Several laboratories have reported that treatment of resting B cells with IFN-γ results in inhibition of B cell activation by anti-Ig, LPS, and BSF-1. This is in contrast to several studies which demonstrate that IFN-γ may be a necessary factor for differentiation of B lymphocytes into antibody-secreting cells.[15,123-124]

Mond et al.[13] demonstrated, using resting B cells, that IFN-γ inhibits the proliferative response to soluble anti-μ or anti-δ antibody. IFN-γ blocked BSF-1 enhanced, soluble anti-

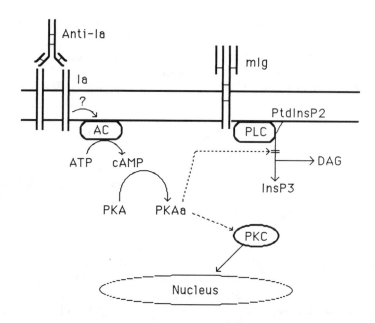

FIGURE 4.   Inhibition of mIg mediated signal transduction following crosslinking of Ia by anti-Ia antibody. Crosslinking of Ia results in an increase in the intracellular concentration of cAMP, presumably through the activation of adenylate cyclase. The increase in cAMP inhibits the formation of DAG and InsP3, while at the same time it induces the translocation of PKC to the nucleus. Presumably, these events are mediated by cAMP-dependent protein kinase.

Ig-mediated proliferation as well. While IFN-γ did not exert a significant effect on anti-Ig-induced blastogenesis, it did suppress hyper-Ia expression. The fact that IFN-γ down-regulates Ia expression indicates that it blocks events associated with activation of the B cell. In contrast to studies using anti-Ig, IFN-γ was found to inhibit blastogenesis and entry into cell cycle, of B cells stimulated with BSF-1.[14] Additionally, IFN-γ was shown to inhibit BSF-1-induced expression of Ia on resting B cells.[125] In these studies, IFN-γ was found to exert its effect on the B cell within 3 h after its addition to culture. Specifically, anti-IFN-γ antibody did not reverse IFN-γ-mediated suppression of activation when added later than 3 h after initiation of culture.

Very little evidence has been presented concerning the mechanism by which IFN-γ induces differentiation of B cells, while at the same time blocking activation. Preliminary studies in the B cell indicate that IFN-γ does not affect the phospholipid/Ca^{2+}-dependent signal transduction cascade utilized by anti-Ig.[126] In support of these findings are the results of Yap et al.[127] and Mills et al.,[128] who demonstrated that treatment of various nonlymphoid cells with IFN-γ does not stimulate an increase in the production of diacylglycerol or inositol trisphosphate.

An alternative second messenger pathway that may be important in mediating the effects of IFN-γ involves the production of prostaglandins, which are known to modulate cAMP levels. Studies in the macrophage have revealed that the combination of PMA and IFN-γ causes a dramatic increase in the production of arachidonic acid metabolites.[129-130] Boraschi et al.[131] also found that IFN-γ and the Ca^{2+} ionophore A23187 act on the macrophage to elicit a large increase in the release of prostaglandin E_2 (PGE_2) which is a particularly potent inducer of cAMP production. These results provide evidence suggesting that activation of IFN-γ, in the presence of activators of PKC, elicits a large increase in the production of prostaglandin. While there is no evidence for an equivalent response to IFN-γ by the B cell, the possibility cannot be excluded. This is especially true in view of the fact that PGE_2 has been shown to inhibit IA induction by BSF-1.[132] Thus, a scenario can be developed in which INFγ causes an increase in the production of prostaglandins in B cells which have received a priming signal such as anti-Ig. The elevation in prostaglandins in turn affects events associated with activation either directly or via stimulation of cAMP. As previously described for Ia binding ligands, an increase in intracellular levels of cAMP could result in the inhibition of activation.

VII. CONCLUSIONS

Studies concerning the molecular mechanisms of signal transduction in resting B cells have begun to unravel the complex nature of events which regulate activation in response to ligands that bind to mIg, the IL-4 receptor, Ia, and the IFN-γ receptor. Signal transduction via mIg has received the most attention to date, and therefore, is the best-defined cascade. Cross-linking of mIg results in phosphoinositide hydrolysis yielding DAG and InsP3. Inositol 1,4,5-trisphosphate mediates mobilization of intracellular Ca^{2+} which acts in concert with DAG to induce translocation and activation of PKC. PKC in turn regulates several poorly defined events which lead to membrane depolarization and transcription of genes encoding c-fos, c-myc, and Ia.

The importance of this cascade is demonstrated by studies which document the ability of phorbol esters and calcium ionophores to synergize in induction of thymidine uptake by B cells, suggesting that under certain circumstances activation of events associated with the mIg signal transduction cascade is sufficient to cause resting B cells to enter the cell cycle. The ability of these pharmacologic agents to induce entry into S phase is presumably due to their prolonged and/or amplified activation of the mIg-associated pathway. This situation is mimicked following stimulation of B cells with high doses of soluble heterologous antibodies, immobilized anti-Ig, or highly polyvalent thymus-dependent type-II antigen. In contrast, interaction of the B cell with thymus-dependent antigen or soluble monoclonal anti-Ig activates the cascade sufficiently to cause an increase in the expression of Ia, but not proliferation. The increase in Ia expression, however, in conjunction with antigen processing and reexpression, leads to an enhanced ability of the B cell to interact productively with antigen-specific, MHC-restricted helper T cells which elaborate several lymphokines that promote proliferation and differentiation. Thus, cross-linking of mIg activates a cascade of events which ultimately enhance the ability of the B cell to mount an immune response.

LPS stimulation of resting B cells results in increased expression of Ia, proliferation, and differentiation into IgM-secreting cells. The ability of LPS to induce these events appears to be due, at least in part, to the direct activation of PKC. Therefore, one might expect that the signal transduction cascades activated by LPS and anti-Ig share a common sequence of events from the point of PKC activation onward which leads to increased transcription of genes encoding Ia and proliferation; however, the ability of LPS to induce B cell differentiation would suggest that there is either a qualitative or quantitative difference between its signaling cascade and that activated by cross-linking of mIg. The ability of LPS to activate a GTP-dependent protein such as N_i or an N_i-like molecule, provides evidence to suggest that this ligand regulates multiple intracellular events which may explain its ability to induce differentiation of resting B cells.

The lymphokine IL-4-like anti-Ig and LPS induces increased expression of Ia by resting B cells. Very little, however, is known about the IL-4 receptor-mediated signal transduction pathway other than the fact that it does not involve any of the early component cell physiologic events which are associated with mIg-mediated activation. The ability of IL-4 to synergize with soluble monoclonal anti-Ig for the induction of B cell proliferation supports the fact that binding of IL-4 to its receptor activates a signal transduction cascade which is qualitatively different. Based on this, it is apparent that particular events associated with activation of the B cell, i.e., increased Ia expression, can be regulated by distinct or convergent signal transduction cascades.

The ability of anti-Ia antibody and IFN-γ to block B cell activation and proliferation is an interesting phenomenon in view of the fact that both Ia and the IFN-γ receptor serve as transducers for signals that promote differentiation of the B cell. This suggests that premature activation (i.e., in resting B cells) of the signal transduction cascades associated with these receptors antagonizes events which mediate activation. While the signal transduction cascade associated with the IFN-γ receptor is unclear, it appears as if neither Ia nor IFN-γ are coupled to PLC activation or mobilization of Ca^{2+}. Cross-linking of Ia by anti-Ia, serving as a surrogate for T cell:B cell interaction, appears to elevate intracellular concentrations of cAMP. Presumably, cAMP affects events associated with B cell activation via cAMP-dependent protein kinase. Studies suggest at least two points in the mIg-induced signal transduction cascade that are affected by increased cAMP levels: phosphoinositide hydrolysis and PKC translocation. Inhibition of one or both of these events is presumably sufficient to block activation mediated by anti-Ig or LPS; however, since IL-4-mediated activation is independent of phosphoinositide hydrolysis or PKC translocation, there may be a point distal to these events which is common to the activation cascades activated by IL-4 and anti-Ig that is antagonized by cAMP. Alternatively, the IL-4 signaling pathway may have one or more points, susceptible to cAMP-mediated inhibition, that are completely distinct.

Thus, it is clear that regulation of B cell activation is a complex process involving several signal transduction cascades which interact with one another on several levels. Complete delineation of these pathways will provide greater insight into the molecular basis of B cell immune regulation.

REFERENCES

1. **Monroe, J. G. and Cambier, J. C.**, Receptor cross-linking by thymus-independent and thymus-dependent antigens induces a rapid decrease in the plasma membrane potential of antigen-binding B lymphocytes, *J. Immunol.*, 131, 2641, 1983.
2. **Cambier, J. C., Monroe, J. G., Coggeshall, K. M., and Ransom, J. T.**, On the mechanisms of transmembrane signaling by membrane immunoglobulin, *Immunol. Today*, 6, 218, 1985.
3. **Finkleman, F. D., Mond, J. J., and Metcalf, E. S.**, Anti-immunoglobulin antibody induction of B lymphocyte activation and differentiation, in *B-Lymphocyte Differentiation*, Cambier, J. C., Ed., CRC Press, Boca Raton, FL, 1986, 41.
4. **Paul, W. E. and Ohara, J.**, B-cell stimulatory factor-1/interleukin-4, *Annu. Rev. Immunol.*, 5, 429, 1987.
5. **Leclercq, L., Bismuth, G., and Theze, J.**, Antigen-specific helper T-cell clone supernatant is sufficient to induce both polyclonal proliferation and differentiation of small resting B lymphocytes, *Proc. Natl. Acad. Sci. U.S.A.*, 81, 6491, 1984.
6. **Leclercq, L., Cambier, J. C., Mishal, Z., Julius, M. H., and Theze, J.**, Supernatant from a cloned helper T cell stimulates most small resting B cells to undergo increased I-A expression, blastogenesis, and progression through cell cycle, *J. Immunol.*, 136, 539, 1986.
7. **Melchers, F. and Andersson, J.**, B cell activation: three steps and their variations, *Cell*, 37, 715, 1984.
8. **Howard, M. E. and Paul, W. E.**, Regulation of B-cell growth and differentiation by soluble factors, *Annu. Rev. Immunol.*, 1, 307, 1983.
9. **Nakanishi, K., Malek, T. R., Smith, K. A., Hamaoka, T., Shevach, E. M., and Paul, W. E.**, Both interleukin 2 and a second T cell-derived factor in EL-4 supernatant have activity as differentiation factors in IgM synthesis, *J. Exp. Med.*, 160, 1605, 1984.
10. **Mond, J. J., Thompson, C., Finkelman, F. D., Farrar, J., Schaefer, M., and Robb, R.**, Affinity-purified interleukin 2 induces proliferation of large but not small B cells, *Proc. Natl. Acad. Sci. U.S.A.*, 82, 1518, 1985.

11. **Swaim, S. L., Howard, M., Kappler, J., Marrack, P., Watson, J., Booth, R., Wetzel, G. D., and Dutton, R. W.,** Evidence for two distinct classes of murine B cell growth factors with activities in different functional assays, *J. Exp. Med.,* 158, 822, 1983.

12. **Bijsterbosch, M. K. and Klaus, G. G. B.,** Crosslinking of surface immunoglobulin and Fc receptors on B lymphocytes inhibits stimulation of inositol phospholipid breakdown via the antigen receptors, *J. Exp. Med.,* 162, 1825, 1985.

13. **Mond, J. J., Finkelman, F. D., Sarma, C., Ohara, J., and Serrate, S.,** Recombinant interferon-γ inhibits B cell proliferative response stimulated soluble but not Sepharose-bound anti-immunoglobulin antibody, *J. Immunol.,* 135, 2513, 1985.

14. **Mond, J. J., Carmman, J., Sarma, C., Ohara, J., and Finkelman, F. D.,** Interferon-γ suppresses B cell stimulation factor (BSF-1) induction of class II MHC determinants on B cells, *J. Immunol.,* 137, 3534, 1986.

15. **Leibson, H. J., Gefter, M., Zlotnik, A., Marrack, P., and Kappler, J.,** Role of γ-interferon in antibody-producing responses, *Nature,* 309, 799, 1984.

16. **Forsgren, S., Pobor, G., Coutinho, A., and Pierres, M.,** The role of I-A/E molecules in B lymphocyte activation. I. Inhibition of lipopolysaccharide-induced responses by monoclonal antibodies, *J. Immunol.,* 133, 2104, 1984.

17. **Sieckman, D. G., Futz, M., Finkelman, F. D., and Mond, J. J.,** Anti-Ia inhibits anti-immunoglobulin induced proliferation of mouse B lymphocytes, *Fed. Proc.,* 41, 423, 1982.

18. **Corley, R. B., LoCascio, N. J., Ovnic, M., and Haughton, G.,** Two separate functions of class II (Ia) molecules: T-cell stimulation and B-cell excitation, *Proc. Natl. Acad. Sci. U.S.A.,* 82, 516, 1985.

19. **Lohmann, S. M. and Walter, U.,** Regulation of the cellular and subcellular concentrations and distribution of cyclic nucleotide-dependent protein kinases, *Adv. Cyclic Nucleotide Protein Phosphorylation Res.,* 18, 63, 1984.

20. **Manalan, A. S. and Klee, C. B.,** Calmodulin, *Adv. Cyclic Nucleotide Protein Phosphorylation Res.,* 18, 227, 1984.

21. **Takai, Y., Kaibuchi, K., and Nishizuka, Y.,** Membrane phospholipid metabolism and signal transduction for protein phosphorylation, *Adv. Cyclic Nucleotide Protein Phosphorylation Res.,* 18, 119, 1984.

22. **Sefton, B. M. and Hunter, T.,** Tyrosine protein kinases, *Adv. Cyclic Nucleotide Protein Phosphorylation Res.,* 18, 195, 1984.

23. **Sibley, D. R. and Lefkowitz, R. J.,** Molecular mechanisms of receptor desensitization using the β-adrenergic receptor-coupled adenylate cyclase system as a model, *Nature,* 317, 124, 1985.

24. **Green, D. A. and Clark, R. B.,** Direct evidence for the role of the coupling proteins in forskolin activation of adenylate cyclase, *J. Cyclic Nucleotide Res.,* 8, 337, 1982.

25. **Clark, R. B.,** Desensitization of hormonal stimuli coupled to regulation of cyclic AMP levels, *Adv. Cyclic Nucleotide Protein Phosphorylation Res.,* 20, 151, 1986.

26. **Ui, M.,** Pertussis toxin as a probe of receptor coupling to inositol lipid metabolism, in *Phosphoinositides and Receptor Mechanisms,* Putney, J. W., Jr., Ed., Alan R. Liss, New York, 1987.

27. **Liebman, P. A. and Sitaramayya, A.,** Role of G protein-receptor interaction in amplified phosphodiesterase activation of retinal rods, *Adv. Cyclic Nucleotide Protein Phosphorylation Res.,* 17, 215, 1984.

28. **Manning, D. R. and Gilman, A. G.,** The regulatory components of adenylate cyclase and transducin: a family of structurally homologous guanine nucleotide-binding proteins, *J. Biol. Chem.,* 258, 7059, 1983.

29. **Hokin, M. R. and Hokin, L. E.,** Enzyme secretion and the incorporation of P[32] into phospholipids of pancreas slices, *Biol. Chem.,* 203, 967, 1953.

30. **Berridge, M. J.,** Inositol trisphosphate and diacylglycerol as second messengers, *Biochem. J.,* 220, 345, 1984.

31. **Streb. H., Irvine, R. F., Berridge, M. J., and Schultz, I.,** Release of Ca^{2+} from a nonmitochondrial intracellular store in pancreatic acinar cells by inositol-1,4,5-trisphosphate, *Nature,* 306, 67, 1983.

32. **Nishizuka, Y.,** The role of protein kinase C in cell surface signal transduction and tumor promotion, *Nature,* 308, 693, 1984.

33. **Anderson, W. B., Estival, A., Tapiovaara, H., and Gopalakrishna, R.,** Altered subcellular distribution of protein kinase C (a phorbol ester receptor). Possible role in tumor promotion and the regulation of cell growth: relationship to changes in adenylate cyclase activity, *Adv. Cyclic Nucleotide Protein Phosphorylation Res.,* 19, 287, 1985.

34. **Denton, R. M.,** Early events in insulin actions, *Adv. Cyclic Nucleotide Protein Phosphorylation Res.,* 20, 293, 1986.

35. **White, M. F., Maron, R., and Kahn, C. R.,** Insulin rapidly stimulates tyrosine phosphorylation of a M_r-185,000 protein in intact cells, *Nature,* 318, 183, 1985.

36. **Maino, V. C., Hayman, M. J., and Crumpton, M. J.,** Relationships between enhanced turnover of phosphatidylinositol and lymphocyte activation by mitogen, *Biochem. J.,* 146, 247, 1975.

37. **Braun, J., Sha'afi, R. I., and Unanue, E. R.,** Crosslinking by ligands to surface immunoglobulin triggers mobilization of intracellular $^{45}Ca^{2+}$ in B lymphocytes, *J. Cell Biol.,* 82, 755, 1979.

38. **Monroe, J. G. and Cambier, J. C.**, B cell activation. I. Anti-immunoglobulin-induced receptor cross-linking results in a decrease in the plasma membrane potential of murine B lymphocytes, *J. Exp. Med.*, 157, 2073, 1983.

39. **Meissner, H. P. and Schmelz, H.**, Membrane potential of beta cells in pancreatic islets, *Pflugers Arch. Eur. J. Physiol.*, 351, 195, 1974.

40. **Wakerly, J. B. and Lincoln, D. W.**, The milk-ejection reflex of the rat: a 20- to 40-fold acceleration in the firing of paraventricular neurons during oxytocin release, *J. Endocrinol.*, 57, 477, 1973.

41. **Monroe, J. G. and Cambier, J. C.**, B cell activation. III. B cell plasma membrane depolarization and hyper-Ia antigen expression induced by receptor immunoglobulin cross-linking are coupled, *J. Exp. Med.*, 158, 1589, 1983.

42. **Monroe, J. G., Niedel, J. E., and Cambier, J. C.**, B cell activation. IV. Induction of cell membrane depolarization and hyper-Ia expression by phorbol diesters suggests a role for protein kinase C in murine B lymphocyte activation, *J. Immunol.*, 132, 1472, 1984.

43. **Berridge, M. J. and Irvine, R. F.**, Inositoltrisphosphate, a novel second messenger in cellular signal transduction, *Nature*, 312, 315, 1984.

44. **Lindsten, T., Thompson, C. B., Finkelman, F. D., Andersson, B., and Scher, I.**, Changes in the expression of B-cell surface markers on complement receptor-positive and complement receptor-negative B-cells induced by phorpbol myristate acetate, *J. Immunol.*, 132, 235, 1984.

45. **Coggeshall, K. M. and Cambier, J. C.**, B cell activation. VI. Effects of exogenous diglyceride and modulators of phospholipid metabolism suggest a central role for diacylglycerol generation in transmembrane signaling by mIg, *J. Immunol.*, 134, 101, 1985.

46. **Coggeshall, K. M. and Cambier, J. C.**, B cell activation. VIII. Membrane immunoglobulins transduce signals via activation of phosphatidylinositol hydrolysis, *J. Immunol.*, 133, 3382, 1984.

47. **Bijsterbosch, M. K., Meade, C. J., Turner, G. A., and Klaus, G. G. B.**, B lymphocyte receptors and polyphosphoinositide degradation, *Cell*, 41, 999, 1985.

48. **Kriz, M. K., Vitetta, E. S., and Sullivan, T. J.**, Changes in phospholipid metabolism during B lymphocyte activation, *J. Immunol.*, 137, 478, 1986.

49. **Ransom, J. T., Harris, L. K., and Cambier, J. C.**, Anti-Ig induces release of inositol 1,4,5-trisphosphate, which mediates mobilization of intracellular Ca^{2+} stores in B lymphocytes, *J. Immunol.*, 137, 708, 1986.

50. **Cambier, J. C. and Harris, L. K.**, Phosphoinositides and transmembrane signaling in the immune system, in *Phosphoinositides and Receptor Mechanisms*, Putney, J. W., Jr., Ed., Alan R. Liss, New York, 1987.

51. **Smith, C. D., Cox, C. C., and Snyderman, R.**, Receptor-coupled activation of phosphoinositide-specific phospholipase C by an N protein, *Science*, 232, 97, 1986.

52. **Carter, H. R. and Smith, A. D.**, Partial purification of a phosphatidylinositol phosphodiesterase isolated from lymphocytes, *Biochem. Soc. Trans.*, 13, 1215, 1985.

53. **Jackowski, S., Rettenmier, C. W., Sherr, C. J., and Rock, C. O.**, A guanine nucleotide-dependent phosphatidylinositol 4,5-diphosphate phospholipase C in cells transformed by the v-fms and v-fes oncogenes, *J. Biol. Chem.*, 261, 4978, 1986.

54. **Harris, L. K. and Cambier, J. C.**, B lymphocyte activation: transmembrane signal transduction by mIg in isolated cell membranes, *J. Immunol.*, 139, 963, 1987.

55. **Cambier, J. C. and Chien, M.**, unpublished data, 1987.

56. **Klaus, G. G. B., Bijsterbosch, M. K., and Holman, M.**, Activation and proliferation signals in mouse B cells. VII. Calcium ionophores are non-mitogenic polyclonal B-cell activators, *Immunology*, 56, 21, 1985.

57. **Ransom, J. T. and Cambier, J. C.**, B cell activation. VII. Independent and synergistic effects of mobilized calcium and diacylglycerol on membrane potential and I-A expression, *J. Immunol.*, 136, 66, 1986.

58. **Klaus, G. G. B., O'Garra, A., Bijsterbosch, M. K., and Holman, M.**, Activation and proliferation signals in mouse B cells. VIII. Induction of DNA synthesis in B cells by a combination of calcium ionophores and phorbol myristate acetate, *Eur. J. Immunol.*, 16, 92, 1986.

59. **Monroe, J. G. and Kass, M. J.**, Molecular events in B cell activation. I. Signals required to stimulate G_0 to G_1 transition of resting B lymphocytes, *J. Immunol.*, 135, 1674, 1985.

60. **Pozzan, T., Arslan, P., Tsien, R. Y., and Rink, T. J.**, Anti-immunoglobulin, cytoplasmic free calcium and capping in B lymphocytes, *J. Cell Biol.*, 94, 335, 1982.

61. **Ransom, J. T., Digiusto, D. L., and Cambier, J. C.**, Single cell analysis of calcium mobilization in anti-immunoglobulin-stimulated B lymphocytes, *J. Immunol.*, 136, 54, 1986.

62. **Cambier, J. C. and Ransom, J. T.**, Molecular mechanisms of transmembrane signaling in B lymphocytes, *Annu. Rev. Immunol.*, 5, 175, 1987.

63. **Partain, K., Jensen, K., and Aldo-Benson, M.**, Inositol phospholipid and intracellular calcium metabolism in B lymphocytes stimulated with antigen, *Biochem. Biophys. Res. Commun.*, 140, 1079, 1986.

64. **Burgess, G. M., Godfrey, P. P., McKinney, J. S., Berridge, M. J., Irvine, R. F., and Putney, J. W.**, The second messenger linking receptor activation to internal Ca release in liver, *Nature*, 309, 63, 1984.

65. **Bijsterbosch, M. K., Rigley, K. P., and Klaus, G. G. B.,** Cross-linking of surface immunoglobulin on B lymphocytes induces both intracellular Ca^{2+} release and Ca^{2+} influx: analysis with Indo-1, *Biochem. Biophys. Res. Commun.,* 137, 500, 1986.

66. **Wilson, A. H., Greenblat, D., Taylor, C. W., Putney, J. W., Tsien, R. Y., Finkelman, F. D., and Chused, T. M.,** The B lymphocyte calcium response to anti-Ig is diminished by membrane immunoglobulin cross-linkage to the Fcγ receptor, *J. Immunol.,* 138, 1712, 1987.

67. **Ransom, J. T. and Cambier, J. C.,** unpublished data, 1987.

68. **Ogawa, Y., Takai, Y., Kawahara, Y., Kimura, S., and Nishizuka, Y.,** A new possible regulatory system for protein phosphorylation in human peripheral lymphocytes. I. Characterization of a calcium-activated, phospholipid-dependent protein kinase, *J. Immunol.,* 127, 1369, 1981.

69. **Ku, Y., Kishimoto, A., Takai, Y., Ogawa, Y., Kimura, S., and Nishizuka, Y.,** A new possible regulatory system for protein phosphorylation in human peripheral lymphocytes. II. Possible relation to phosphatidylinositol turnover induced by mitogens, *J. Immunol.,* 127, 1375, 1981.

70. **Cambier, J. C., Justement, L. B., Newell, M. K., Chen, Z. Z., Harris, L. K., Sandoval, V. M., Klemsz, M. J., and Ransom, J. T.,** Transmembrane signals and intracellular "second messengers" in the regulation of quiescent B-lymphocyte activation, *Immunol. Rev.,* 95, 37, 1987.

71. **Chen, Z. Z., Coggeshall, K. M., and Cambier, J. C.,** Translocation of protein kinase C during membrane immunoglobulin-mediated transmembrane signaling in B lymphocytes, *J. Immunol.,* 136, 2300, 1986.

72. **Nel, A. E., Wooten, M. W., Landreth, G. E., Goldschnidt-Clermont, P. J., Stevenson, H. C., Miller, P. J., and Galbraith, R. M.,** Translocation of phospholipid/Ca^{2+}-dependent protein kinase in B-lymphocytes activated by phorbol ester or cross-linking of membrane immunoglobulin, *Biochem. J.,* 233, 145, 1986.

73. **Chen, Z. Z. and Cambier, J. C.,** unpublished data, 1986.

74. **Lapetina, E. G., Billah, M. M., and Cuatrecasas, P.,** The phosphatidylinositol cycle and the regulation of arachidonic acid production, *Nature,* 292, 367, 1981.

75. **Billah, M. M., Lapetina, E. G., and Cuatrecasas, P.,** Phosphatidylinositol-specific phospholipase C of platelets: association with 1,2-diacylglycerol-kinase and inhibition by cyclic-AMP, *Biochem. Biophys. Res. Commun.,* 90, 92, 1979.

76. **Hornbeck, P. and Paul, W. E.,** Anti-immunoglobulin and phorbol ester induce phosphorylation of proteins associated with the plasma membrane and cytoskeleton in murine B lymphocytes, *J. Biol. Chem.,* 261, 14817, 1986.

77. **Newell, M. K. and Cambier, J. C.,** unpublished data.

78. **Braun, J. and Unanue, E. R.,** Surface immunoglobulin and the lymphocyte cytoskeleton, *Fed. Proc.,* 42, 2446, 1983.

79. **Nel, A. E., Landreth, G. E., Goldschmidt-Clermont, P. J., Tung, H. E., and Galbraith, R. M.,** Enhanced tyrosine phosphorylation in B lymphocytes upon complexing of membrane immunoglobulin, *Biochem. Biophys. Res. Commun.,* 125, 859, 1984.

80. **Harrison, M. L., Low, P. L., and Geahlen, R. L.,** T and B lymphocytes express distinct tyrosine protein kinases, *J. Biol. Chem.,* 259, 9348, 1984.

81. **Earp, H. S., Austin, K.S., Gillespie, G. Y., Buessow, S. C., Davies, A. A., and Parker, P. J.,** Characterization of distinct tyrosine-specific protein kinases in B and T lymphocytes, *J. Biol. Chem.,* 260, 4351, 1985.

82. **Earp, H. S., Austin, K. S., Buessow, S. C., Dy, R., and Gillespie, G. Y.,** Membranes from T and B lymphocytes have different patterns of tyrosine phophorylation, *Proc. Natl. Acad. Sci. U.S.A.,* 81, 2347, 1984.

83. **Nel, A. E., Navailles, M., Rosberger, D. F., Landreth, G. E., Goldschmidt-Clermont, P. J., Baldwin, G. J., and Galbraith, R. M.,** Phorbol ester induces tyrosine phosphorylation in normal and abnormal human B lymphocytes, *J. Immunol.,* 135, 3448, 1985.

84. **Mizuguchi, J., Beaven, M. A., Hu Li, J., and Paul, W. E.,** Phorbol myristate acetate inhibits anti-IgM-mediated signaling in resting B cells, *Proc. Natl. Acad. Sci. U.S.A.,* 83, 4474, 1986.

85. **Mizuguchi, J., Yong-Yong, J., Nakabayaschi, H., Huang, K.-P., Beaven, M. A., Chused, T., and Paul, W. E.,** Protein kinase C activation blocks anti-IgM-mediated signaling in BAL17 B lymphoma cells, *J. Immunol.,* 139, 1054, 1987.

86. **Cambier, J. Chen, Z. Z., Pasternak, J., Ransom, J., and Sandoval, V.,** Ligand-induced desensitization of B-cell membrane immunoglobulin-mediated Ca^{2+} mobilization and protein kinase C translocation, *Proc. Natl. Acad. Sci. U.S.A.,* 85, 6493, 1988.

87. **Leeb-Lundberg, L. M., Cotecchia, F. S., Lomasney, J. W., Debernardis, J. F., Lefkowitz, R. J., and Caron, M. G.,** Phorbol esters promote a1-adrenergic receptor phosphorylation and receptor uncoupling from inositol phospholipid metabolism, *Proc. Natl. Acad. Sci. U.S.A.,* 82, 5651, 1985.

88. **Cheng, H.-L., Blattner, F. R., Fitzmaurice, L., Mushinski, J. F., and Tucker, P. W.,** Structure of genes for membrane and secreted IgD heavy chains, *Nature,* 296, 410, 1982.

89. **Howard, M., Farrar, J., Hilfiker, M., Johnson, B., Takatsu, K., Hamaoka, T., and Paul, W. E.,** Identification of a T cell-derived B cell growth factor distinct from interleukin 2, *J. Exp. Med.*, 155, 914, 1982.

90. **Stein, P., DuBois, P., Greenblatt, D., and Howard, M.,** Induction of antigen-specific proliferation in affinity-purified small B lymphocytes: requirement for BSF-1 by type 2 but not type 1 thymus-independent antigens, *J. Immunol.*, 136, 2080, 1986.

91. **Roehm, N. W., Leibson, H. J., Zlotnik, A., Kappler, J., Marrack, P., and Cambier, J. C.,** Interleukin-induced increase in Ia expression by normal mouse B cells, *J. Exp. Med.*, 160, 679, 1984.

92. **Noelle, R., Krammer, P. H., Ohara, J., Uhr, J. W., and Vitetta, E. S.,** Increased expression of Ia antigens on resting B cells: an additional role for B-cell growth factor, *Proc. Natl. Acad. Sci. U.S.A.*, 81, 6149, 1984.

93. **Noelle, R. J., Kuziel, W. A., Maliszewski, E. M., Vitetta, E. S., and Tucker, P. W.,** Regulation of the expression of multiple class II genes in murine B cells by B cell stimulatory factor-1 (BSF-1), *J. Immunol.*, 137, 1718, 1986.

94. **Klemsz, M. J., Justement, L., Palmer, E., and Cambier, J. C.,** B cell activation. IX. Different expression control mechanisms are operative in anti-Ig and BSF-1 induction of increased Ia mRNA and surface expression, submitted for publication, 1989.

95. **Klemsz, M. J., Justement, L., Palmer, E., and Cambier, J. C.,** Anti-immunoglobulin and BSF-1 mediated induction of c-myc and c-fos mRNA expression, submitted for publication, 1989.

96. **Noma, Y., Sideras, P., Naito, T., Begstedt-Lindquist, S., Azuma, C., Severinson, E., Tanabe, T., Kinashi, T., Matsuda, F. Yaioti, Y., and Honjo, T.,** Cloning of cDNA encoding the murine IgG1 induction factor by a novel strategy using SP6 promoter, *Nature*, 319, 640, 1986.

97. **Lee, F., Yokota, T., Otsuka, T., Meyerson, P., Villaret, D., Coffman, R., Mosmann, T., Rennick, D., Roehm, N., Smith, C., Zlotnik, A., and Arai, K.-I.,** Isolation and characterization of a mouse interleukin cDNA clone that expresses B-cell stimulatory factor 1 activities and T-cell and mast-cell stimulating activities, *Proc. Natl. Acad. Sci. U.S.A.*, 83, 2061, 1986.

98. **Park, L. S., Friend, D., Grabstein, K., and Urdal, D. L.,** Characterization of the high-affinity cell-surface receptor for murine B-cell-stimulatory factor-1, *Proc. Natl. Acad. Sci. U.S.A.*, 84, 1669, 1987.

99. **Ohara, J. and Paul, W. E.,** Receptors for B-cell stimulatory factor-1 expressed on cells of haematopoietic lineage, *Nature*, 325, 537, 1987.

100. **Howard, M.,** personal communication, 1987.

101. **Mizuguchi, J., Beaven, M. A., Ohara, J., and Paul, W. E.,** BSF-1 action on resting B cells does not require elevation of inositol phospholipid metabolism of increased [Ca^{2+}], *J. Immunol.*, 137, 2215, 1986.

102. **Justement, L., Chen, Z., Harris, L., Ransom, J., Sandoval, V., Smith, C., Rennick, D., Roehm, N., and Cambier, J.,** BSF1 induces membrane protein phosphorylation but not phosphoinositide metabolism, Ca^{2+} mobilization, protein kinase C translocation, or membrane depolarization in resting murine B lymphocytes, *J. Immunol.*, 137, 3664, 1986.

103. **O'Garra, A., Warren, D. J., Holman, M., Popham, A. M., Sanderson, C. J., and Klaus, G. G. B.,** Effects of cyclosporine on responses of murine B cells to T cell-derived lymphokines, *J. Immunol.*, 137, 2220, 1986.

104. **Kay, J. E., Benzie, R. T. C. R., and Borghetti, A. F.,** Effects of cyclosporine A on lymphocyte activation by the calcium ionophore A23187, *Immunology*, 50, 441, 1983.

105. **Justement, L. B., Newell, M. K., and Cambier, J. C.,** unpublished data, 1986.

106. **Newell, M. K. and Cambier, J. C.,** unpublished data, 1987.

107. **Cambier, J. C., and Chen, Z. Z.,** Diacylglycerol, calcium cAMP and cGMP mediate qualitatively distinct protein kinase C translocation events in normal B lymphocytes, in *Lymphocyte Activation and Differentiation*, Mani, J. C. and Dornand, J., Eds., Walter de Gruyter, Berlin, 1988, 56.

108. **Cambier, J. C.,** unpublished data, 1986.

109. **Justement, L. B. and Cambier, J. C.,** unpublished data, 1987.

110. **Morrison, D. C. and Ryan, J.L.,** Bacterial endotoxins and host immune responses, *Adv. Immunol.*, 28, 293, 1979.

111. **Castagna, M., Takai, Y., Kaibuchi, K., Sano, K., Kikkawa, U., and Nishizuka, Y.,** Direct activation of calcium-activated, phospholipid-dependent protein kinase by tumor-promoting phorbol esters, *J. Biol. Chem.*, 257, 7847, 1982.

112. **Wightman, P. D. and Raetz, R. H.,** The activation of protein kinase C by biologically active lipid moieties of lipopolysaccharide, *J. Biol. Chem.*, 259, 10048, 1984.

113. **DeFranco, A. L., Gold, M. R., and Jakway, J. P.,** B-lymphocyte signal transduction in response to anti-immunoglobulin and bacterial lipopolysaccharide, *Immunol. Rev.*, 95, 161, 1987.

114. **Jakway, J. P., Usinger, W. R., Gold, M. R., Mishell, R. I., and DeFranco, A. L.,** Growth regulation of the B lymphoma cell line WEHI-231 by anti-immunoglobulin, lipopolysaccharide, and other bacterial products, *J. Immunol.*, 137, 2225, 1986.

115. **Jakway, J. P. and DeFranco, A. L.,** Pertussis toxin inhibition of B cell and macrophage responses to bacterial lipopolysaccharide, *Science,* 234, 734, 1986.
116. **Niederhuber, J. E., Frelinger, J. A., Dugan, E., Coutinho, A., and Schreffler, D. C.,** Effects of anti-Ia serum on mitogenic responses. I. Inhibition of the proliferative response to B cell mitogen, LPS, by specific anti-Ia sera, *J. Immunol.,* 115, 1672, 1975.
117. **Forsgren, S., Martinez, C., and Coutinho, A.,** The role of I-A/E molecules in B-lymphocyte activation. II. Mechanism of inhibition of the responses to lipopolysaccharide by anti-I-A/E antibodies, *Scand. J. Immunol.,* 25, 225, 1987.
118. **Newell, M. K., Justement, L. B., Lehman, K., Caldwell, K., Cooper, D. M. F., and Cambier, J. C.,** Do Class II major histocompatibility molecules function as signal transducers during B lymphocyte activation?, in *Major Histocompatibility Genes and Their Roles in Immune Function,* David, C. S., Ed., Plenum Press, New York, 1987, 531.
119. **Cambier, J. C.,** unpublished data, 1987.
120. **Chen, Z. Z., McGuire, J. C., Leach, K. L., and Cambier, J. C.,** Transmembrane signaling through B cell MHC class II molecules: anti-Ia antibodies induce protein kinase C translocation to the nuclear fraction, *J. Immunol.,* 138, 2345, 1987.
121. **Chen, Z. Z. and Cambier, J. C.,** unpublished data, 1987.
122. **Cambier, J. C., Newell, M. K., Justement, L. B., McGuire, J. C., Leach, K. L., and Chen, Z. Z.,** Membrane IA binding ligands induce increased intracellular cAMP which mediates the transient association of protein kinase C with the nucleus of B lymphocytes, *Nature,* 327, 629, 1987.
123. **Sidman, C. L., Marshall, J. D., Schultz, L. D., Gray, P. W., and Johnson, H.,** γ-Interferon is one of several direct B-cell maturing lymphokines, *Nature,* 309, 801, 1984.
124. **Sherris, D. I. and Sidman, C. L.,** Distinction of B cell maturation factors from lymphokines affecting B cell growth and viability, *J. Immunol.,* 136, 994, 1986.
125. **Rabin, E. M., Mond, J. J., Ohara, J., and Paul, W. E.,** Interferon-γ inhibits the action of B cell stimulatory factor (BSF)-1 on resting B cells, *J. Immunol.,* 137, 1573, 1986.
126. **Cambier, J. C.,** unpublished data, 1987.
127. **Yap, W. H., Teo, T. S., and Tan, Y. H.,** An early event in the interferon-induced transmembrane signaling process, *Science,* 234, 355, 1986.
128. **Mills, G. B., Hannigan, G., Stewart, D., Mellors, A., Williams, B., and Gelfand, E. W.,** Interferons do not signal cells through rapid alterations in phosphatidylinositide hydrolysis, cytoplasmic free calcium, or cytoplasmic alkalinization, *Prog. Clin. Biol. Res.,* 202, 357, 1985.
129. **Hamilton, T. A., Rigsbee, J. E., Scott, W. A., and Adams, D. O.,** γ-Interferon enhances the secretion of arachidonic acid metabolites from murine peritoneal macrophages stimulated with phorbol diesters, *J. Immunol.,* 134, 2631, 1985.
130. **Celada, A. and Schreiber, R. D.,** Role of protein kinase C and intracellular calcium mobilization in the induction of macrophage tumoricidal activity by interferon-γ, *J. Immunol.,* 137, 2373, 1986.
131. **Boraschi, D., Censini, S., Bartalini, M., and Tagliabue, A.,** Regulation of arachidonic acid metabolism in macrophages by immune and non-immune interferons, *J. Immunol.,* 135, 502, 1985.
132. **Polla, B. S., Poljak, A., Ohara, J., Paul, W. E., and Glimcher, L. H.,** Regulation of class II gene expression: analysis in B cell stimulatory factor 1-inducible murine pre-B cell lines, *J. Immunol.,* 137, 3332, 1986.

Chapter 7

LYMPHOID GROWTH FACTORS: GENE REGULATION AND BIOCHEMICAL MECHANISMS OF ACTION

William L. Farrar, Annick Harel-Bellan, and Douglas K. Ferris

TABLE OF CONTENTS

I. INTRODUCTION

The biochemical and molecular basis of higher organisms' responses to mechanical or chemical insult have been conserved evolutionarily. The adaptable vertebrate immune system is a highly mobile and diffuse physiological organization which responds to both benevolent and malevolent interactions with the environment; however, the functional cellular and chemical mediators which control the biological response still maintain strong phenotypic identities with those found in the most primitive unicellular organisms. Even the mechanical processes of protection or assimilation of nutrients observed in *Paramecium* are similar to systems highly studied in cells of monocyte/macrophage hematopoietic lineages. The rise of multicellular organism interactions which have evolved into reciprocating specialized functions is a process developed from the evolutionary pressure of synergism and adaptability.

Complex organisms evolved, it is presumed, by the interaction of unicellular organisms in ways which provided biochemical advantages for survival. For example, as oxygen levels increased due to biochemical conversion in the atmosphere and soil, those organisms with oxidative metabolisms obtained a selective advantage to survive in terrestrial or oxygen-rich environments. Organisms which maintained a synergistic relationship with other organisms/ organelles which maintained oxidative tolerance therefore survived. It is in this manner that the evolution of mitochondria in eukaryotes is envisioned.

Similarly, the evolution of organismal defense is intrinsic to survival through biochemical synergism. In addition to physical barriers and internal mechanisms of cellular defense/ survival, the secretion of chemical agents produced by the organism can modify the microenvironment to be deleterious to other competing organisms. Conversely, organisms which could survive and perhaps flourish in the presence of secreted metabolites coexisted, synergized, and were capable of forming heterogeneous cellular populations. The biochemical nature of secreted substances from microorganisms, which have biological modifying activity, is limited to two fundamentally distinct chemical structures, organic and polypeptide. Among the most rigorously studied in the context of environmental immunity against intruding cellular populations are the cyclic planar ring organics (antibiotics) and polypeptides broadly referred to as toxins. These two classes of chemical substances have served in the phylogenetic evolution of microorganisms as the principal mediators of extracellular control of the environmental niche. The chemical forms and mechanisms of actions of toxins and antibiotics have been maintained and have evolved broader roles in the control of the intercellular environment. In vertebrates, the chemical class structures are conserved in polypeptide hormones and autocoids (prostaglandins, leukotrienes, etc.) which regulate virtually all known cellular physiological systems. Therefore, microorganismal "immunity" maintains three general features analogous to the mammalian immune system which are controlled by extracellular chemical signals. These are toxic inhibition of noncompatible alien organisms (nonself), environmental synergism with compatible organisms (self), and extreme potential for genetic variability and adaptation (genetic recombination).

The vertebrate immune "survival" system maintains the same fundamental cellular and biochemical constituent elements which govern the survival and adaptive responses of microorganisms. Heterogenous cellular constituents (immunocytes) interact in a synergistic and reciprocal manner to insure mutual survival. The cellular constituents are programmed by genetic recombination to recognize "self" and "nonself". Control of population interaction is dictated by both extracellular chemical signals and recognition molecules (receptors) on the surface of cellular membranes. The biochemical nature of these molecular elements is still either organic (i.e., prostaglandins) or protein (i.e., cytokines, receptors, histocompatibility structures). Defenses against nonself or invading organisms include physical interaction and degradation (monocytes/macrophages) and biochemical attack such as antibody/complement or cytolysis by production of toxic substances. These mechanisms of immunity in the mammal are highly reminiscent of those survival mechanisms in micro-organisms previously discussed.

The communication network of the immune system is regulated by cell to cell recognition. Such interactions cause the production of a class of regulatory molecules collectively referred to as cytokines. Cytokines, like all hormones and "informational substances", transfer their instructions to a cell by interacting with a molecular antennae (receptor). This interaction causes a series of biochemical transformations in which the initial nature of the chemical interaction, namely ligand-receptor, is translated into another form of chemical substances to which the cell now responds. As suggested in the preceding introduction, not only are the organization and biochemical nature of external signals conserved, so are the internal signals generated at the membrane. In fact, far greater homology exists within phylogeny concerning the intracellular biochemical constituents which govern cellular viability or responses to extracellular stimuli. This chapter discusses in some detail the biochemical and molecular events that occur upon cytokine stimulation of target cells and describes the extraordinary consensus biochemical structures that have been evolutionarily conserved among the simplest microorganisms and mammalian tissues.

II. GENERAL FEATURES OF SIGNAL TRANSDUCTION

Signal transduction is the biochemical process by which ligand-receptor interactions simplify and amplify a series of chemical signals which activate a myriad of enzymatic activities that regulate cell metabolism and macromolecular synthesis. A limited repertoire of signals generated at the membrane has been observed with a wide variety of hormones, neurotransmitters, or "informational substances". The number of second messengers is surprisingly small and remarkably universal. Two major signal pathways are now known. One employs cyclic adenosine monophosphate (cAMP) and the other calcium ions and the phosphoinositide species, inositol triphosphate (IP_3) and diacylglycerol. The paths have many common features (Figure 1). Both utilize specific protein recognition sites (receptors) which bind with high affinity (kDa = 10^{-9} to $10^{-12} M$) informational substances, which may have peptic or organic structures. In order for the signal to be initiated, the informational substance (ligand) must bind the receptor outside the plasma membrane with sufficient affinity to engage the interaction of a guanosine triphosphate (GTP)-binding protein with the receptor within the transmembrane structure.

The GTP-binding protein (G protein) is activated by binding GTP and then "transducing" the external information to an amplifying system, adenylate cyclase (AC), for cAMP-coupled transduction and phospholipase C (PLC) for phosphoinositol coupled systems. The amplifier enzymes convert precursor molecules, usually with energy-rich phosphate groups, into second messengers. In the case of adenylate cyclase, adenosine triphosphate (ATP) is converted into cAMP, whereas PLC hydrolyzes phosphatidylinositol 4,5-bisphosphate (PIP_2) into IP_3 which stimulates the release of intracellular stores of Ca^{2+}, effecting the activation of Ca^{2+}-dependent kinases such as Ca^{2+} calmodulin-dependent protein kinase. Diacylglycerol stimulates the activation of a phospholipid-dependent protein kinase, protein kinase C (PKC). The result of the activation of these kinase systems is to regulate the function of specific substrate proteins. Both pathways can be mimicked by pharmacological analogs. Stable derivatives of cAMP can readily penetrate the cell and activate protein kinase A (PKA). Release of intracellular Ca^{2+} and Ca^{2+} influx can be irreversibly achieved by the addition of Ca^{2+} ionophores (ionomycin, A23187) to cell cultures. Likewise, a potent class of tumor promoters, phorbol esters, can penetrate the cell membrane and activate PKC. These pharmacological stimulants have proven useful in cause-effect experimentation to elucidate the roles of the discrete second messengers on cellular functions and gene expression. It is noteworthy that none of the analogs are reversible and (at best) only approximate physio-

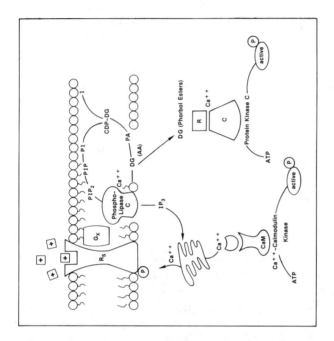

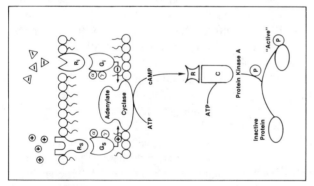

EXTERNAL SIGNAL (Informational Substance)	
RECEPTOR (Molecular Recognition Site)	
TRANSDUCER	
AMPLIFIER	
PHOSPHORYLATED PRECURSOR	
SECOND MESSENGER	
EFFECTOR MOLECULE	
ACTIVATION SUBSTRATE	
BIOCHEMICAL MOBILIZATION	

FIGURE 1.   Second messenger system.

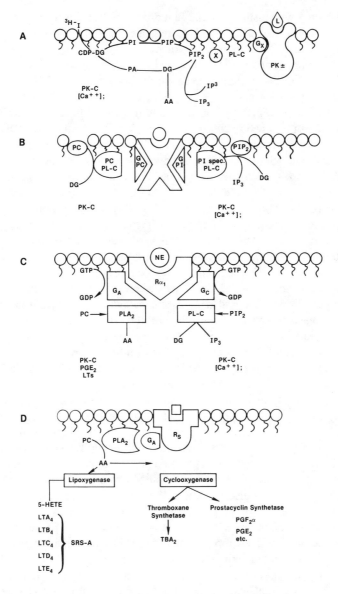

FIGURE 2. Phospholipid catabolic pathways.

logical conditions of second messengers, and are particularly refractory to normal feedback regulatory mechanisms evoked by physiological stimuli.

III. PHOSPHOLIPID DEGRADATION AND ION FLUX

One major means by which external substances transduce and convert biochemical information is the hydrolysis of membrane phospholipids. Unlike the adenylate cyclase system, phospholipid second messengers are cannabalized from the plasma membrane itself. Not only is the lipid structure of the plasma membrane a substrate for second messenger generation for a variety of adrenergic and muscarinic hormones, but it is also the target of many toxins and venoms. There are many ways the hydrolysis of lipids can occur in response to external stimuli (Figure 2). Each pathway is unique in that it may produce different and/

or common metabolites with distinct cellular functions. The "classical" phosphatidylinositol pathway is cyclic and utilizes a G-protein to regulate the stimulatory receptor interaction with the amplifier enzyme, PLC (Figure 2A) which hydrolyses PIP_2 into IP_3 and diacyglycerol (DG). These bifurcating second messengers effect the release of intracellular Ca^{2+}, causing a transient rise in $[Ca^+]i$, and DG participates in the activation of PKC.

More recently, alternative pathways have been discovered which have led to the generation of DG independent of PIP_2 hydrolysis. Besterman et al.[1] have demonstrated the rapid formation of DG from phosphatidylcholine (Figure 2B). This formation of DG occurred in the presence of platelet-derived growth factor (PDGF), previously believed to generate DG only from PIP_2. The generation of DG from PC does not produce IP_3 and would not stimulate changes in $[Ca^{2+}]i$, even though PKC would be activated. PLA_2, the enzyme responsible for cleavage of PC into arachidonic acid (AA), appears to be linked with α_1-adrenergic receptors.[2] This implies that both major hydrolysis pathways for phospholipids are modulated by G-proteins specific for unique amplifier enzyme systems (Figure 2C). What is particularly important is the observation that *cis*-fatty acids (AA, oleic, etc.) have been shown to activate PKC without additional phospholipids or Ca^{2+}.[3] This suggests the provocative notion that PKC may also be activated by mechanisms which do not generate DG and uncouples what was previously thought to be a strict relationship between PIP_2 hydrolysis and PKC activation.

Among the various phospholipid degradation pathways known, the arachidonic acid pathway has been most rigorously studied (Figure 2D). AA formed by the action of PLA_2 on phosphatidylcholine can be additionally modified by two distinct enzyme (amplifier) systems. The cyclooxygenase pathway synthesizes thromboxanes and the prostaglandins. The lipoxygenase system forms the various leukotriene isomers. All of these lipid products have potent physiological effects or hormone-like actions.

Since many hormones have been shown to stimulate these various phospholipid degradative pathways, they are obviously a potential target for activators of lymphoid cells and lymphokine action. The activation of PIP_2 hydrolysis as a means of transmembrane signaling has been most seriously indicated in the activation of resting T and B lymphocytes. Both lectins and antibody to the T3-antigen receptor complex have been shown to cause PIP_2 hydrolysis, increased $[Ca^{2+}]i$, and PKC activation.[4-7] Cross-linking of immunoglobulin M (IgM) with antibody in B cells also leads to a similar activation biochemistry as that seen with T cell mitogens.[8] The role of phospholipid hydrolysis for cytokines is less clear. Although potent agents which cross-link membrane receptors elicit increased phosphoinositide formation, the subtle effects of polypeptide ligands have been more difficult to detect. Mills et al.[9] reported that interleukin-2 (IL-2) does not stimulate phosphatidylinositol (PI) hydrolysis in T cells, whereas under serum-free conditions in which cells were washed and deprived of IL-2 and restimulated, PIP_2 hydrolysis was observed by Bonvini et al.[10] In neither case was an α_1-adrenergic stimulant used as a positive control. PHA is hardly representative of a hormonal stimuli, but is often used as a positive control for PI hydrolysis in T lymphocytes. Neither IL-1 nor BSF-1 have been shown to stimulate PIP_2 hydrolysis.[11,12] IL-1 has been shown to stimulate prostaglandin E_2 (PGE_2) synthesis in monocytes, however, arguing the possibility that PLA_2 activation may occur in that tissue type. The ability of most cytokines to affect other lipid degradative pathways as suggested in Figure 2 has not been substantively addressed. Since many studies have used ^3H-inositol as tracer label (Figure 2A), alternative phospholipid degradative pathways would be undetected.

The data regarding ion flux in cytokine-stimulated cells also remain conflicting. Changes in $[Ca^{2+}]i$ have not been seen in lymphocytes immediately washed from IL-2 and restimulated.[13] Under similar conditions IL-2 induced Na^+/H^+ antiport activation.[14] The conclusions from both studies suggested that neither changes in $[Ca^{2+}]i$ or intracellular alkalinization were required for IL-2-stimulated growth.[15] The lack of a requirement for Na^+/H^+ antiporter activity for IL-2-stimulated events seen in those experiments contrasts

TABLE 1
Intrinsic Kinase

Receptor	Size (kDa)	Activity	Ref.
EGF	170	Yes	94
PDGF	180	Yes	95
Insulin			
α-Chain	135	Yes	96
β-Chain	90	Yes	
NGF	103	?	97
IGF-1	α-2	Yes	98
	β-2		
Bombesin	115	Probably	99
IL-2	55—58	No	67
IL-3	55 & 75	?	100
G-CSF	30	?	100
GM-CSF	51	?	101
M-CSF, CSF 1	165	Yes	102

with the studies of Pouyssegur and colleagues.[16,17] These studies have shown that cytoplasmic pH is a key determinant to serum-stimulated proliferation of fibroblasts. IL-2 has been shown to stimulate ATPase dep-Na^+/K^+ exchange which is inhibited by ouabain.[18] Both depletion of K^+ from medium and ouabain treatment inhibited the proliferative response. The relative roles of specific phospholipase pathways and ion flux remain somewhat equivocal for cytokine action. The examination of PC degradation as a means of providing DG or *cis*-fatty acids for PKC activation is relatively uninvestigated. On the other hand, more sensitive analysis of PI hydrolysis may be necessary to detect changes evoked by growth factors.

IV. GROWTH FACTOR RECEPTORS AND TYROSINE KINASES

A variety of intracellular events take place in growth factor-stimulated cells prior to cell division. Some of the earliest occurrences, such as tyrosine phosphorylation, calcium mobilization, phospholipid turnover, cellular alkalinization, and PKC activation and translocation may be involved in transduction of the growth factor signal.

While the importance of protein phosphorylation in regulating cellular metabolism has been well established, its precise role in growth factor-induced signal transduction is unclear. Since the discovery in 1980 that the transforming gene product of the Rous sarcoma virus (RSV) was a tyrosine kinase,[19] a variety of viral oncogenes and their cellular counterparts, the protooncogenes, have been demonstrated to possess tyrosine kinase activity.[20-22] The members of this family of protooncogenes are transmembrane proteins consisting of, at minimum, an external receptor portion, a transmembrane section, and a cytoplasmic catalytic site. Included within this group are the epidermal growth factor (EGF) receptor, PDGF receptor, the insulin receptor, and the insulin-like growth factor (IGF-1) receptor.[22] Other growth factor receptors may also possess tyrosine kinase activity, but it is clear from inspection of Table 1 that all of the currently indentified receptors with kinase activity are fairly large proteins. When the appropriate growth factor is bound to a receptor bearing tyrosine kinase activity, the catalytic site becomes activated. First, the enzyme autophosphorylates on one or more tyrosine residues, then begins phosphorylating both membrane bound and cytosolic substrate proteins.[22] In the case of the EGF receptor, both autophosphorylation on tyrosine and phosphorylation on serine or threonine by a different kinase (or kinases) alters the activity of the receptor and its affinity for EGF.[23,24] The cell surface expression of the EGF, PDGF and insulin receptors, as well as a variety of other receptors, including the transferrin receptor and T-cell antigen receptor complex (T3-Ti complex), is reduced by a process of receptor-mediated endocytosis following either ligand binding or treatment by phorbol esters, known activators of PKC.[23,25-28] In certain instances, internalized receptors are eventually recycled to the cell surface. The down-regulation of receptors, mediated in some cases through phosphorylation, is currently thought to be a fairly general phenomenon and may be important in carrying out some of the biological effects of growth factors and hormones.[29] For instance, it has been reported that EGF, PDGF, and nerve growth factor (NGF) are all specifically bound to chromatin following receptor internalization and that proteins antigenically similar to the respective receptors were also bound at the same locations.[28]

The tyrosine phosphorylation patterns of cellular proteins in virally transformed cells have been compared to those of the uninfected cells both before and after serum and growth factor stimulation. Prominently labeled proteins of 36 and 42 kDa have been identified in chicken embryo fibroblasts (CEF) transformed by avian erythroblastosis virus (AEV) or RSV.[30,31] The 42 kDa protein was also phosphorylated on tyrosine in uninfected CEF after EGF treatment. Although phosphorylation of the 36 kDa protein on tyrosine could not be demonstrated in EGF-treated CEF cells it has been reported in a human cell line A431 that expresses high levels of the EGF receptor.[32] While these results and others like them are interesting, they are restricted to phenomenology. With the exception of the growth factor receptors themselves, three glycolytic enzymes,[33] and lipocortin,[34] the biochemical functions of the proteins phosphorylated on tyrosine *in situ* are mostly unknown. However, regarding proteins phosphorylated *in vitro* using partially purified materials, several interesting reports have appeared that describe phosphorylation of protein phosphatase 1, transducin and DNA topoisomerase by pp60 V-src, the insulin receptor, and a 75-kDa cellular tyrosine kinase, respectively.[35-37]

V. PROTEIN KINASE C

A calcium- and phospholipid-dependent protein kinase, known as protein kinase C (PKC), was described in 1979 by Nishizuka and his co-workers.[38] First isolated from rat brain, PKC has since been found in a wide variety of tissues and species, although the highest levels are associated with neural and lymphoid cells. *In vivo*, PKC is regulated by diacylglycerol, a product of PI hydrolysis by PLC.[39] In general it appears that when PI hydrolysis is stimulated, PKC binds diacylglycerol and translocates from the cytosol to the plasma membrane. There, in the presence of membrane phospholipids and calcium, PKC begins phosphorylating protein substrates.

Two types of evidence suggest that PKC is involved in signal transduction pathways leading to growth and proliferation. The effects of phorbol ester tumor promoters have been studied. These compounds are not directly tumorigenic, but the ability of primary carcinogens to cause tumors in animals is greatly potentiated by various phorbol esters. The biologically active phorbol esters bind to a single type of intracellular receptor with high affinity, and it is now known that the receptor is PKC.[39-43] Phorbol-12-myristate-13-acetate (PMA), or 12-*O* tetradecanoyl phorbol-13 bind PKC, and directly activate the enzyme. Therefore, it is thought that the tumor-promoting effects of phorbol esters must be due to the activities of PKC.[39]

A variety of stimuli cause the turnover of PIs and the release of diacylglycerol. To those interested in growth regulation, however, the finding that several growth factors induce PI hydrolysis is particularly noteworthy because it suggests that activation of PKC is one consequence of ligand/growth factor receptor interaction.[44] More direct evidence of the involvement of PKC in growth-related signal transduction has come from previous work in our laboratory, as well as others, that has shown rapid activation and translocation of PKC in response to phorbol ester or growth factor stimulation of quiescent cells.[39,45,46]

The proteins phosphorylated in response to phorbol esters or growth factor stimulation have been examined in several systems. Although the EGF receptor is a tyrosine kinase, the phosphorylation of the receptor on serine and threonine residues has been described. The phosphorylation of EGF-R induced by PMA results in decreased affinity of the receptor for EGF and also in the removal of the receptor from the cell surface.[23,47-49]

Using two-dimensional gel electrophoresis, we have examined the proteins phosphorylated in several growth factor-dependent murine lymphoid and myeloid cell lines following stimulation with the appropriate growth factor or DG. We found that stimulation with DG induced rapid phosphorylation of a 68-kDa protein (p68) in each of the four cell lines tested and the same protein was also phosphorylated in response to growth factors.[50] There was, however, an intriguing exception to the general finding that p68 phosphorylation was induced in all cells responding to an appropriate growth factor. One of the cell lines (NSF 60.8) can proliferate in response to either GM-CSF or G-CFS, but p68 phosphorylation was only induced by G-CSF. This finding suggests the existence of an alternate pathway involving protein phosphorylation that leads to cell growth. While p68 is the predominant protein phosphorylated in these cells in response to phorbol esters, its biochemical function is still unknown. In addition to p68, a protein of 30 kDa was also phosphorylated in response to IL-2 or DG, while phosphorylation of p60 and p80 was only stimulated by IL-2.

More recently, Ishii and co-workers[51] have described the IL-2-dependent phosphorylation of proteins of 67 and 63 kDa in human T-lymphocytes, that may be the human homologs of the murine proteins p68 and p60 described above. Due to the different techniques used for the first dimension separation (pH 3.5 to 10 nonequilibrating pH gradient gel electrophoresis used by us, vs. pH 5 to 8 isoelectric focusing), it is uncertain how similar in charge these proteins are.

Whetton and his co-workers[53] showed that PKC phosphorylates the hexose transport protein in the IL-3-dependent cell line, FDC-P1, both *in vitro* and *in situ* in response to TPA or IL-3. More recently, it has been reported that TPA and a calcium ionophore can replace the maintenance requirement for IL-3 in these cells. They suggest that the increased glucose transport resulting from phosphorylation of the transport protein in response to TPA/ionophore or IL-3 is important to both the survival and proliferation of FDC-P1 cells.[53]

Phosphorylation of cellular proteins induced by IL-1 and BSF-1 has been reported. Matsushima et al.[54] have shown that recombinant IL-1α stimulates the phosphorylation of a 65-kDa protein in dexamethasone-treated monocytes. BSF-1 has also been shown to stimulate phosphorylation of a 44-kDa protein in membranes isolated from B lymphocytes.[12] Neither ligand has been shown to stimulate Ca^{2+} influx or PI hydrolysis.[11] The approximate sizes of both receptors (<80 kDa) suggests that neither will contain a tyrosine kinase activity. The only cytokine receptor to date recognized to contain tyrosine kinase activity is that for CSF-1.[55] In fact, the putative receptor has been shown to be homologous to the v-*fms* oncogene.[56] No cellular targets of the kinase have been identified.

VI. G PROTEINS

While it is certain that protein phosphorylation is a fundamental mechanism in several different signal transduction pathways leading to growth and proliferation, many of the details are obscure. Recently, much attention has been given to a family of GTP-binding proteins known as G proteins whose members include G_i and G_s, the well-known modulators of AC activity; G_o, a protein of unknown function; transducin; an outer rod retinal protein; and the transforming products of the *ras* genes.[57,58] The functions that are known for G proteins involve linking membrane bound receptors to effector enzymes. The effector can, by this mechanism, potentially be regulated by any receptor capable of interacting with the proper G protein. Two G proteins, G_i and G_s, can interact with AC to either stimulate its cAMP synthesizing activity (G_s), or inhibit it (G_i). The intracellular levels of cAMP, and consequently, the activity of the cAMP-dependent kinase are therefore, in large measure, determined by the interactions of G_s and G_i with AC.[57]

Recent evidence suggests that G proteins are also involved in regulating phospholipase C hydrolysis of phosphatidylinositol to produce inositol 1,4,5-triphosphate (IP$_3$) and diacylglycerol.[59-61] Both of these products are important intracellular second messengers, IP$_3$ causing increases in intracellular Ca^{2+}, and diacylglycerol activating PKC.[62]

Work in our laboratory has shown that IL-2, the primary growth factor for antigen or lectin primed T lymphocytes, stimulates both rapid turnover of PI and translocation of PKC from the cytosol to the plasma membrane, effects that could be mimicked by the addition of phorbol esters to the cells.[46] In addition, we had observed that PGE, which stimulates the accumulation of cAMP in a variety of lymphocytes, inhibited the proliferative response of IL-2-dependent CT6 cells.[63] The inhibition of proliferation by PGE was dose-dependent and could be overcome by increasing amounts of IL-2. Treatment of CT6 with either IL-2 or PMA also caused a marked inhibition of basal and PGE-stimulated AC activity. Further, we found that the addition of purified PKC to CT6 membrane preparations also inhibited AC activity.[63]

Since the intracytoplasmic region of the IL-2 receptor is too small to function as a kinase,[64] we speculated that a G protein might be involved in transducing IL-2 effects on PI hydrolysis, PKC activation, and in overcoming the effects of PGE. When membranes isolated from quiescent IL-2-dependent cells were treated with IL-2, a rapid rise in GTP binding and hydrolysis was observed, thus suggesting the involvement of a G protein in the IL-2 signal transduction apparatus.[65]

Because the addition of purified PKC to isolated membranes caused the inhibition of AC activity, we attempted to determine whether PKC might be phosphorylating either G_i or G_s. We used cholera toxin (CT) and pertussis toxin (PT) to ^{32}P-ADP-ribosylate the α subunits of G_s and G_i, respectively. When the migration of these labeled proteins was compared with PKC substrates on two-dimensional analysis it appeared that PKC did not phosphorylate either of the α subunits *in situ*.[66] It is still possible that PKC phosphorylates either the β or γ subunits of G_i or G_s or, alternatively, that it modifies AC directly. A recent report, however, describes the multisite phosphorylation of the D-GP-bound α subunit of transducin by PKC and the insulin receptor kinase.[36]

VII. S6 RIBOSOMAL PHOSPHORYLATION

The proliferation of cells requires the synthesis of new proteins, some of which (histones, etc.), are directly required in the processes of mitosis and cell division. Agents that block protein synthesis also block the initiation of DNA synthesis and the requirement for new synthesis extends through S and G2. When quiescent cells are stimulated by serum and growth factors, the S6 protein of the 40s ribosomal subunit is rapidly phosphorylated. This phosphorylation is associated with the formation of polysomes and increased initiation of protein synthesis.[67]

The binding of EGF, PDGF, or insulin stimulates the intrinsic tyrosine kinase activity associated with the receptors for these factors. The ribosomal S6 protein is phosphorylated on serine, however, so it is clearly not a direct substrate of receptors expressing tyrosine kinase activity.[68] PI turnover has been linked to the activation of the PDGF, EGF, and insulin receptors, but it is not clear whether the linkage involves a G protein.[44,69-71] It is possible that several growth factor receptors phosphorylate *in situ* certain intermediates of the inositol cycle, as has been shown *in vitro* for pp60v-src.[72] Regardless what the precise mechanism is, however, DG is produced and PKC is activated in cells responding to those growth factors.

Tryptic peptide gel patterns of S6 phosphorylated *in situ*, in response to serum or PMA, are identical to each other, but different from digest patterns produced from S6 phosphorylated *in vitro* by purified PKC.[73] In addition, an S6 kinase has been identified that is stimulated in lysates of EGF or serum-treated cells.[74] This S6 kinase activity is not responsive to cyclic nucleotides of Ca^{2+} and phospholipids. These observations indicate that although PKC activation is required for S6 phosphorylation in serum- or EGF-treated cells, it is not directly responsible.

We have examined S6 phosphorylation in IL-2-dependent CT6 cells. Although the initial signal transduction mechanism may be different than that involved in cells responding to EGF-R and similar receptors (since the IL-2 receptor, unlike the EFG receptor, has no intrinsic kinase activity), S6 was phosphorylated in response to IL-2 or 1-oleyl-2-acetylgly-cerol (OAG), a synthetic, direct activator of PKC. As had been found in other systems, an S6 kinase activity was present in cell lysates that was separable from PKC. Tryptic digests of S6 phosphorylated *in vitro* by partially purified S6 kinase free of demonstrable PKC activity were compared to digests of S6 phosphorylated either *in situ*, in response to IL-2, or *in vitro* by purified PKC. Our analysis indicated that PKC was not directly involved in physiological S6 phosphorylation, although activation of PKC was required.

VIII. Ti/T3 ANTIGEN RECEPTOR COMPLEX PHOSPHORYLATION AND TRANSMEMBRANE SIGNALING

The clonally specific, MHC restricted, proliferative response of mature T lymphocytes is initiated by interaction of the heterodimeric Ti antigen receptor with antigen. This interaction is required for the expression of both IL-2 and the IL-2 receptor. The functional elegance of this requirement is that T lymphocyte clones that have not been exposed to their specific antigen are incapable of binding and responding to IL-2 produced by other T lymphocytes clonally expanding in response to different antigens. While the biological response of T cells to antigens or lectins is thoroughly characterized, the biochemical mechanisms invoved are not well understood.

The antigen receptor consists of idiotypic, disulfide linked α- and β-chains.[75] The five polypeptides of the murine T3 antigen (gp26, gp21, p25, p21, p16) are noncovalently associated with the antigen receptor.[76] Recent work has shown that, as is the case for a variety of receptors, ligand binding or activation of PKC by phorbol esters induces phosphorylation of components of the receptor complex as well as selective loss of the complex from the cell surface.[27,76-82] Activators of PKC induced serine phosphorylation of the murine (and human homologs) T3 p25 and gp21 chains.[27,82,83] Antigen or lectin activation also induced serine phosphorylation of murine p23 and gp21 as well as both serine and tyrosine phosphorylation of p21.[76]

Recently,[84] the phosphorylation of pp60c-src following stimulation of T cells by monoclonal antibodies to T3 has been described. Soluble anti-T3 antibodies blocked the proliferative response of the cells while antibodies bound to a solid substrate induced both IL-2 production and proliferation. The significance of the phosphorylation of pp60c-src induced by anti-T3 antibodies is uncertain, however, since both soluble and substrate-bound antibodies caused apparently identical phosphorylation.

IX. STRESS PROTEINS

A number of agents including heat, transition metals, glucose deprivation, and ethanol induce the synthesis of various members of a set of cellular proteins known collectively as stress proteins.[85] The most prominent members of the stress proteins have molecular weights of about 70 and 90 kDa and have been described in organisms ranging from bacteria to

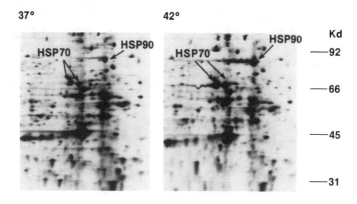

FIGURE 3.   The effects of heat shock on synthesis of HSP70 and HSP90.
Quiescent human T cells were either (A) maintained at 37° for 1 h or (B) heat
shocked at 42°. The labeled proteins were separated by pH 3.5 to 10 isoelectric
focusing in the first dimension followed by 7.5% SDS-PAGE in the second
dimension.

mammals.[86] The importance of the 70 kDa stress protein and its isoforms is indicated by
the highly conserved sequences at both the nucleic acid and protein levels.[87-89] While the
biochemical functions of heat shock proteins are not well understood, induction of their
sythesis by mild heat shock or ethanol has been correlated with increased cell survival during
subsequent harsh treatment.[86] Recently, the induction and intracellular location of heat shock
proteins during the growth of mammalian cells was investigated. Wu and Morimoto[90] found
that HSP70 RNA was induced at maximal levels 12 to 18 h after serum stimulation of
quiescent HeLa and human embryonic kidney cells. Using a monoclonal antibody, Welch
and Feramisco[91] have found that HSP70 is present in the cytosol and nuclei of cells. Following
heat shock both cytoplasmic and nuclear staining increased with some nuclear staining
associated with nucleoli. Milarski and Morimotol[92] found that HSP70 mRNA increased 10-
to 15-fold upon entry into S phase and declined by late S phase. They also reported that
during the S phase HSP70 is localized to the nucleus, while during G_1 and G_2 it was diffusely
distributed in both the nucleus and the cytoplasm. The probable involvement of HSP70 in
growth promotion is also indicated by experiments showing induction of HSP70 by trans-
acting immortalizing proteins of DNA tumor viruses.[93]

We have examined the patterns of HSP70 and HSP90 synthesis in quiescent, IL-2-
dependent, human T lymphocytes following heat shock or IL-2 stimulation. Both HSP70
and HSP90 were strongly induced by heat shock (Figure 3). After 3 h of IL-2 stimulation
(Figure 4), the rate of HSP70 synthesis was triple that of the control cells and by the 6th
hour had decreased to double that of the controls. The synthetic rate of HSP90, in contrast,
did not increase until after 3 h of IL-2 stimulation. By the 6th hour, IL-2-stimulated HSP90
synthesis was almost double that in the control cells. In other experiments we have seen
induction of HSP70 mRNA and HSP70 protein synthesis as early as 1 h following treatment
of quiescent T cells with IL-2 (data not shown).

X. LYMPHOKINES REGULATE GENE EXPRESSION

A few minutes after cytoplasmic activation by a growth factor, the signal is transduced
to the nucleus. Nuclear activation can be monitored by drastic quantitative and qualitative
changes in the transcriptional activity of the cell. Activation signals, whether mitogens or
lymphokines, induce the appearance of new messages in the cytoplasm that are undetectable
during G_0 and early G_1. Several of the growth factor- or mitogen-activated genes have been

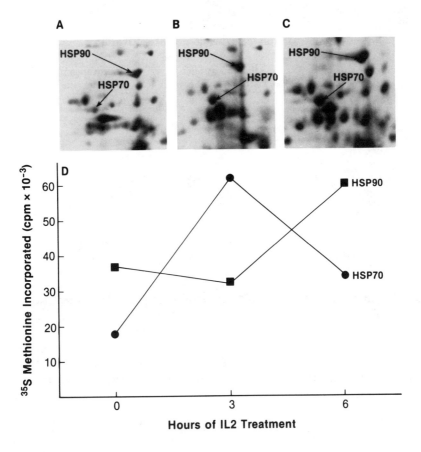

FIGURE 4. The effect of IL-2 stimulation on HSP70 and HSP90 synthesis. Quiescent human T cells were stimulated with IL-2 for either (A) 0 (control), (B) 3, or (C) 6 h. The labeled proteins were separated by pH 3.5-10 isoelectric focusing followed by 7.5% SDS-PAGE. (D) HSP70 and HSP90 were exercised from the gels shown in panels A through C and ^{35}S-methionine incorporated into each protein was determined by liquid scintillation counting.

identified in lymphocytes. Some are tissue specific genes and some are "consensus genes" that are activated by growth factors in every tissue studied, from fibroblasts to nerve cells, including thyroid cells, lymphoid, and myeloid cells.

XI. ACTIVATION OF TISSUE SPECIFIC GENES: IL-2, IL-2 RECEPTOR α-CHAIN AND γ-INTERFERON

The proliferation of resting (G$_o$ blocked) T lymphocytes requires two sequential signals,[104] the first signal being given by an antigen, which binds to the antigen-specific receptor (and can be mimicked *in situ* by the use of lectins such as PHA or concanavalin A, Con A), and the second signal being IL-2. Major events induced by the first signal include *de novo* synthesis of IL-2 and IL-2 receptor. In a second step, the interaction between IL-2 and its receptor allows the cell to proceed further in the cell cycle toward the S phase. The major changes in gene expression during these two phases of activation are listed in Table 2. Expression of IL-2 and IL-2 receptor genes have been studied using cDNA probes corresponding to IL-2[105-108] and TAC antigen,[64,109-113] a molecule which has by itself a low affinity for IL-2,[114] but is believed to be at least part of a high affinity receptor,[115] and which has recently been renamed the IL-2 receptor α-chain.[116-118] Activation of resting peripheral

TABLE 2
Genes Modulated During T Cell Activation

	Mitogen activation of resting T lymphocytes	IL-2 activation of T lymphoblasts
IL-2	+ +	−
IL-2 receptor α	+ + +	
α-IFN	+ +	
T-fr	+ +	
c-*fos*	+ [a,b]	+
c-*myc*	+ + +	+ + +
c-*myb*	+ +	+ +
c-*abl*	+	−
N-*ras*	+	−

[a]   − = not modulated; + = modulated.
[b]   The number of + indicating the apparent level of induction; blank space: not determined.

T lymphocytes by PHA induces the rapid expression of IL-2 and IL-2 receptor α messages, the induction of IL-2 receptor α message preceding, in some studies, the appearance of IL-2 message.[119,120] Whereas IL-2 messages appear as a homogenous population of 1 kb transcripts,[121,122] IL-2 receptor α messages are detected as a heterologous population of 3.5 and 1.5 kb. In the second step of activation, following the interaction between IL-2 and its receptor, transcription of IL-2 receptor is triggered again. In fact, IL-2 induces the biosynthesis of its own receptor.[123-126]

XII. ACTIVATION OF "CONSENSUS" GENES

Mitogens, as well as lymphokines, induce the activation of several genes in T lymphocytes,[119,120,127] B lymphocytes,[127] and myeloid cells[128,129] that are not restricted to immunological tissues, but rather seem to be involved in the proliferation of several (if not all) systems. Among those, the oncogenes are of special interest. Oncogenes were first described as the genes responsible for target cell transformation in the genome of transforming viruses, mostly retroviruses.[130]   In fact, it has rapidly been shown that each of these genes has a normal cellular counterpart, the so-called protooncogenes. Relationships between oncogenes and growth factors were described early in the course of the study of these genes. With relation to the subcellular localization and to the functional properties of their polypeptide products, these genes can be classified into three categories:[126] (1) oncogenes which are structurally related to growth factors (no lymphokine-related oncogene has been described), (2) oncogenes which are related to growth factor receptors or signal transducing proteins (the product of the *fms* gene, for example, is homologous to the extracellular domain of the CSF-1 receptor,[131] a receptor for a lymphokine which is a macrophage specific growth factor) and (3) nuclear protooncogenes, such as c-*myc*, c-*fos*, c-*myb*, or p53. Interestingly, the link betweeen oncogenes and growth factor-induced proliferation also occurs at the level of these nuclear protooncogenes, since these genes are silent in a resting cell and their expression is activated upon triggering by a growth factor, as has been well documented in fibroblasts.[127,132-134] Induction of c-*myc* in mitogen stimulated resting T cells was first described by Kelly et al.[127] in the murine system, and has been observed in human resting T cells upon activation by a mitogen[119,135] and in IL-2-dependent cells either from human[135] or mouse origin.[136,137] These observations have been extended to cerebrospinal fluid (CSF)-dependent myeloid cell lines,[128,129] thymocytes,[138] and B lymphocytes activated by B cell-specific mitogens.[127] In all these systems, activation signals induced the rapid expression of

TABLE 3
Comparison of the Effects of Physiological (Growth Factors) and Pharmacological (Protein Kinase Agonist) Ligands on Nuclear Protooncogene Modulation in Synchronized, Early G_1 Blocked Cells

		GF[a]	PKC	PKA	GF + PKC	GF + PKA	PKC + PKA
CSF	c-fos	+[b]	+	+	+	+ +	+ + + +
	c-myc	+ + + +	+ +	−	+ + + +	+ +	+
IL-2	c-fos	+		+		+ +	
	c-myc	+ + + +		−		+ / −	
	c-myb	+ + +		+ +		+ +	

a   GF = growth factor; PKC = activation of protein kinase C by PMA; PKA = activation of protein kinase A by 8-Br-cAMP.

b   The number of + indicates the level of mature message detected on Northern blot performed using standard procedures.

c-*fos* and c-*myc*. Induction of c-*fos* occurred within minutes and was very transient, returning to undetectable levels after 1 h of contact with the activating molecule. c-*myc* transcript also appeared very rapidly, but continued to accumulate with a peak around 6 h after stimulation. c-*myc* and p53 messages were also induced, although at later time points.[119,139] Nuclear protooncogene induction seems, therefore, to be a common feature in mitogen as well as lymphokine activation.

XIII. INTRACYTOPLASMIC SIGNALS RESPONSIBLE FOR GENE MODULATION BY LYMPHOKINES

The intracytoplasmic biochemical pathways which transduce the activation signal from the membrane to the nucleus and induce the modulation of gene expression are now the object of numerous studies. Results on the involvement of protein kinases are summarized in Table 3. PMA, a pharmacological activator of PKC, has recently been show to induce steady-state levels of IL-2[140] and IL-2 receptor α[141,142] messages in resting human T cells. PMA is also able to induce c-*fos* and c-*myc* in resting normal PBL,[127,135,143] in thymocytes[138] in quiescent (growth factor deprived) IL-2 dependent cell lines[136] and CSF-dependent myeloid cell lines,[129] as well as in serum-deprived fibroblasts.[144,145] In fibroblasts, PMA triggers the expression of the same genes as PDGF.[146] These results strongly suggest the participation of PKC in induction of these messages. However, several lines of evidence suggest that PKC is not the only enzymatic activity involved in this induction. In fibroblasts apparently deprived of PKC activity by a long exposure to PMA, growth factors are still able to induce a low level of proliferation[147] as well as c-*fos* and c-*myc*[146] messages. Experiments to address this question in lymphoid or myeloid cells are now in progress, but it is clear that PKC activation by the usual dosages of PMA does not result in levels of induction of c-*myc* steady-state levels comparable to those observed with growth factors. Pharmacological activation of the cAMP dependent PKA, another unique kinase employed to internally transduce signals by several hormones,[148] exerts a strong antiproliferative effect in lymphokine dependent cell lines. Nevertheless, 8-Br-cAMP was able to induce a c-*fos* message to levels comparable to those observed with growth factors in IL-2-dependent[169] and CSF-dependent[129] murine cell lines. 8-Br-cAMP, when added together with the growth factor, was able to superinduce steady-state levels of c-*fos* mRNA. 8-Br-cAMP was also able to induce IL-2 receptor α and c-*myc* message in IL-2 dependent T cell lines. In contrast, 8-Br-cAMP was not able to induce c-*myc* by itself in either system, and in fact, inhibited the growth factor induced c-*myc* message in both systems. This observation indicates that although c-*fos* and c-*myc* are always induced together by growth factors, the intracellular pathways resulting in c-*fos* and c-*myc* steady-state mRNAs induction may be different. Alternate pathways for c-*fos* and c-*myc* induction could include ionic signals. It has been shown that c-*fos* can be induced through a potassium channel[150] or through a Ca^{2+} channel[143] agonist. Tyrosine kinases could also play a role in this activation pathway. Addition of IL-2 to quiescent (blocked in early G_1 phase) IL-2-dependent murine T cell lines induces the phosphorylation of a set of proteins which are not phosphorylated by pharmacological activation of PKC using PMA.[151]

The use of "nuclear run off", a recently developed technique allowing measurement of the actual rate of transcription of a specific gene, has clearly shown that in lymphoid and myeloid cell lines,[120,152] as well as in quiescent fibroblasts,[133] the transcription of c-*fos*, c-*myc*, and c-*myb* genes was activated within minutes by the addition of growth factors. This transcriptional activation was also observed for IL-2, IL-2 receptor α, and γ-interferon genes in resting human PBL upon activation by PHA.[120] Transcriptional activation is regulated in eukaryotic genes at the level of the 5' flanking region of the genes, where *cis*-regulatory elements (enhancers) bind transactivating proteins. The 5' flanking regions of IL-2, IL-2 receptor α, and γ-interferon genes seem to share a consensus sequence,[153] which could account for their tissue specificity demonstrated at the transcriptional level, at least for interferon.[154] Several lines of evidence indicated that they can also be activated independently, indicating the existence of other regulatory elements, specific for each gene.

The "missing link" between cytoplasmic activation of PKC and transcriptional activation of specific genes could include the phosphorylation of DNA-binding transactivating proteins by PKC itself or by a substrate of this enzyme. Such a phosphorylation is suspected in the regulatory process of immunoglobulin genes. Transcriptional initiation is not the only step where gene expression is regulated. For example, in the case of c-*myc* gene, a block to elongation of the transcript seems to be responsible for the disappearance of mature c-*myc* in differentiating, growth arrested, myelomonocytic human cell lines,[155] Superinduction of IL-2 mRNA,[122] c-*fos*, or c-*myc* messages[156,119,183] in the presence of inhibitors of protein synthesis such as cycloheximide is currently explained by stabilization of the mature message,[132] since cycloheximide does not enhance the rate of transcription of these genes.[120] In fact, c-*fos* and c-*myc* messages both have interesting structural properties in regard to stability of the message.[157,158]

Interestingly, cycloheximide, contrary to its effects on c-*fos* and c-*myc*, inhibits the induction of the late activated genes c-*myb*, N-*ras*, and the transferrin receptor in PHA activated human PBL.[120] Nuclear run-off analysis has shown that at least for the transferrin receptor, this inhibition occurs at the level of gene transcription.[120] This indicates that the transcriptional activation of these "late phase" genes necessitates the synthesis of a protein encoded by one or the other of the "early" genes.

XIV. STUDIES ON THE FUNCTION OF c-*myc* PROTEIN

Due to the universal, early, tightly regulated expression and nuclear localization of their products, nuclear protooncogenes are thought to be part of the cellular proliferation control system; however, the functional role of these proteins is unclear. Although c-*myc* protein expression is a common feature of cells progressing in G_1 phase toward the S phase, c-*myc* expression is not restricted to actively proliferating cells. In fact, resting human T lymphocytes stimulated by PHA express c-*myc* after 30 min of stimulation. At this point, no IL-2 is available in the medium and the S phase does not occur until 2 d later. c-*myc* has also been shown to be induced by EGF in fibroblasts (A431 cell subclones), whether EGF induces or blocks the proliferation of the subclone.[159] c-*myc* is also induced by differentiating agents which exert an antiproliferative effect in B cell lines.[160] A strict correlation between c-*myc*

TABLE 4
Effect of Microinjection of Anti-c-*myc* Protein Antibodies on IL-2-Induced Thymidine Incorporation by Murine IL-2-Dependent T cell CTB6

Antibodies microinjected	IL-2 activation	% of labeled nuclei
−	−	8
−	+	54
Anti-c-*myc*	+	5
OKT4	+	22

Note: CTB6 cells were synchronized in early G_1 by IL-2 deprivation overnight, allowed to adhere on Cell-Tak (Biopolymers, Inc.) treated coverslip, and microinjected with anti-c-*myc* affinity purified rabbit polyclonal antibodies (Oncor) (1 mg/ml) or OKT 4 monoclonal antibody (Ortho) (1 mg/ml). Immediately after microinjections, coverslips were transferred in medium containing 100 U/ml of recombinant IL-2 (Cetus) (+) or no IL-2 (−) and thymidine was added simultaneously (120 Ci/mmol, Amersham). After 18 h, coverslips were washed and processed for autoradiography.

expression and proliferation is therefore not established. To our knowledge, there are very few studies on the functional role of c-*myc* protein. It is known to be a nuclear protein[161-163] and is suspected to be a DNA-binding protein.[164] c-*myc* protein could be involved in the DNA synthesis process, since antibodies directed against the protein seems to inhibit DNA replication and not RNA transcription in isolated nuclei.[165]

The situation for c-*fos* is even more controversial. Although c-*fos* is induced by proliferative signals and constitutive expression of c-*fos* protein can commit a cell to transformation,[166] c-*fos* expression has often been associated with differentiation rather than with proliferation.[156,166-168] In fact, c-*fos* message can be induced, or even superinduced, by antiproliferative signals, such as 8-Br-cAMP, a pharmacological activator of PKA.[129,159] To our knowledge, no study addressing the question of c-*fos* function has been performed, although it has been proposed that c-*fos* protein may modulate the transcription of other genes.

An obvious way to demonstrate the involvement of a protein in a process is to specifically block its function and demonstrate that the blockade inhibits the studied process. This method has been widely employed in the study of metabolic pathways in prokaryotic organisms, in which the rapid division rate allows the derivation of deletion or thermosensitive mutants. Unfortunately, this technology is hardly applicable to eukaryotic cells. Following are the results of experiments designed to specifically block the expression of nuclear protooncogenes and to study the effect of such an inhibition on cellular proliferation.

XV. MICROINJECTION OF ANTI-c-*myc* ANTIBODIES

Cells from a murine IL-2-dependent cell line (CTB6) were blocked in the G_1 phase of the cell cycle by IL-2 deprivation and microinjected with identical volumes of an anti-c-*myc* protein antibody or anti-T4 (OKT 4) antibody as a control. IL-2 was then added to the cultures which were simultaneously ³H-thymidine pulsed and subsequently autoradiographed in order to monitor their ability to synthesize DNA. Results of such an experiment are shown in Table 4. In nonmicroinjected cells, 54% of the nuclei were labeled in the presence of IL-2, whereas only 8% of the nuclei were positive when IL-2 was omitted. In IL-2-stimulated cells microinjected with anti-c-*myc* antibodies, only 5% of the nuclei were labeled. When anti-T4 antibodies were used as a control, such a drastic drop in the percent of labeled nuclei was not observed, since 22% of the nuclei were still able to incorporate ³H-thymidine. (The decrease of positive nuclei in these microinjected control cells most probably correspond to a nonspecific effect of microinjection by itself.) The result of this experiment suggests that c-*myc* protein is necessary for the entry in S phase.

XVI. INHIBITION OF c-*myc* PROTEIN BIOSYNTHESIS BY ANTISENSE OLIGONUCLEOTIDES

A new approach to achieve the specific inhibition of protein function has recently arisen from studies of gene regulation in the bacteria. The Ompc gene expression, for example, is regulated (at least in part) by the physiological transcription of "antisense" RNA, which is transcribed from the complementary noncoding strand of the gene. The antisense RNA is believed to block the expression of the gene by hybridizing with the normal message *in situ* and preventing its translation into polypeptide.[169] This discovery prompted the successful trials of artificial inhibition of specific protein synthesis in eukaryotic cells by the introduction of a relevant antisense into the cell.[166,170] As depicted in Figure 5, a convenient way to introduce such antisense RNAs is to transfect the cells with plasmids in which the gene has been flipped in relation to the promoter in such a way that the transcribed strand in the plasmid is the no coding, complementary strand. This technique allows the creation of permanently transfected clones. One of the major caveats of the technique is that a 100-fold excess of the antisense has to be reached in order to achieve a significant inhibition of protein synthesis.[171] The promoter regulating the transcription of the antisense message, therefore, has to be chosen carefully. This technique has, nevertheless, been used to block the expression of an interferon-inducible gene, 2-5A synthetase, showing that the enzymatic activity was necessary to achieve viral protection.[172] When attempting to block genes which are putatively necessary for cell proliferation, the problem is complicated by the fact that the inhibition must be inducible; therefore, one needs potent and stringent inducible promoters. Such a strategy has been successfully employed in fibroblasts by Holt et al.[173] These authors have introduced in NIH-3T3 cells an antisense c-*fos* plasmid under the promoter of the virus MMTV. They have been able to induce the transcription of the antisense message with dexamethasone and have shown that the induction inhibited proliferation. In lymphoid or myeloid cell lines, attempts to use the same strategy are impaired by the fact that the efficiency of transfection is usually very low, combined with the fact that dexamethasone is by itself inhibitory for the proliferation of these cells. For these reasons, we and others have attempted to use synthetic antisense oligonucleotides to block the expression of nuclear protooncogenes. Oligonucleotides have been successfully used to specifically block the expression of viral proteins in virus-infected cells,[174-178] most probably by inhibiting the translation of the message as indicted by *in vitro* studies.[179] Neckers et al.[180] have used a 15 mer oligonucleotide complementary to the very beginning of the second exon of the human c-*myc*. Resting peripheral human T cells were simply incubated with the purified oligomer. These authors have shown that this simple incubation was able to specifically prevent the induction of c-*myc* protein by PHA (no effect was observed on late G_1 phase-induced proteins such as the IL-2 receptor α-chain) and demonstrated that this inhibition prevented the cells from entering S phase. We have extended this observation to IL-2 induced proliferation on IL-2 dependent human T cells using a similar oligonucleotide. We have first shown a time course association of ³²P-labeled oligonucleotide with the cells with a plateau reached at 2 h of incubation (data not shown). Associated radioactivity seemed to be intracellular, as assessed by autoradiography (data not shown). Figure 6 shows a dose-dependent inhibition of IL-2-induced proliferation of synchronized, growth arrested normal human T cells by the addition of antisense oligonucleotide. Such an inhibition was not observed using a control sense-strand oligonucleotide. Figure 6 also shows that the inhibition was more easily achieved on PHA-

133

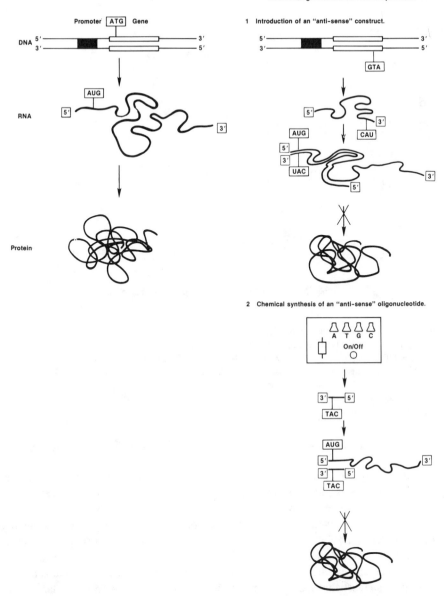

FIGURE 5. Two strategies to specifically block gene expression, using the antisense technology. The left panel of the figure shows the physiological process of gene expression with a schematic view of transcription and transduction. The right panel shows two possible strategies to block specifically the expression of a gene, using the introduction of an antisense plasmid (upper panel) or synthetic deoxyoligonucleotides (lower panel).

induced proliferation of resting T cells than on IL-2-induced proliferation of G_1 blocked T cells.

This technology will help us determine which proteins are really necessary in the proliferation process. Furthermore, it is hoped that it will allow us to elucidate the role of these proteins. The use of chemically modified, and thus rendered nuclease resistant, oligonucleotides could extend the applications to stable constitutive gene products such as protein kinases, for example, making possible the elucidation of intracellular pathways responsible for signal transduction.

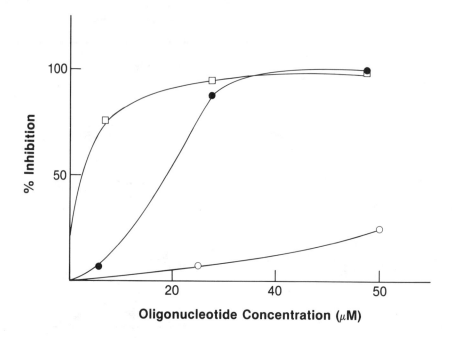

FIGURE 6.   Dose dependent inhibition of thymidine incorporation by antisense c-*myc* 15 mer deoxyoligonucleotide. Human resting peripheral T cells (-□-), or human PHA preactivated IL-2-dependent T lymphoblasts synchronized by a 24-h period of IL-2 deprivation (-●-), were incubated 2 h with the indicated dose of an antisense c-*myc* deoxyoligonucleotide corresponding to the 5′ end of exon 2 (-□-, -●-) or with the corresponding sense oligonucleotide as a control (-○-). IL-2 (recombinant IL-2 from Cetus, 100 U/ml) was added together with ³H-thymidine. Cultures were harvested 18 h later.

XVII. PERSPECTIVES AND SUMMARY

The various aspects of signal transduction and regulation of gene transcription for IL-2 are schematically summarized in Figure 7. Since growth is the universal characteristic of living organisms and its regulation crucial to the propagation and survival of the species, it is not surprising that growth factors and their signal transduction mechanisms are highly conserved. Analysis of genes for insulin, vasopressin, calcitonin, and growth hormone demonstrate that not only are these genes highly conserved and ancient, but they also exhibit evidence of nonallelic evolution, since it is assumed that growth factor mutations are lethal. Studies to date suggest that the biochemical elements of vertebrate intracellular communication originated in unicellular microbes and are highly conserved; evolution changed the anatomy and complexity of regulation of the extracellular signals, but the basic components, i.e., the growth factor and second messengers such as cAMP, remain virtually unchanged.

Particularly striking is the observation that IL-2 stimulates heat shock proteins (HSPs) (Figure 4). The response to heat shock is universal. It has been observed in every organism in which it has been sought, from eubacteria, soybeans, and man. Our demonstration that a growth factor also regulates the expression of HSPs offers the intriguing hypothesis that the process of growth by cellular activation utilizes a set of ancient genes which originated as a response to cellular stress.

Do growth mechanism(s) utilize primitive biochemical processes evolved from stress/shock stimuli? It appears that this is the case. The heat-shock response is found in almost every cell and tissue type of multicellular organism, in explanted tissues, and in cultured cells.[86] The ubiquity of the response and remarkable conservation of some of the genes

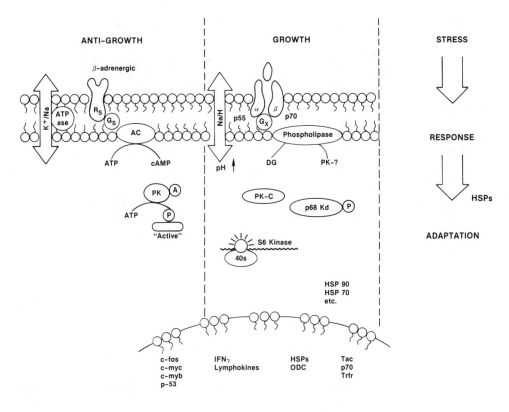

FIGURE 7. Summary of IL-2 signal transduction.

attests to their importance. The relative importance of individual HSPs can be tested with oligonucleotide antisense as we have shown for the c-*myc* gene.

It is noteworthy that recent studies investigating the genomic structures of the IL-2 receptor and interferons have suggested homologous sequence relationships to a number of proteins with diverse biological activity. Extensive protein sequence analysis of the complement proteins, human C2, factor B, and C4BP has been performed. The cDNA coding for all or part of each of the proteins has been cloned and complete amino acid sequences can be predicted for human C2, C4BP, factor B, Cl, and mouse H. On examination of all these sequences it is apparent that each protein contains repeating homology units of approximately 60 amino acids which conform to a consensus sequence having a framework of highly conserved residues. These structurally homologous complement proteins are also functionally related as they all interact with C3b and C4b during the complement activation cascade. The repeating units also occur in unrelated proteins including C1 receptor, β_2 glycoprotein 1, blood clotting factor XIII and the IL-2 receptor.[181] This suggests that the IL-2 receptor may be related to a super-family of structurally related proteins which may have descended from an ancestral 60 amino acid structure.

Interferons have evolved from an extraordinarily ancient antiviral defense used by plants and animals. The postulated ancestral gene would have given rise directly to antiviral factors in plants and γ-interferon in animals in response to continued parasitism by viral particles. Interestingly, the cholera toxin B subunit gene has some remarkable homology with γ-interferon. The family of α-interferons appear to have arisen from the recent amplification of the β-interferon gene.[182] The ancestor of the α- and β-interferon genes may have originally been formed as a processed pseudogene from an mRNA of the intervening sequence containing the γ-interferon gene. During this evolutionary process, α- and β-interferon began to evolve new functions. γ-Interferon, in fact, has functional properties equivalent to IL-1 and can apparently participate in the activation of cytolytic T cells and immunoglobulin secretion.

Clearly, from the brief discourse presented here, a new perspective of the nature of extracellular messengers which regulate the immune response is emerging from information obtained from structure-function studies of biological mediators. Basic information is relatively scarce, limited by phylogenetic sequence information of the regulatory molecules. L-2, a model represented here, utilizes a number of highly conserved biochemical systems by which its receptor communicates with cellular signals. The same biochemical elements are found in prokaryotes. It is not surprising that evolution has maintained remarkable conservation in the chemical nature of the signals and mechanisms of action which control intercellular communication.

Finally, with the efforts of molecular biology, the phylogenetic relationship of proteins with ancestral genes may elucidate fundamental aspects of genetic evolution and the role of pseudogenes in the evolution of protein function and diversity.

REFERENCES

1. **Besterman, J. M., Duronio, V., and Cuatrecasas, P.,** Rapid formation of diacylglycerol from phosphatidylcholine: a pathway for generation of a second messenger, *Proc. Natl. Acad. Sci. U.S.A.,* 83, 6785, 1986.
2. **Burch, R. M., Luini, A., and Axehod, J.,** Phospholipase A_2 and phospholipase C are activated by distinct GTP-binding proteins in response to $\alpha^2$1-adrenergic stimulation in FRTL5 thyroid cells, *Proc. Natl. Acad. Sci. U.S.A.,* 83, 7201, 1986.
3. **Murakami, K., Chan, S. Y., and Routtenberg, A.,** Protein kinase C activation by cis-fatty acid in the absence of Ca^{2+} and phospholipids, *J. Biol. Chem.,* 261, 15424, 1986.
4. **Imboden, J. B. and Stobo, J. D.,** Transmembrane signalling by the T cell antigen receptor, *J. Exp. Med.,* 161, 446, 1985.
5. **Weiss, A., Imboden, J., Shoback, D. and Stobo, J.,** T3-dependent activation results in an increase in cytoplasmic free calcium, *Proc. Natl. Acad. Sci. U.S.A.,* 81, 4169, 1984.
6. **Tsien, R. Y., Pozzan, T., and Rink, T. J.,** T-cell mitogens cause early changes in cytoplasmic free Ca^{2+} and membrane potential in lymphocytes, *Nature,* 295, 68, 1982.
7. **Farrar, W. L. and Ruscetti, F. W.,** Association of protein kinase C activation with IL 2 receptor expression, *J. Immunol.,* 136, 1266, 1986.
8. **Cambier, J. C., Justement, L. B., Newell, M. K., Chen, Z. Z., Harris, L. K., Sandoval, V. M., Klemsa, M. J. and Ransom, J. T.,** Transmembrane signals and intracellular second messengers in the regulation of quiescent B-lymphocyte activation, *Immunol. Rev.,* 95, 37, 1987.
9. **Mills, G. B., Stewart, D. J., Mellors, A., and Gelfand, E. W.,** Interleukin 2 does not induce phosphatidylinositide hydrolysis in T cells: evidence against signalling through phosphatidylinositide hydrolysis, *J. Immunol.,* 136, 3019, 1986.
10. **Bonvini, E., Ruscetti, F. W., Ponzoni, M., Hoffman, T., and Farrar, W. L.,** Interleukin 2 rapidly stimulates synthesis and breakdown of polyphosphoinositides in interleukin-2-dependent murine T-cell lines, *J. Biol. Chem.,* 262, 4160, 1987.
11. **Abrahams, R. T., Ho, S. N., Baina, T. J., and McKean, D. J.,** Transmembrane signalling during interleukin 1-dependent T cell activation, *J. Biol. Chem.,* 262 (6), 2719, 1987.
12. **Justement, L., Chen, Z. Z., Harris, L. K., Ransom, J. T., Sandoval, V. S., Smith, C., Rennick, D., Roehm, N., and Cambier, J.,** BSF1 induces membrane protein phosphorylation but not phosphoinositide metabolism. Ca^{++} mobilization, protein kinase C translocation, or membrane depolarization in resting murine B lymphocytes, *J. Immunol.,* 137, 3664, 1986.
13. **Mills, G. B., Cheung, R. K., Grinstein, S., and Gelfand, E. W.,** Interleukin 2-induced lymphocyte proliferation is independent of increases in cytosolic-free calcium concentrations, *J. Immunol.,* 134, 2431, 1985.
14. **Mills, G. B., Crague, E. J., Gelfund, E. W., and Grinstein, S.,** IL 2 induces a rapid increase in intracellular pH through activation of a Na^+/H^+ anti-port, *J. Biol. Chem.,* 260, 12500, 1984.

15. **Gelfand, E. W., Mills, G. B., Cheung, R. K., Lee, W. W. J., and Grinstein, S.,** Transmembrane ion fluxes during activation of human T lymphocytes: role of Ca^{2+}, Na^+/H^+ exchange and phospholipid turnover, *Immunol. Rev.,* 95, 60, 1987.

16. **L'Allemain, G., Franchi, A., Cragoe, E. J., and Pouyssegur, J.,** Blockade of the Na^+/H^+ antiport abolishes growth factor-induced DNA synthesis in fibroblasts, *J. Biol. Chem.,* 259, 4313, 1984.

17. **Pouyssegur, J., Franchi, A., L'Allemain, G., and Paris, S.,** Cytoplasmic pH, a key determinant of growth factor-induced DNA synthesis in quiescent fibroblasts, *FEBS Lett.,* 190, 115, 1985.

18. **Redondo, J. M., Rivas, A. L., and Fresno, M.,** Activation of the Na^+/K^+-ATPase by interleukin 2, *FEBS Lett.,* 206, 199, 1986.

19. **Collett, M. S., Purchio, A. F., and Erickson, R. L.,** Avian sarcoma virus-transforming protein, pp60[src], shows protein kinase activity specific for tyrosine, *Nature,* 285, 167, 1980.

20. **Kolata, G.,** Is tyrosine the key to growth control?, *Science,* 219, 377, 1983.

21. **Hunter, T.,** The proteins of oncogenes, *Sci. Am.,* V251(2), 70, 1984.

22. **Hunter, T. and Cooper, J. A.,** Protein—tyrosine kinases, *Annu. Rev. Biochem.,* 54, 897, 1985.

23. **Cochet, C., Gill, G. N., Mersenhelder, J., Cooper, J. A., and Hunter, T.,** C-kinase phosphorylates the epidermal growth factor receptor and reduces its epidermal growth factor-stimulated tyrosine protein kinase activity, *J. Biol. Chem.,* 259, 2553, 1984.

24. **Weber, W., Bertics, P. J., and Gill, G. N.,** Immunoaffinity purification of the EGF receptor: stoichiometry of EGF binding and kinetics of self-phosphorylation, *J. Biol. Chem.,* 259, 14631, 1984.

25. **Lee, L.S. and Weinstein, I. B.,** Mechanism of tumor promoter inhibition of cellular binding of epidermal growth factor, *Proc. Natl. Acad. Sci. U.S.A.,* 76, 5168, 1979.

26. **Jacobs, S., Sahyoun, N. E., Saltiel, A. R., and Cuatrecasas, P.,** Phorbol esters stimulate the phosphorylation of receptors for insulin and somatomedin C, *Proc. Natl. Acad. Sci. U.S.A.,* 80, 6211, 1983.

27. **Cantrell, D. A., Davies, A. A., and Crumpton, M. J.,** Activators of protein kinase C down-regulate and phosphorylate the T_3/T-cell antigen receptor complex of human T lymphocytes, *Proc. Natl. Acad. Sci. U.S.A.,* 82, 8158, 1985.

28. **Rakowicz-Szvlczynska, E. M., Rodeck, V., Herlyn, M., and Koprowski, H.,** Chromation binding of epidermal growth factor, nerve growth factor and platelet-derived growth factor in cells bearing the appropriate surface receptors, *Proc. Natl. Acad. Sci. U.S.A.,* 83, 3728, 1986.

29. **Sibley, D. R., Strasser, R. H., Benovic, J. L., Daniel, K., and Lefkowitz, R. J.,** Phosphorylation/dephosphorylation of the β-adrenergic receptor regulates its functional coupling to adenylate cyclase and subcellular distribution, *Proc. Natl. Acad. Sci. U.S.A.,* 83, 9408, 1986.

30. **Radke, K. and Martin, G. S.,** Transformation by Rous sarcoma virus: effects of src gene expression on the synthesis and phosphorylation of cellular polypeptides, *Proc. Natl. Acad. Sci. U.S.A.,* 76, 5212, 1979.

31. **Gilmore, T., Declue, J. E., and Martin, G. S.,** Tyrosine kinase activity associated with the v-erb-b gene product, in *Cancer Cells 3/Growth Factors and Transformation,* Publ. No. 25, Cold Spring Harbor Laboratory, Cold Spring Harbor, NY, 1985, 33.

32. **Hunter, T. and Cooper, J.,** Epidermal growth factor induces rapid tyrosine phosphorylation of proteins in A 431 human tumor cells, *Cell,* 24, 741, 1981.

33. **Cooper, J., Reiss, N., Schwartz, R., and Hunter, T.,** Three glycolytic enzymes are phosphorylated on tyrosine in cells transformed by Rous sarcoma virus, *Nature,* 302, 218, 1983.

34. **Pepinsky, R. B. and Sinclair, L. K.,** Epidermal growth factor dependent phosphorylation of lipocortin, *Nature,* 321, 81, 1986.

35. **Johansen, J. W. and Ingebritsen, T. S.,** Phosphorylation and inactivation of protein phosphatase 1 by pp60[v-src], *Proc. Natl. Acad. Sci. U.S.A.,* 83, 207, 1986.

36. **Zick, Y., Sagi-Eisenberg, R., Pines, M., Giernhick, P., and Spiegel, A. M.,** Multisite phosphorylation of the α subunit of transducin by the insulin receptor kinase and protein kinase C, *Proc. Natl. Acad. Sci. U.S.A.,* 83, 9294, 1986.

37. **Tse-Dinh, Y. C., Wong, T. W., and Goldberg, A. R.,** Viral and cell-encoded tyrosine protein kinases inactivate DNA topoisomerases *in vitro, Nature,* 312, 785, 1984.

38. **Takai, Y., Kishimoto, A., Iwasn, Y., Kavahara, Y., Mori, T., and Nishizuka, Y.,** Calcium-dependent activation of a multifunctional protein kinase by membrane phospholipids, *J. Biol. Chem.,* 254, 3692, 1979.

39. **Nishizuka, Y.,** The role of protein kinase C in cell surface signal transduction and tumor promotion, *Nature,* 308, 693, 1984.

40. **Driedger, P. E. and Blumberg, P. M.,** Specific binding of phorbol ester tumor promoters, *Proc. Natl. Acad. Sci. U.S.A.,* 77, 567, 1980.

41. **Castoyna, M., Takai, Y., Kaibnchi, K., Sano, K., Kikkawa, V., and Nishizuka, Y.,** Direct activation of calcium-activated, phospholipid-dependent protein kinase by tumor-promoting phorbol esters, *J. Biol. Chem.,* 257, 7848, 1982.

42. **Ashendel, C. L., Staller, J. M., and Boutwell, R. K.,** Protein kinase activity associated with a phorbol ester receptor purified from mouse brain, *Cancer Res.,* 43, 4333, 1983.

43. **Niedel, J. E., Kuhn, L. J., and Vanderback, G. R.,** Phorbol diester receptor co-purifies with protein kinase C, *Proc. Natl. Acad. Sci. U.S.A.,* 80, 36, 1983.

44. **Sawyer, S. T. and Cohen, S.,** Enhancement of calcium uptake and phosphatidylinositol turnover by epidermal growth factor in A 431 cells, *Biochemistry,* 20, 6280, 1981.

45. **Farrar, W. L., Thomas, P. T., and Anderson, W. B.,** Altered cytosol/membrane enzyme redistribution on interleukin 3 activation of protein kinase C, *Nature,* 315, 235, 1985.

46. **Farrar, W. L. and Anderson, W. B.,** Interleukin 2 stimulates association of protein kinase C with plasma membrane, *Nature,* 315, 233, 1985.

47. **Shoyab, M., De Larco, J. E., and Todaro, G. J.,** Biologically active phorbol esters specifically alter affinity of epidermal growth factor membrane receptors, *Nature,* 279, 387, 1979.

48. **Salomon, D. S.,** Inhibition of epidermal growth factor binding to mouse embryonal carcinoma cells by phorbol esters mediated by specific phorbol ester receptors, *J. Biol. Chem.,* 256, 7958, 1981.

49. **Iwashita, S. and Fox, C. F.,** Epidermal growth factor and potent phorbol tumor promoters induce epidermal growth factor receptor phosphorylation in a similar but distinctively different manner in human epidermoid carcinoma A 431 cells, *J. Biol. Chem.,* 259, 2559, 1984.

50. **Evans, S. W., Rennick, D., and Farrar, W. L.,** Multilineage hematopoietic growth factor interleukin 3 and direct activators of protein kinase C stimulate phosphorylation of common substrates, *Blood,* 68, 906, 1986.

51. **Ishii, T., Kohno, M., Nakamura, M., Hinuma, Y., and Sugamura, K.,** Characterization of interleukin 2-stimulated phosphorylation of 67 and 63 kDa proteins in human T-cells, *Biochem. J.,* 242, 211, 1987.

52. **Witters, L. A., Vater, C. A., and Lienhard, G. E.,** Phosphorylation of the glucose transporter *in vitro* and *in vivo* by protein kinase C, *Nature,* 315, 27, 1985.

53. **Whetton, A. D., Heyworth, C. M., and Dexter, T. M.,** Phorbol esters activate protein kinase C and glucose transport and can replace the requirement for growth factor in interleukin-3-dependent multipotent stem cells, *J. Cell Sci.,* 84, 93, 1986.

54. **Matsushima, K., Akahoshi, T., and Oppenheim, J. J.,** Phosphorylation of a cytosolic 65 KDa protein in response to interleukin 1 in normal human mononuclear cells preincubated with glucocorticoids, *Fed. Proc.,* 46(3), 767, 1987.

55. **Yeung, Y. G., Jubinsky, P. T., Sengupta, A., Yeung, D. C. Y., and Stanley, E. R.,** Purification of the colony-stimulating factor 1 receptor and demonstration of its tyrosine kinase activity, *Proc. Natl. Acad. Sci. U.S.A.,* 84, 1268, 1987.

56. **Shen, C. J., Rettenmier, C. W., Sscca, R., Roussel, M. F., Look, A. T., and Stanley, E. R.,** The c-fms proto-oncogene product is related to the receptor for the mononuclear phagocyte growth factor CSF-1, *Cell,* 41, 665, 1985.

57. **Gilman, A. G.,** G proteins and dual control of adenylate cyclase, *Cell,* 36, 577, 1984.

58. **Gibbs, J. B., Sigol, I. S., Poe, M., and Scolnick, E. M.,** Intrinsic GTPase activity distinguishes normal and oncogenic ras p21 molecules, *Proc. Natl. Acad. Sci. U.S.A.,* 81, 5704, 1984.

59. **Blackmore, P. F., Bocckino, S. B., Waynick, L. E., and Exton, J. H.,** Role of a guanine nucleotide-binding regulatory protein in the hydrolysis of hepatocyte phosphatidylinositol 4,5-bisphosphate by calcium-mobilizing hormones and the control of cell calcium, *J. Biol. Chem.,* 260(7), 14477, 1985.

60. **Fleischman, L. F., Chahwala, S. B., and Cantley, L.,** Ras-transformation of cells: altered levels of phosphatidylinositol 4,5-bisphosphate and catabolites, *Science,* 231, 407, 1986.

61. **Benjamin, C. W., Tarpley, W. G., and Gorman, R. R.,** Loss of platelet-derived growth factor-stimulated phospholipase activity in NIH-3T3 cells expressing the EJ-ras oncogene, *Proc. Natl. Acad. Sci. U.S.A.,* 84, 546, 1987.

62. **Majerus, P. W., Connolly, T. M., Deckmyn, H., Ross, T. S., Bross, T. E., Ishii, H., Bansal, V. S., and Wilson, D. B.,** The metabolism of phosphoinositide-derived messenger molecules, *Science,* 234, 1519, 1986.

63. **Beckner, S. K. and Farrar, W. L.,** Interleukin 2 modulation of adenylate cyclase: potential role of protein kinase C, *J. Biol. Chem.,* 261(7), 3043, 1986.

64. **Leonard, W. J., Depper, J. M., Crabtree, G. R., Rudikoff, S., Pumphrey, J., Robb, R. J., Krönke, M., Svetlik, P. B., Peffer, N. J., Waldman, T. A., and Greene, W. C.,** Molecular cloning and expression of cDNA for the human interleukin 2 receptor, *Nature,* 311, 623, 1984.

65. **Evans, S. W., Beckner, S. K., and Farrar, W. L.,** Interleukin 2 stimulates specific GTP binding and hydrolysis activities in lymphocyte membrane, *Nature,* 325, 166, 1987.

66. **Farrar, W. L., Cleveland, J. L., Beckner, S. K., Bonvini, E., and Evans, S. W.,** Biochemical and molecular events associated with interleukin 2 regulation of lymphocyte proliferation, *Immunol. Rev.,* 92, 49, 1986.

67. **Thomas, G. J., Martin-Perez, J., Siegmann, M., and Otto, A. M.,** Effect of serum, EGF, PGF$_2\alpha$ and insulin on S6 phosphorylation and the initiation of protein and DNA synthesis, *Cell,* 30, 235, 1982.

68. **Maller, J. L., Foulkes, J. G., Erikson, E., and Baltimore, D.,** Phosphorylation of ribosomal protein S6 on serine after microinjection of the Abelson murine leukemia virus, tyrosine-specific protein kinase into Xenopus oocytes, *Proc. Natl. Acad. Sci. U.S.A.,* 82, 272, 1984.

69. **Habenicht, A. J. R., Glomset, J. A., King, W. C., Nist, C., Mitchell, C. D., and Ross, R.,** Early changes in phosphatidylinositol and arachidonic acid metabolism in quiescent Swiss 3T3 cells stimulated to divide by platelet-derived growth factor, *J. Biol. Chem.,* 256, 12329, 1981.

70. **Rozengurt, E., Rodriguez-Pena, M. and Smith, K. H.,** Phorbol esters, phospholipase C, and growth factors rapidly stimulate the phosphorylation of a M_r 80,000 protein in intact quiescent 3T3 cells, *Proc. Natl. Acad. Sci. U.S.A.,* 80, 7244, 1983.

71. **Collins, M. K. L., Sinnett-Smith, J. W., and Rozengurt, E.,** Platelet-derived growth factor treatment decreases the affinity of the epidermal growth factor treatment decreases the affinity of the epidermal growth factor receptors of Swiss 3T3 cells, *J. Biol. Chem.,* 258, 11689, 1983.

72. **Suginoto, Y., Whitman, M., Cantley, L. C., and Erikson, R. L.,** Evidence that the Rous sarcoma virus transforming gene product phosphorylates phosphatidylinositol and diacylglycerol, *Proc. Natl. Acad. Sci. U.S.A.,* 81, 2117, 1984.

73. **Blenis, J., Spivack, J. G., and Erikson, R. L.,** Phorbol ester, serum and Rous sarcoma virus transforming gene product induce similar phosphorylations of ribosomal protein S6, *Proc. Natl. Acad. Sci. U.S.A.,* 81, 6408, 1984.

74. **Novak-Hofer, I. and Thomas G.,** An activated S6 kinase in extracts from serum and epidermal growth factor-stimulated Swiss 3T3 cells, *J. Biol. Chem.,* 259, 5995, 1984.

75. **Marrack, P. and Kappler, J.,** The antigen-specific, major histocompatibility complex-restricted receptor on T cells, *Adv. Immunol.,* 38(1), 30, 1986.

76. **Samelson, L. E., Patel, M. D., Weissman, A. M., Harford, J. B., and Klausner, R. D.,** Antigen activation of murine T cells induces tyrosine phosphorylation of a polypeptide associated with the T cell antigen receptor, *Cell,* 46, 1083, 1986.

77. **Reinherz, E. L., Meuer, S., Fitzgerald, K. A., Hussey, R. E., Levine, H., and Schlossman, S.,** Antigen recognition by human T lymphocytes is linked to surface expression of the T3 molecular complex, *Cell,* 30, 735, 1982.

78. **Meuer, S. C., Fitzgerald, K. A., Hussey, R. E., Hodgdon, J. C., Schlossman, S., and Reinherz, E. L.,** Clonotypic structures involved in antigen-specific human T cell function, *J. Exp. Med.,* 157, 705, 1983.

79. **Zanders, E. Lamb, J., Feldman, M., Green, N., and Beverley, P.,** Tolerance of T-cell clones is associated with membrane antigen changes, *Nature,* 303, 625, 1983.

80. **Truneh, A., Albert, F., Goldstein, P., and Schmitt-Verhulst, A. M.,** Early steps of lymphocyte activation bypassed by synergy between calcium ionophores and phorbol ester, *Nature,* 313, 318, 1985.

81. **Ando, I., Hariri, G., and Wallace, D.,** Tumor promoter phorbol esters induce unresponsiveness to antigen and expression of interleukin 2 receptor on T cells, *Eur. J. Immunol.,* 15, 196, 1985.

82. **Samelson, L. E., Harford, J., Schwartz, R. H., and Klausner, R. D.,** A 20-kDa protein associated with the murine T-cell antigen receptor is phosphorylated in response to activation by antigen or by concanavalin A, *Proc. Natl. Acad. Sci. U.S.A.,* 82, 1969, 1985.

83. **Samelson, L. E., Davidson, W. F., Morse, H. C., III, and Klausner, R. D.,** Abnormal tyrosine phosphorylation on T-cell receptor in lymphoproliferative disorders, *Nature,* 324, 18, 1986.

84. **Ledbetter, J. A., Gentry, L. E., June, C. H., Rabinovitch, P.S., and Purchio, A. F.,** Stimulation of T cells through the CD3-T-cell receptor complex: role of cytoplasmic calcium, protein kinase C translocation, and phosphorylation of pp60[c-src] in the activation pathway, *Mol. Cell. Biol.,* 7, 650, 1987.

85. **Lanks, K. W.,** Modulators of the eukaryotic heat shock response, *Exp. Cell Res.,* 165, 1, 10, 1986.

86. **Subjeck, J. R. and Shyy, T.-T.,** Stress protein systems of mammalian cells, *Am. J. Physiol.,* 250(C1), C17, 1986.

87. **Lowe, D. G., Fulford, W. D., and Moran, L. A.,** Mouse and *Drosophila* genes encoding the major heat shock protein (hsp70) are highly conserved, *Mol. Cell. Biol.,* 3, 1540, 1983.

88. **Hunt, C. and Morimoto, R. J.,** Conserved features of eukaryotic *hsp70* genes revealed by comparison with the nucleotide sequence of human hsp70, *Proc. Natl. Acad. Sci. U.S.A.,* 82, 6455, 1985.

89. **Wu, B., Hunt, C., and Morimoto, R.,** Structure and expression of the human gene encoding major heat shock protein HSP70, *Mol. Cell. Biol.,* 5, 330, 1985.

90. **Wu, B. J. and Morimoto, R. I.,** Transcription of the human *hsp70* gene is induced by serum stimulation, *Proc. Natl. Acad. Sci. U.S.A.,* 82, 6070, 1985.

91. **Welch, W. J. and Feramisco, J. R.,** Nuclear and nucleolar localization of the 72,000-dalton heat shock protein in heat-shocked mammalian cells, *J. Biol. Chem.,* 259, 4501, 1984.

92. **Milarski, K. L. and Morimoto, R. I.,** Expression of human HSP70 during the synthetic phase of the cell cycle, *Proc. Natl. Acad. Sci. U.S.A.,* 83, 9517, 1986.

93. **Wu, B. J., Hurst, H. C., Jones, N. C., and Morimoto, R. I.,** The E1A 13S product of adenovirus 5 activates transcription of the cellular human HSP70 gene, *Mol. Cell. Biol.,* 6, 2994, 1986.

94. **Cohen, S., Vshiro, H., Stoscheck, C., and Chinkers, M.,** A native 170,000 epidermal growth factor receptor-kinase complex from shed plasma membrane vesicles, *J. Biol. Chem.,* 257, 1523, 1982.

95. **Frackelton, A. E., Tremble, P. M., and Williams, L. T.,** Evidence for the platelet-derived growth factor-stimulated tyrosine phosphorylation of the platelet-derived growth factor receptor, *in vivo, J. Biol. Chem.,* 259, 7909, 1984.

96. **Petruzzelli, L., Herrera, R., and Rosen, O. M.,** Insulin receptor is an insulin-dependent tyrosine protein kinase: co-purification of insulin binding and protein kinase activities to homogeneity from human placenta, *Proc. Natl. Acad. Sci. U.S.A.,* 81, 3327, 1984.

97. **Green, S. H. and Greens, L. A.,** A single M_r ~103,000 ^{125}I-β-nerve growth factor-affinity-labeled species represents both the low and high affinity forms of the nerve growth factor receptor, *J. Biol. Chem.,* 261, 15316, 1986.

98. **Jacobs, S., Kull, F. C., Jr., Earp, H. S., Svoboda, M. E., Van Wyk, J. J., and Cuatrecasas, P.,** Somatomedin-C stimulates the phosphorylation of the β-subunit of its own receptor, *J. Biol. Chem.,* 258(16), 4581, 1983.

99. **Cirillo, D. M., Guadino, G., Naldini, L., and Comoglio, P. M.,** Receptor for bombesin and associated tyrosine kinase activity, *Mol. Cell. Biol.,* 6, 4641, 1986.

100. **Clark, S. C. and Kamen, R.,** The human hematopoietic colony-stimulating factors, *Science,* 236, 1229, 1987.

101. **Walker, F. and Burgess, A. W.,** Specific binding of radioiodinated granulocyte-macrophage colony-stimulating factor to hemopoietic cells, *EMBO J.,* 4, 933, 1985.

102. **Shen, C. J., Rettenmier, C. W., Sacca, R., Roussel, M. F., Look, A. T., and Stanley, E. R.,** The c-fms proto-oncogene product is related to the receptor for the mononuclear phagocyte growth factor CSF-1, *Cell,* 41, 665, 1985.

103. **Morgan, C. J. and Stanley, E. R.,** Chemical cross-linking of the mononuclear phagocyte-specific growth factor CSF-1 to its receptor at the cell surface, *Biochem. Biophys. Res. Commun.,* 119, 35, 1984.

104. **Smith, K. A.,** T cell growth factor, *Immunol. Rev.,* 51, 337, 1981.

105. **Taniguchi, T., Matsui, H., Fujita, T., Takaoka, C., Kashima, N., Yoshimoto, R., and Hamuro, J.,** Structure and expression of a cloned cDNA for human interleukin 2, *Nature,* 302, 1983.

106. **Devos, R. and Plaetinck, G.,** Molecular cloning of human interleukin 2 cDNA and its expression in *E. coli, Nucl. Acids Res.,* 11, 4307, 1983.

107. **Yokota, T., Arai, N., Alle, F., Rennick, D., Mosman, T., and Arai, K.,** Isolation of a mouse Interleukin 2 cDNA clone that expresses T cell growth factor activity after transfection of monkey cells; use of cDNA expression vector for identifying T cell derived lymphokine gene, *Lymphokine Res.,* 3, 283, 1984.

108. **Holbrook, N. J., Smith, K. A., Fornace, A. J., Comeau, C. M., Wiskocil, R. L., and Crabtree, G. R.,** T cell growth factor: complete nucleotide sequence and organization of the gene in normal and malignant cells, *Proc. Natl. Acad. Sci. U.S.A.,* 81, 1634, 1984.

109. **Nakaido, T., Shimizu, N., Ishida, N., Sabe, H., Teshigawara, K., Maeda, M., Uchiyama, T., Yodoi, J., and Honjo, T.,** Molecular cloning of cDNA encoding human IL 2 receptor, *Nature,* 311, 623, 1984.

110. **Cosman, D., Ceretti, D. P., Larsen, A., Park, L., March, C., Dower, S., Gillis, S., and Urdal, D.,** Cloning, sequence and expression of human interleukin 2 receptor, *Nature,* 321, 768, 1984.

111. **Shimizu, A., Kondo, S., Takeda, S., Diamantstein, T., Nikaido, T., and Honjo, T.,** Nucleotide sequence of mouse interleukin 2 receptor cDNA and its comparison with the human interleukin 2 receptor sequence, *Nucl. Acids. Res.,* 13, 1505, 1985.

112. **Miller, J., Malek, T. R., Leonard, W. J., Greene, W. C., Shevach, E. M., and Germain, J. I.,** Nucleotide sequence and expression of a mouse interleukin 2 receptor cDNA, *J. Immunol.,* 134, 4212, 1985.

113. **Ishida, N., Kanamori, M., Noma, T., Nikaido, T., Sabe, H., Suzuki, N., Shimizu, A., and Honjo, T.,** Molecular cloning and structure of the human interleukin 2 receptor gene, *Nucl. Acids. Res.,* 13, 7579, 1985.

114. **Greene, W. C., Robb, R. J., Svetlik, P. B., Rusk, C. M., Depper, J. M., and Leonard, W. J.,** Stable expression of cDNA encoding the human interleukin 2 receptor in eukaryotic cells, *J. Exp. Med.,* 162, 363, 1985.

115. **Robb, R. J. and Greene, W. C.,** Direct demonstration of the identity of T cell growth factor binding protein and the Tac antigen, *J. Exp. Med.,* 158, 1332, 1983.

116. **Sharon, M., Klausner, R. D., Cullen, B. R., Chizzonite, R., and Leonard, W. J.,** Novel interleukin 2 subunit detected by cross-linking under high affinity conditions, *Science,* 234, 859, 1986.

117. **Robb, R. J., Rusk, C. M., Yodoi, J., and Greene, W.C.,** Interleukin 2 binding molecule distinct from the Tac protein: analysis of its role in formation of high affinity receptors, *Proc. Natl. Acad. Sci. U.S.A.,* 84, 2002, 1987.

118. **Teshigawara, K., Wang, H. M., Kato, K., and Smith, K. A.,** Interleukin 2 high-affinity receptor expression requires two distinct binding proteins, *J. Exp. Med.,* 165, 223, 1987.

119. **Reed, J. C., Alpers, J. D., Nowell, P. C., and Hoover, R. G.,** Sequential expression of proto-oncogenes during lectin stimulated mitogenesis of normal human lymphocytes, *Proc. Natl. Acad. Sci. U.S.A.,* 83, 3982, 1986.

120. **Krönke, M., Leonard, W. J., Depper, J. M., and Greene, W. C.,** Sequential expression of genes involved in human T lymphocytes growth and differentiation, *J. Exp. Med.,* 161, 1593, 1985.

121. **Efrat, S., Pilo, S., and Kaempfer, R.,** Kinetics of induction and molecular size of mRNAs encoding human interleukin 2 and γ interferon, *Nature,* 297, 236, 1982.

122. **Efrat, S. and Kaempfer, R.,** Control of biologically active interleukin 2 messenger RNA formation in induced human lymphocytes, *Proc. Natl. Acad. Sci. U.S.A.,* 9, 2601, 1984b.

123. **Welte, K., Andreef, M., Platzer, E., Holloway, B. Y., Rubin, M. A., Moore, S., and Mertelsmann, R.,** Interleukin 2 regulates the expression of TAC antigen on peripheral blood T lymphocytes, *J. Exp. Med.,* 60, 1390, 1984.

124. **Smith, K. A. and Cantrell, D. A.,** Interleukin 2 regulates its own receptor, *Proc. Natl. Acad. Sci. U.S.A.,* 82, 864, 1985.

125. **Depper, J. M., Leonard, W. J., Drogula, M., Krönke, M., Waldmann, T. A., and Greene, W. C.,** Interleukin 2 (IL 2) augments transcription of IL 2 receptor gene, *Proc. Natl. Acad. Sci. U.S.A.,* 82, 4230, 1985.

126. **Harel-Bellan, A., Bertoglio, J., Quillet, A., Marchiol. C., Wakazugi, H., Mishall, Z., and Fradelizi, D.,** Interleukin 2 (IL 2) up regulates its own receptor on a subset of human unprimed peripheral blood lymphocytes and triggers their proliferation, *J. Immunol.,* 136, 2463, 1986.

127. **Kelly, K., Cochran, B. H., Stiles, C. C., and Leder, P.,** Cell specific regulation of the c-*myc* gene by lymphocyte mitogenes and PDGF, *Cell,* 35, 603, 1983.

128. **Conscience, J. F., Verrier, B., and Martin, G.,** Interleukin 3 dependent expression of the c-*fos* and c-*myc* proto-oncogenes in hemopoietic cell lines, *EMBO J.,* 5, 317, 1986.

129. **Harel-Bellan, A. and Farrar, W. L.,** Modulation of proto-oncogene expression by colony stimulating factors and activators of protein kinase in murine myeloid cell lines, *J. Cell Biochem.,* 38, 145, 1988.

130. **Bishop, J. M.,** Viral oncogenes, *Cell,* 42, 23, 1985.

131. **Sherr, C. J., Rettenmier, C. W., Sacca, R., Roussel, M. F., Look, A. T. and Stanley, E. R.,** The c-*fms* proto-oncogene is related to the receptor for the mononuclear phagocyte growth factor, CSF_1, *Cell,* 41, 665, 1985.

132. **Kruijer, W., Cooper, J. A., Hunter, T., and Verma, I. M.,** Platelet-derived growth factor induces rapid but transient expression of the c-*fos* gene and protein, *Nature,* 312, 711, 1984.

133. **Greenberg, M. E. and Ziff, E. B.,** Stimulation of 3T3 cells induces transcription of c-*fos* proto-oncogene, *Nature,* 311, 433, 1984.

134. **Müller, R., Bravo, R., Burckhardt, J., and Curran, T.,** Induction of c-*fos* gene and protein by growth factors precedes activation of c-*myc*, *Nature,* 312, 716, 1984.

135. **Reed, J. C., Nowell, P. C., and Hoover, R. G.,** Regulation of c-*myc* mRNA levels in normal human lymphocytes by modulators of cell proliferation, *Proc. Natl. Acad. Sci. U.S.A.,* 82, 4221, 1985.

136. **Reed, J. C., Sabbath, D. E., Hoover, R. G., and Preystowski, M. B.,** Recombinant interleukin 2 regulates level of c-*myc* mRNA in a cloned murine T lymphocyte, *Mol. Cell. Biol.,* 5, 3361, 1985.

137. **Cleveland, J. L., Rapp, U. R., and Farrar, W. L.,** IL 2 regulated growth of cytotoxic T lymphocytes: role of c-*myc* and oncogenes in normal cells in their malignant variants, *J. Immunol.,* 138, 3495, 1987.

138. **Moore, J. P., Todd, J. A., Hesketh, T. R., and Metcalfe, J. C.,** c-*fos* and c-*myc* gene activation, ionic signals, and DNA synthesis in thymocytes, *J. Biol. Chem.,* 261, 8158, 1986.

139. **Stern, J. B. and Smith, K. A.,** Interleukin 2 induction of T cell G_1 progression and c-*myc* expression, *Science,* 233, 203, 1986.

140. **Farrar, J. J., Benjamin, W. K., Hilfiker, M. L., Howard, M., Farrar, W. L., and Fuller-Farrar, J.,** The biochemistry, biology and role of IL 2 in the induction of cytotoxic T cell and antibody forming cell response, *Immunol. Rev.,* 63, 129, 166, 1982.

141. **Shakelford, D.A. and Trowbridge, I. S.,** Induction of expression and phosphorylation of the human interleukin 2 receptor by a phorbol ester, *J. Biol. Chem.,* 259, 11706, 1984.

142. **Depper, J. M., Leonard, W. J., Krönke, M., Naguchi, D., Cunningham, R. E., Waldmann, T. A., and Greene, W. C.,** Regulation of interleukin 2 receptor expression: effects of phorbol ester, phospholipase C and reexposure to lectin or antigen, *J. Immunol.,* 133, 3054, 1984.

143. **Grausz, J. D., Fradelizi, D., Dautry, F., Monier, R., and Lehn, P.,** Modulation of c-*fos* and c-*myc* mRNA levels in normal human lymphocytes by calcium ionophore A 23187 and phorbol ester, *Eur. J. Immunol.,* 16, 1217, 1986.

144. **Coughlin, S. R., Lee, W. M. F., Williams, P. W., Giels, G. M., and Williams, L. T.,** c-*myc* gene expression is activated by agents that activate protein kinase C and does not account for the mitogenic effect of PDGF, *Cell,* 43, 243, 1985.

145. **McCaffrey, P., Ran, W., Campisi, J., and Rosner, M. R.,** Two independent growth factor generated signals regulate c-*fos* and c-*myc* mRNA level in Swiss 3T3 cells, *J. Biol. Chem.,* 262, 1442, 1987.

146. **Rabin, M. S., Doherty, P. J., and Gottesman, M. M.,** The tumor promoter phorbol-12-myristate 13 acetate induces a program of altered gene expression similar to that reduced by platelet derived growth factor and transforming oncogenes, *Proc. Natl. Acad. Sci. U.S.A.,* 83, 357, 1986.

147. **Pasti, G., Lacal, J. C., Warren, B. S., Aaronson, S. A., and Blumberg, P. M.,** Loss of mouse fibroblast cell response to phorbol esters restored by microinjected protein kinase C, *Nature,* 324, 375, 1986.

148. **Berridge, M. J.,** Inositol tris phosphate and diacylglycerol as second messengers, *Biochem. J.,* 220, 345, 1984.

149. **Farrar, W. L., Evans, S. W., Rapp, V. R., and Cleveland, J. L.,** Effect of anti-proliferative cyclic AMP on interleukin 2 stimulated gene expression, *J. Immunol.,* 139, 2075, 1987.

150. **Morgan, J. I. and Curran, T.,** Role of ion flux in the control of c-*fos* expression, *Nature,* 321, 702, 1986.

151. **Evans, S. W., Rennick, D., and Farrar, W. L.,** Identification of a signal transduction pathway shared by haematopoetic growth factors with diverse biological activity, *Biochem. J.,* 244, 683, 1987.

152. **Farrar, W. L., Evans, S. W., Ruscetti, F. W., Bonvini, E., Young, H., and Birchenall-Sparks, M.,** Biochemical and molecular events associated with interleukin 2 regulation of lymphocyte proliferation, in *Leukocyte in Host Defense,* Oppenheim, J. J. and Jacobs, D., eds., 1986, 49.

153. **Fujita, T., Shibuya, H., Ohashi, T., Yamanishi, K., and Taniguchi, T.,** Regulation of human interleukin 2 gene: functional DNA sequences in the 5' flanking region for the gene expression in activated T lymphocytes, *Cell,* 46, 401, 1986.

154. **Young, H. A., Dray, J. F., and Farrar, W. L.,** Expression of transfected human interferon γ DNA: evidence for cell specific regulation, *J. Immunol.,* 136, 4700, 1986.

155. **Bentley, D. L. and Groudine, M.,** A block to elongation is largely responsible for decreased transcription of c-*myc* in differentiated HL 60 cells, *Nature,* 321, 702, 1986.

156. **Müller, R. and Wagner, E. F.,** Differentiation of F9 teratocarcinoma stem cells after transfer of c-*fos* proto-oncogene, *Nature,* 311, 438, 1984.

157. **Rabbits, P. H., Forster, A., Stinson, M. A., and Rabbits, T. H.,** Truncation of exon 1 from the c-*myc*, gene results in prolonged c-*myc* mRNA stability, *EMBO J.,* 4, 3727, 1985.

158. **Miller, A. D., Curran, T., and Verma, I. M.,** c-*fos* protein can induce cellular transformation: a novel mechanism of activation of a cellular oncogene, *Cell,* 36, 51, 1984.

159. **Bravo, R., Burckhardt, J., Curran, T., and Müller, R.,** Stimulation and inhibition of growth by EGF in different A 631 cell clones is accompanied by the rapid induction of c-*fos* and c-*myc* protooncogenes, *EMBO J.,* 4, 1193, 1985.

160. **Larsson, L. G., Gray, H. E., Totterman, T., Peterson, U., and Nilson, K.,** Drastically increased expression of *myc* and *fos* proto-oncogenes during *in vitro* differentiation of chronic lymphocytic leukemia cells, *Proc. Natl. Acad. Sci. U.S.A.,* 84, 223, 1987.

161. **Eisenman, R. N., Tachibana, C. Y., Abrams, H. D., and Hann, S. R.,** V-*myc* and c-*myc* encoded proteins are associated with the nuclear matrix, *Mol. Cell. Biol.,* 5, 114, 1985.

162. **Evan, G. I. and Hancock, D. C.,** Studies on the interaction of the human c-*myc* protein with cell nuclei p62 c-*myc* as a member of a discrete subset of nuclear proteins, *Cell,* 43, 253, 1985.

163. **Persson, H., Gray, H. E., Godeau, F., Braunhut, S., and Bellvè,** Multiple growth-associated nuclear proteins immunoprecipitated by antisera raised against human c-*myc* peptide antigens, *Mol. Cell. Biol.,* 6, 942, 1986.

164. **Watt, R. A., Shatzman, A. R., and Rosenberg, M.,** Expression and characterization of the human c-*myc* DNA binding protein, *J. Mol. Cell. Biol.,* 5, 448, 1985.

165. **Studzinski, G. P., Brelvi, Z. S., Feldman, S. C., and Watt, R. A.,** Participation of c-*myc* protein in DNA synthesis of human cells, *Science,* 234, 467, 1986.

166. **Curran, T. and Morgan, J. I.,** Superinduction of c-*fos* by nerve growth factor in the presence of peripherally active benzodiazepines, *Science,* 229, 1265, 1985.

167. **Shuin, T., Billings, P. C., Lillehaug, J. R., Patierno, S. R., Roy-Burman, P., and Landolph, J. R.,** Enhanced expression of c-*myc* and decreased expression of c-*fos* proto-oncogenes in chemically and radiation-transformed C3H/10T1/2ce8 mouse embryo cell lines, *Cancer Res.,* 46, 5302, 1986.

168. **Leibowitch, M. P., Leibowitch, S. A., Hillion, J., Guillie, M., Schmitz, A., and Harel, J.,** Possible role of c-fos, c-N-ras and c-mos proto-oncogenes in muscular development, *Exp. Cell Res.,* 170, 80, 1987.

169. **Green, P. J., Pines, O., and Inouye, M.,** The role of antisense RNA in gene regulation, *Annu. Rev. Biochem.,* 55, 569, 1986.

170. **Izant, J. G. and Weintraub, H.,** Inhibition of thymidine kinase gene expression by anti-sense RNA: a molecular approach to genetic analysis, *Cell,* 36, 1007, 1984.

171. **Izant, J. G. and Weintraub, H.,** Constitutive and conditional suppression of exogenous and endogenous genes by anti-sense RNA, *Science,* 229, 345, 1985.

172. **De Benedetti, A., Pytel, B. A., and Baglioni, C.,** Loss of (2'-5') oligoadenylate synthetase activity by production of antisense RNA results in lack of protection by interferon from viral infections, *Proc. Natl. Acad. Sci. U.S.A.,* 84, 658, 1987.

173. **Holt, J. T., Venkat, G. T., Moulton, A. D., and Nienhuis, A. W.,** Inducible production of a c-*fos* antisense RNA inhibits 3T3 cell proliferation, *Proc. Natl. Acad. Sci. U.S.A.,* 83, 4794, 1986.

174. **Zamecnik, P. C., Goodchild, J., Taguchi, Y., and Sarin, P. S.,** Inhibition of replication and expression of human T-cell lymphotropic virus type III in cultured cells by exogenous synthetic oligonucleotides complementary to viral RNA, *Proc. Natl. Acad. Sci. U.S.A.,* 83, 4143, 1986.

175. **Stephenson, M. L. and Zamecnik, P. C.,** Inhibition of Rous sarcoma viral RNA translation by a specific oligodeoxyribonucleotide, *Proc. Natl. Acad. Sci. U.S.A.,* 75, 285, 1978.

176. **Zamecnik, P. C. and Stephenson, M. L.,** Inhibition of Rous sarcoma virus replication and cell transformation by a specific oligodeoxynucleotide, *Proc. Natl. Acad. Sci. U.S.A.,* 75, 280, 1978.

177. **Smith, C. C., Aurelian, L., Reddy, M. P., Miller, P. S., and Ts'o, P. O. P.,** Antiviral effect of an oligo(nucleoside methylphosphonate) complementary to the splice junction of herpes simplex virus type 1 immediate early pre-mRNAs 4 and 5, *Proc. Natl. Acad. Sci. U.S.A.,* 83, 2787, 1986.

178. **Lemaitre, M., Bayard, B., and Lebleu, B.,** Specific antiviral activity of a poly(L-lysine)-conjugated oligodeoxyribonucleotide sequence complementary to vesicular stomatitis virus N protein mRNA initiation site, *Proc. Natl. Acad. Sci. U.S.A.,* 84, 648, 1987.

179. **Kawasaki, E. S.,** Quantitative hybridization-arrest of mRNA in *Xenopus* oocytes using single-stranded complementary DNA or oligonucleotide probes, *Nucl. Acids Res.,* 13, 4991, 1985.

180. **Neckers, L. M., Schwak, G., Wickstrom, E., Peuznick, D., and Heikkila, R.,** Role of c-*myc* in lymphocyte mitogenesis: studies with an anti-sense oligonucleotide, *Fed. Proc.,* 3, 742, 1987.

181. **Reid, K. B. M., Bentley, D. R., Campbell, R. D., Chung, L. P., Sim, R. P., Kristensen, T., and Tack, B. F.,** Complement system proteins which interact with C3b or C4b, *Immunol. Today,* 7, 230, 1986.

182. **Carter, W. A., Swartz, H., and Gillespie, D. H.,** Independent evolution of antiviral and growth modulating activities of interferon, *J. Biol. Res. Models,* 4, 447, 1985.

183. **Harel-Bellan, A.,** unpublished observations.

Chapter 8

INTERLEUKIN-1 AND ITS BIOLOGICALLY RELATED CYTOKINES

Charles A. Dinarello

TABLE OF CONTENTS

I. INTRODUCTION

Interleukin-1 (IL-1) is the term for two polypeptides (IL-1α and IL-1β) that possess a wide spectrum of immunologic and nonimmunologic activities. Although both forms of IL-1 are distinct gene products, they recognize the same receptor and share the same biological properties. IL-1 is produced in response to infection, microbial toxins, inflammatory agents, products of activated lymphocytes, complement, and clotting components. Its name as an interleukin, which means "between" leukocytes, is somewhat inappropriate because IL-1 is synthesized by both leukocytic and nonleukocytic cells; furthermore, IL-1 effects are not restricted to leukocytes but rather are manifested in nearly every tissue. Nevertheless, the term "interleukin" is often used for lack of a better system of nomenclature. To date, the primary amino acid sequences for eight molecules of human origin have been reported (IL-1α, IL-1β, IL-2 through IL-7); most of these molecules share some biological activities.

There are other polypeptides for which the primary human amino acid sequences are known but are not called interleukins. IL-1 is the prototype of a group of biologically potent polypeptides with molecular weights between 10,000 and 30,000 Da. Because these substances are produced by a variety of cells and act on many different cell types, there is a growing acceptance of the terms "cytokines" rather than "lymphokines" or "monokines" for these polypeptides. Of the various cytokines, several share the ability to stimulate or augment cell proliferation, initiate the synthesis of new proteins in a variety of cells, and induce the production of inflammatory metabolites. Although several exist, IL-1 is biologically similar to tumor necrosis factor (TNF), lymphotoxin, IL-6, fibroblast growth factor (FGF), platelet-derived growth factor (PDGF), and transforming growth factor-beta (TGFβ). Although monocytes and macrophages are, in fact, sources of these cytokines, some are prominent products of platelets, fibroblasts, keratinocytes, and endothelial cells. In general, the various cytokine polypeptides possess diverse biological properties, most of which are associated with either host responses to various disease states or participate as part of a pathological process.

IL-1 was originally described in the 1940s as a heat-labile protein found in acute leukocytic exudate fluid which, when injected into animals or humans, produced fever. This material was a small protein (10,000 to 20,000 Da) and was called endogenous pyrogen.[7] In the 1970s it was shown that 30 to 50 ng/kg of homogeneous endogenous pyrogen produced monophasic fever in rabbits.[47,173] No amino acid sequence for endogenous pyrogen was known, but studies demonstrated that endogenous pyrogen did more than cause fever. When injected into animals it induced hepatic acute phase protein synthesis, caused decreases in plasma iron and zinc levels, produced neutrophilia, stimulated serum amyloid A protein synthesis, and augmented T-cell responses to mitogens and antigens *in vitro*.[43,103] The multiple biological activities of endogenous pyrogen, particularly its ability to affect immunocompetent cells, resulted changing its name to IL-1. The name IL-1 now includes several substances originally named for their biological activities, but following data generated with recombinant IL-1 or compared to N-terminal amino acid sequences, these are identical to IL-1. These are leukocytic endogenous mediator,[103] lymphocyte activating factor,[79] mononuclear cell factor,[117] catabolin,[212] osteoclast activating factor,[41] and hemopoietin-1.[165,167]

The various cytokines listed above are for the most part structurally distinct with the exception of IL-1α/IL-1β and fibroblast growth factor. IL-1α and IL-β, despite distinct primary amino acids sequences, are structurally related as shown by molecular modeling, crystallographic analysis, and receptor recognition. A similar case exists for TNF and lymphotoxin. In addition, IL-1β is structurally related to fibroblast growth factors (acidic form) and shares the growth-promoting properties of these molecules.[242] TNF and IL-1 induce nearly identical biological effects, particularly those associated with systemic and local inflammatory as well as destructive joint disease,[19,36,44,117] but share only 3% primary amino acid structure. Receptors for IL-1 and TNF are distinct.

Considerable interest has focused on IL-1, TNF, and IL-6 as mediators of systemic "acute phase" responses. Injecting experimental animals with either IL-1 or TNF results in fever, hypozincemia, hypoferremia, increased hepatic acute phase proteins synthesis, and other manifestations of the response. IL-6 induces fever and hepatic acute phase protein synthesis. Recent evidence suggests that IL-6, like IL-1 and TNF, is present in human body fluids associated with inflammatory and febrile diseases. This chapter focuses on IL-1, but the related cytokines, TNF and IL-6, are also discussed particularly as these molecules share biological properties with IL-1.

II. INTERLEUKIN-1 STRUCTURE

Two forms of IL-1 have been cloned; IL-1β was cloned from human blood monocytes[8] and IL-1α was cloned from the mouse macrophage line P388D.[136] Subsequent to the description of cDNAs to these two forms, IL-1β has been cloned in the cow, rabbit, rat, and mouse and IL-1α in the human, rat, and rabbit, It is unclear whether more than these two gene products exist for IL-1. IL-1β is the prominent form of IL-1 and the amount of IL-1β mRNA found in activated cells is usually 10- to 50-fold greater than the α form. In addition, culture supernates and various human body fluids contain more IL-1β than the α form. However, several studies have shown that IL-1β is readily secreted from activated cells, whereas IL-1α remains cell associated.

Originally identified as a pI 7 (IL-1β) and pI 5 (IL-1α) species on isoelectric focusing, the two forms of IL-1 are initially synthesized as 31,000 Da precursor polypeptides and share only small stretches of amino acid homology (26% in the case of the two human IL-1 forms). Neither form contains a signal peptide sequence which would indicate a cleavage site for the N-terminus. This fact makes IL-1 a highly unique substance. Other cytokines such as TGF and TNF have clearly identifiable signal peptide sequences. Lacking a clear signal peptide, a considerable amount of the IL-1 that is synthesized remains cell associated.[124] In fact, membrane-associated IL-1 is biologically active and may be the form which participates in activating lymphocytes, particularly in lymphoid tissue where lymphocytes form rosettes around macrophages.[121] "Membrane-bound" IL-1 is also active on nonlymphocyte target cells. The steps involved in transcription, translation, and "processing" of IL-1 are discussed below.

Within the various animal species of IL-1β, the primary amino acid sequences are conserved in the range of 75 to 78%, whereas the α sequences are in the range of 60 to 70%; between the β and α IL-1 within each species, conserved amino acid homologies are only 25%. The entire human genes for each IL-1 form have also been cloned.[31,75] Each gene

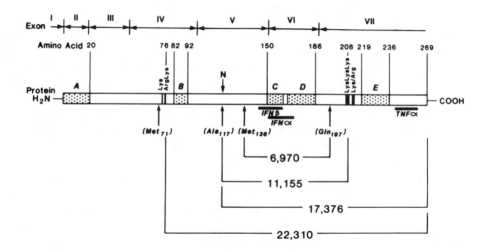

FIGURE 1.   Structure of IL-1β. The top line depicts the 7 exons of the human IL-1β gene (adapted from Reference 31). The bar represents the IL-1β precursor protein with the stipled areas showing the amino acid homologous regions with IL-1α (adapted from Reference 9). The amino acid numbers are shown as are likely trypsin-like cleavage sites. The predicted size of these IL-1 fragments are shown (adapted from Reference 10).

contains seven exons coding for the processed IL-1 mRNA and raise the possibility of alternate RNA processing. The gene for human IL-1β is located on chromosome 2[254] and the gene for mouse IL-1α is also on chromosome 2. The existence of other IL-1 forms (as separate gene products or the result of processed mRNA) has recently been introduced in studies on IL-1 from Epstein-Barr virus infected human B cells;[202] however, it remains to be shown whether these latter cells produce a different IL-1 gene product or that post-translational processing results in IL-1 of different molecular weights and charges. The N-terminal amino acid sequence reported for B cell IL-1[202] is unrelated to the N-termini of IL-1β or -α. Recently, a T cell factor with physical characteristics similar to those of the human B cell IL-1 has been shown to possess the identical N-terminal amino acids.[239] This T cell factor is biologically related to IL-1 in that it induces the p55/TAC antigen on T cells. The factor is derived from human adult T cell lymphotropic virus-1 transformed T cell lines. It appears that the IL-2R-inducing lymphokine is the same as B cell IL-1.

When the amino acid sequences of the two IL-1 forms are compared, only four small regions of amino acid homologies exist. These have been identified and called regions A-E[9] (see Figure 1); since regions A and B are contained in the precursor sequence which is missing in the mature IL-1 form, the important regions of homology for the two mature IL-1 forms are located in the carboxyl C-D and E regions. These regions may represent a putative "active site" of the IL-1 molecule which would explain the observation that although the two forms are structurally distinct, they share the same spectrum of multiple biological properties and recognize the same receptor. Of interest to the evolution of iL-1 is that the C-D region of IL-1-β/α homology is coded by the entire VIth exon and this region also contains some limited amino acid homology with interferon-alpha-2 (IFN-α2) and IFN-β1. There is also a small (3%) region of amino acid homology with TNF, but this region does not correspond to the IL-1-β/α homologous regions.

Since both mature forms of IL-1 recognize the same cell receptor and both forms possess the same biological properties, attention has focused on the concept that the C-D contains the minimal structural requirements for receptor activation. Several peptides have been produced either by synthetic[4] or recombinant DNA methods.[208] Although these IL-1 peptides have some biological activity, the specific activities are low and they do not block the receptor binding of the mature peptide. Antibodies to this C-D region do not block the activity of the mature IL-1β peptide on a variety of target cells whereas antibodies to synthetic C-terminal and N-terminal peptides do reduce biological actvity.[153] These data support other studies (see below), suggesting that both the N- and the C-terminal amino acids are involved in receptor binding events.

Small molecular weight peptides at 4 and 2 kDa, with IL-1 immunoreactive and biological activity, have been consistently isolated from human body fluids.[28,50,111] These small molecular weight peptides have been observed in preparatons of recombinant IL-1 and appear to be generated by trypsin sensitive sites. The amino acid sequence of human IL-1β contains several cleavage sites for serine proteases which would generate peptides of various molecular weights. These are illustrated in Figure 1. There is a 6970 Da peptide which contains the C-D region and generated by serine proteases. There is also a 5488 Da C-terminal peptide generated at the lysine-lysine-lysine site which could represent the active C-terminal fragment.[185] Inhibitors of serine proteases prevent the appearance of this and other small molecular weight immunoreactive IL-1 peptides in supernates of human monocytes.[10] Recently, an endopeptidase which is membrane-bound and is involved with degradation of neuropeptides has been shown to destroy the biological activity of IL-1β.[193]

Human IL-1β has recently been crystallized and its tertiary structure analyzed at a resolution of 3.0 Å.[198] The molecule that was crystallized had an N-terminus at alanine 117 and hence represents a 17.5 kDa processed form. This is the dominant form found in extracellular fluids. The three dimensional structure revealed 12 β-strands forming a complex of hydrogen bonds. Computerized molecular modeling of IL-1 from the primary sequence also revealed a similar structure.[33] The basic structure is similar to a tetrahedron the interior of which is filled with hydrophobic side chains. The overall folding of the 12 β-strands is similar to that found in the soybean trypsin inhibitor. The interior of the IL-1β is strongly hydrophobic with no charged amino acids in the interior. The histidine at position 147 is on the surface of the molecule and when this amino acid is substituted by site-specific mutation, a corresponding loss of biological and receptor binding activity takes place.[144] The N-terminal mutations have also yielded altered biological and receptor binding data,[97] suggesting that N-terminal amino acids, seemingly the result of limited proteolysis by serine proteases,[54] play an important role in either stabilizing the tertiary structure or by direct interaction with receptor binding domains. Studies on the active site of IL-1 have been carried out using antibodies directed against different synthetic peptides and assessing their ability to neutralize the immunostimulatory as well as inflammatory properties of the whole IL-1.[153,203]

Fibroblast growth factors have been shown to stimulate fibroblast and endothelial cell proliferation, smooth muscle cell proliferation, and angiogenesis, properties similar to those of IL-1. Like IL-1, these molecules exist in two forms, acidic (pI 5) and basic (pI 8). Bovine brain-derived acidic and basic FGFs have significant amino acid homologies with the IL-1β[242] and to a lesser degree with IL-1α. The stretches of IL-1 and FGF amino acid homologies are distributed throughout the sequences; however, analysis of the IL-1 sequence in the C-D region (see above) with that of the FGFs does not reveal any particular homology in this region. Nevertheless, the amino acid sequence similarities between the two IL-1 forms and the two forms of FGF support the observation that some biological properties are shared, particularly their ability to induce cell proliferation. It is unknown whether IL-1 binding to fibroblasts is displaced by FGFs. Other growth factors such as TGF (β and α) and PDGF do not have any structural homologies to IL-1 or TNF at the level of amino acid sequences. In addition, the receptors to these cytokines appear distinct. It seems likcly that these different cytokines bring about similar biological changes because they induce similar postreceptor cellular signals.

III. GENE EXPRESSION, SYNTHESIS,
AND PROCESSING OF IL-1

A critical aspect of understanding IL-1 gene expression in a variety of cells is the exquisite sensitivity of some IL-1-producing cells to the effects of endotoxins (bacterial lipopolysaccharides). This is particularly the case with human blood monocytes which will produce IL-1 when stimulated by concentrations of endotoxin as low as 5 to 10 pg/ml. Routine tissue culture media contain orders of magnitude greater amounts of endotoxin. It is often difficult to assess gene expression in some experiments since IL-1 transcription can easily be stimulated by routine laboratory culture media. In order to demonstrate increases in IL-1 mRNA, some investigators have used 10 μg/ml of endotoxin to show stimulation of IL-1 transcription over that of the "unstimulated" control.[108] Therefore, in many studies, IL-1β transcription has already taken place during the preparation and early culture of monocyte/macrophages. Adherence to glass and some plastic surfaces can serve as a stimulus of RNA synthesis. If one carefully separates human blood mononuclear cells on endotoxin-free Ficoll-Hypaque and avoids activating cells by adherence or endotoxin-contaminated culture media, there is no IL-1 mRNA present in unstimulated cells and no IL-1 protein is translated, including both intracellular and extracellular compartments.[221]

Transcription of IL-1 mRNA is rapid in stimulated cells; in both human macrophage cell lines as well as in human blood mononuclear cells, endotoxin stimulated IL-1β RNA transcription can be observed within 15 min.[70,71] In human cultured endothelial and smooth muscle cells, a similar rapid increase has been reported.[126,127] Transcription increases and reaches peak levels in 3 to 4 h and then levels off for several hours before decreasing. Transcription of IL-1α appears to be under tighter control in that inhibitors of protein synthesis are sometimes required to observe IL-1α RNA.[127] In fact, the total amount of IL-1β mRNA increases and is maintained at higher levels when inhibitors of protein synthesis are used.[70] During endotoxin stimulation, transcriptional repressors are translated (or activated by phosphorylation) and these either suppress further transcription or increase mRNA degradation.

In addition to a tight control over transcription, IL-1 is translated by a mechanism which is poorly understood. For example, human monocytes can be stimulated by adherence to glass surfaces and still not translate any of the mRNA into IL-1 protein. In fact, the level of mRNA following adherence to glass or cellulosic membranes can be as high as that following endotoxin stimulation and yet no IL-1 protein is produced in the absence of another stimulant, in most cases endotoxin. This requirement for a second signal for translation is similar to the case for ferritin biosynthesis in which cells contain high levels of mRNA but require iron to stimulate translation. Of course, endotoxin and similar stimulants serve the dual purpose of initiating transcription as well as translation. IL-1 itself serves to stimulate both transcription and translation of IL-1.[52,253] Corticosteroids, when added to cells before they are stimulated, prevent both transcription and translation;[114] however, if corticosteroids are added after IL-1 mRNA is present, there is no evidence of decreased transcription and most of the effect is on translation.[108]

Prostaglandins and prostacyclins have no effect on transcription but prevent translation.[114,118] Blocking cyclooxygenase results in increased production of IL-1 protein, particularly when cells are stimulated by agents which increase prostaglandin E (PGE) synthesis. In these situations, reduction of PGE and prostacyclin (PGI) by cyclooxygenase inhibitors removes the suppressive effect of the arachidonate metabolites. This effect may represent the artifact of *in vitro* cultured cells since PGE accumulates under these conditions, whereas *in vivo*, efficient mechanisms exist to rapidly remove PGE metabolites. The mechanism of PGE-induced suppression of IL-1 translation appears to be via the induction of cyclic adenosine monophosphate (cAMP).[113] The addition of PGE and dibutyl cAMP or PGE and theophylline augments the suppression. It is unclear exactly how increased cAMP affects the translation of IL-1 protein but studies show no effect on IL-1β mRNA when cAMP degradation is prevented by inhibitors of phosphodiesterase.

Despite the lack of a signal peptide, IL-1 is found in the supernates of stimulated monocytes and macrophages. Other cells producing IL-1, for example, endothelial cells, keratinocytes, smooth muscle cells, and renal mesangial cells, transcribe large amonts of IL-1 mRNA and translate IL-1 protein, but a considerable amount of the IL-1 remains intracellular as the precursor molecule (31 kDa).[10,157] The amount of IL-1 that is "secreted" depends upon the cell type and the conditions of stimulation. The monocyte/macrophage appears to be the cell best equipped to "secrete" IL-1. These cells contain polyadenylated RNA coding for IL-1β at concentrations as high as 2 to 5% of the total poly A after adherence and stimulation by endotoxin. Most of the IL-1β mRNA transcribed is translated under these conditions. Using radioimmunoassays or enzyme-linked assays, studies indicate that as much as 100 fg of IL-1 is synthesized per human monocyte (or 100 ng/10^6 monocytes) during the 24 h following stimulation.[64,133] Although the amount of mRNA coding for IL-1α is approximately 20 to 50% less than IL-1β in these cells,[39] there is more total (cell-associated plus extracellular) IL-1α protein produced following endotoxin stimulation.[64-66]

The reason for this discrepancy between the amount of IL-1α mRNA and the amount of IL-1α protein translated remains unclear. One possibility is that a considerable amount of the IL-1β mRNA is never translated, whereas translation of the IL-1α RNA is highly efficient. An alternative explanation is that the mRNA for IL-1β is more rapidly degraded than that for IL-1α. Control of IL-1 translation is affected by other cytokines. IL-1-induced IL-1 production (eithr IL-1β-induced IL-1α or IL-1α-induced IL-1β) is suppressed by IFN-γ, whereas IFN-γ augments the amount of IL-1 synthesized following endotoxin or TNF stimulation.[81] Posttranscriptional suppression of IL-1 synthesis is observed in cells treated with PGE$_2$ and is a cAMP-dependent mechanism;[113] corticosteroids can suppress IL-1 synthesis when added before transcription[114] as well as after transcription.[108]

As depicted in Figure 2, activators of cells for IL-1 synthesis also trigger the events leading to increased prostaglandins and leukotrienes. As mentioned above, prostaglandins suppress IL-1 translation; however, leukotrienes appear to augment IL-1 production. This has been shown by adding LTB-4 to human monocytes and stimulating IL-1 production.[207] Agents that block the lipoxygenase pathway of arachidonate metabolism leading to formation of leukotrienes also reduce IL-1 production.[49,118] Similar studies demonstrate that this series of events also occurs in macrophages producing TNF. Recent evidence supports the importance of lipoxygenase products in the production of IL-1. In human volunteers taking eicosapentaenoic acid fatty acid dietary supplements, there is a 70% reduction in the ability of their mononuclear cells to synthesize IL-1β and IL-1α in vitro.[66] A similar observation was made for TNF. The mechanism probably involves the ability of these omega-3 fatty acid precursors to be metabolized to LTB-5 rather than LTB-4. LTB-5 competes with LTB-4 for receptor occupancy. It is unclear at which stage the lipoxygenase metabolites act on IL-1 production. Since one can add a lipoxygenase inhibitor 1 to 2 h after cell stimulation without affecting the amount of IL-1 synthesized, it appears that lipoxygenase metabolites are involved with early events such as transcription.

The first translation product of IL-1 is the 31 kDa precursor. This can be found mostly in the intracellular pool. The intracellular pool also contains other molecular weight fragments of IL-1 at 22 and 17 kDa, but it is not clear whether these occur as a result of artifactual proteolysis during specimen preparation.[10] The localization of cell-associated IL-1 (as compared to extracellular IL-1) is almost entirely cytoplasmic. Using antibody staining or radioimmunoassays, the data consistently indicate that cell-associated IL-1β is primarily in the cytosol, not in the endoplasmic reticulum, Golgi, or plasma membrane fraction.[232,234] Despite the failure to measure IL-1 in the plasma membrane fractions, several studies have shown IL-1β staining on the cell surface.[72] Lysosomal localization appears to be important

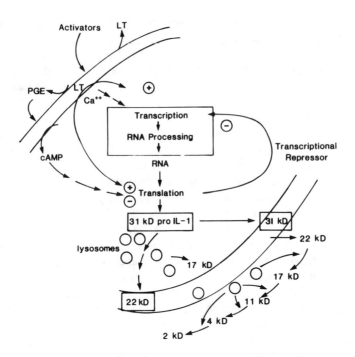

FIGURE 2.   Activation of a monocyte leading to the transcription, translation, processing, and secretion of IL-1. Activators stimulate several changes in cell membrane lipids and intracellular signals. PGE, leukotrienes (LT), calcium, and cAMP are shown with their respective role as enhancers or suppressors of IL-1 production. The effect of a transcriptional repressor is shown (adapted from Reference 70). The 31 kDa IL-1 precursor is found mostly intracellularly in the cytosol but also in the plasma membrane (IL-1α) and associated with lysosomes. A 22 kDa peptide (see Figure 1) is also associated with the three compartments. The extracellular generation of the mature 17.5 kDa IL-1 peptide and its fragments are shown.

for the processing and secretion of IL-1.[12,232] Studies on the localization of IL-1α also indicate a similar predominance in the cytosol,[234] but others have demonstrated IL-1α associated with the plasma membrane.[17] IL-1α is also phosphorylated and it is unclear how this contributes to its cellular localization.[115]

There is a 22 kDa form which can be isolated from the intracellular pool and the extracellular fluid. The 22 kDa IL-1 is also thought to be an intermediate form which may be located transiently in the membrane. The 31 kDa IL-1 precursor is immunoprecipitated by anti-IL-1α where it is biologically active as an inducer of hepatic acute phase protein synthesis.[17] Most of the IL-1 found in the extracellular fluid, however, is the "mature" 17.5 kDa peptide with an N-terminus at position 117 (alanine) for the IL-1β precursor[248] and at position 113 (serine) for the human IL-1α. Smaller peptide fragments of these mature peptides have been found in monocyte supernates and the appearance of these peptides can be reduced in the presence of serine protease inhibitors.[10] Elastase and plasmin have been implicated as monocyte proteases which cleave IL-1 into its 17.5 kDa mature fragment.[157] This and other various subfragments are biologically active and are routinely found in human plasma, urine, peritoneal, pleural, and joint fluids. As shown in Figure 2, smaller peptides with molecular weights at 22, 17, 11, 6, 4, and 2 kDa are found in the extracellular fluid of stimulated human monocytes and may correspond to the potential cleavage sites depicted in Figure 1.

The mechanism of IL-1 cleavage is thought to be via lysosomal enzymes.[12] There is a correlation between the amount of processed 17.5 kDa mature IL-1 found in the extracellular fluid and the type of stimulus used to activate the monocyte or macrophage. Particles such as *Staphylococcus epidermidis* or zymosan induce large amounts of IL-1 that are mostly mature and extracellular. These stimulators are also potent inducers of lysosomal exocytosis. Other stimulators such as low-dose (50 to 100 pg/ml) of bacterial endotoxins induce approximately equal amounts of intra- and extracellular IL-1β, whereas IL-1α is nearly entirely cytosolic. Adherence to plastic or glass surfaces in the absence of endotoxins induce mRNA for IL-1β but no detectable IL-1 protein. Small amounts of endotoxin rapidly induce translation of this mRNA.[221] However, most commercial tissue culture media or sera contain sufficient endotoxin concentrations (10 to 50 pg/ml) to stimulate cell-associated IL-1, including membrane-bound IL-1 which is biologically active.[121] Thus, it is likely that most cultures containing monocyte/macrophages have active cell-associated IL-1 despite a failure to demonstrate extracellular IL-1.

IV. THE BIOLOGICAL EFFECTS OF IL-1

The expression of recombinant IL-1 has been accomplished and, in general, there does not seem to be any difference in the spectrum of biological activities of either form. IL-1β is vulnerable to oxidation, and thus biological specific activities of IL-1β can be lower than those of IL-1α which is highly stable. If IL-1β is purified under nondenaturing conditions, it is equipotent with the α form in a variety of *in vivo* and *in vitro* assays. The binding of either IL-1β or IL-1α to various cells in receptors binding assays is blocked by each form.[110] Both recombinant human IL-1β and -α augment T, B, and natural killer (NK) cell responses. The ability of IL-1 to activate immunocompetent cells seems unique to the group of cytokines which affect cellular growth and proliferation; FGF, PDGF, and TGF have either no effect on immunocompetent cells, or in the case of TGFβ, are potent immunosuppressive agents.[107] Both forms of IL-1 induce systemic acute phase responses including fever, hepatic acute phase protein synthesis, neutrophilia, hypoferremia, hypozincemia, increased levels of hormones, and sleep. At higher doses, IL-1 induces hypotension and a shock-like state.[182] Some biological properties reported for natural IL-1 have not been confirmed with either recombinant form. These include the ability of IL-1 to cause neutrophil superoxide production and degranulation *in vitro*[78] and to induce muscle proteolysis *in vitro*.[85,166] Others, however, do show an effect of recombinant IL-1β on muscle proteolysis,[32] particularly a fragment of IL-1 generated from the recombinant IL-1β form. It appears the effects of IL-1 on neutrophils are due to its ability to augment the biological effects of other neutrophil activators such as the chemotactic peptides. There are receptors for IL-1 on neutrophils[201] and IL-1 acts as a cofactor or permissive factor for the activity of f-met-leu-phe. Recombinant human IL-1, however, directly stimulates basophil[88,238] and eosinophil degranulation of histamine and arylsulfatase,[194] respectively.

The multiple biological activities of IL-1 have been studied in terms of *in vivo* and *in vitro* effects. In patients with bacterial infection, injury, or chronic inflammatory disease, IL-1 may account for a majority of observed acute phase changes. It is difficult to study such subjective symptoms as headache, myalgias, arthralgias, and lassitude in animal models, but the potency (10^{-12} to 10^{-15} M) of IL-1 in inducing release of PGE_2 from fibroblasts, synovial, and other cells suggests that these symptoms are likely mediated by increased levels of IL-1.

A. EFFECTS ON HEPATIC PROTEIN SYNTHESIS
Hepatic proteins which change during acute phase responses include clotting factors, complement components, fibrinogen, haptoglobin, ceruloplasmin, and others. In addition, there are increases in hepatic proteins generally not synthesized in health but in association

with infection, injury, or other pathological processes. IL-1, TNF, and hepatocyte stimulating factor (now identified as the same molecule as IFN-β2 and B cell stimulating factor-2 or IL-6) play important roles in regulating the synthesis of hepatic proteins. The cytokine-induced increases in normal hepatic proteins is usually in the range of 2- to 3-fold, but the synthesis of pathological proteins can increase 100- to 1000-fold. Two such proteins, serum amyloid A (SAA) protein and C-reactive protein are classical "acute phase reactants", and serve as markers of disease. SAA contributes to the development of secondary amyloidosis.

IL-1 induces hepatocytes to synthesize a spectrum of acute phase proteins; these include SAA,[199] fibrinogen,[80] complement components, and various clotting factors. At the same time, albumin levels decrease. Studies have shown that IL-1 regulates the synthesis of these and other hepatic acute phase proteins at the level of mRNA transcription. In isolated hepatocytes, IL-1 decreases the transcription of RNA coding for albumin, increases transcription of factor B, initiates SAA mRNA synthesis, but has no effect on gene expression of a control protein, actin. Other proteins have been studied in hepatic cell line cultures (HepG2 and Hep3B), and in picomolar ranges, IL-1 stimulates the biosynthesis of complement protein C3 and α_1-antichymotrypsin.[188] There is also a modest stimulation of α_1-acid glycoprotein and inter-α_1-trypsin inhibitor synthesis. In addition to decreased albumin transcription, hepatic cells exposed to IL-1 synthesize less transferrin. In hepatic cells lines, IL-1 does not increase the expression of C-reactive protein (CRP), although the intravenous injection of recombinant IL-1 does result in elevated CRP levels after 24 h. In murine fibroblasts transfected with cosmid DNA bearing the genes for C2 and factor B, IL-1 stimulated the expression of factor B, but did not affect synthesis of C2.[189]

IL-1 has other effects on liver metabolism. It depresses the activity of liver cytochrome P450-dependent drug metabolism in mice,[80] and this observation may explain the impaired drug clearance and excretion in patients with infections and fever. The response of the liver to IL-1 also includes the synthesis of metalloproteins which bind serum iron and zinc and account for the hypozincemia and hypoferremia induced by IL-1. Bacteria and tumor cells require large amounts of iron for cell growth, particularly at elevated temperatures, and the ability of the host to remove iron from tissue fluids seems to be a fundamental host defense mechanism.

B. EFFECTS OF IL-1 ON ENDOTHELIAL CELLS

Of its many biological properties, IL-1-induced changes in endothelial cells relate directly to the initiation and progression of pathological lesions in vascular tissue. From a physiological viewpoint, IL-1 activates human endothelial cells *in vitro* to synthesize and release PGI$_2$, PGE$_2$, and platelet activating factor.[38,210] A 10-fold increase in PGI$_2$ release is observed with concentrations of IL-1 in the femtomolar range. Although arachidonate metabolites increase blood flow, IL-1 also orchestrates a cascade of cellular and biochemical events that lead to vascular congestion, clot formation, and cellular infiltration. One of these initiating steps involves the ability of IL-1 to alter endothelial cell plasma membranes so that neutrophils, monocytes, and lymphocytes adhere avidly.[21] Endothelial cells need be exposed to IL-1 for 1 h or less in order to increase their adhesiveness. The action of IL-1 in this process appears to be related to the interaction of the leukocyte glycoprotein complex called "leukocyte function antigen" with a fibroblast and endothelial cell surface molecule called "intercellular adhesion molecule-1". Within 1 h following IL-1 exposure, endothelial cells increase their expression of intercellular adhesion molecule-1.[62] Patients with defective leukocyte function antigen expression have repeated bouts of bacterial infection. In addition to activating endothelial cell-leukocyte adhesion, IL-1 also increases the binding and lysis by NK cells by a variety of tumor targets and is chemotactic for monocytes and lymphocytes. Consistent with the effects of IL-1 on leukocyte chemotaxis and adherence to endothelial cells, IL-1 injected intradermally causes the accumulation of neutrophils, and IL-1 can

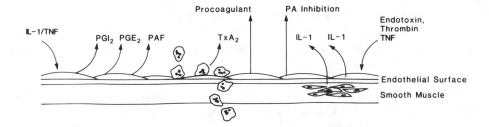

FIGURE 3.   IL-1 and TNF effects on vascular tissue. PAI indicates plasminogen activator inhibitor.

substitute for endotoxin in either limb of the local Schwartzman reaction. This latter property is most apparent using the combination of IL-1 and TNF.[169]

IL-1 increases endothelial cell surface procoagulant activity[20] and production of a plasminogen activator inhibitor.[174] These events lead to activation of thrombin in the initiation of clotting. Taken together, these effects would decrease blood flow in vessels and increase the accumulation of leukocytes and platelets. Since IL-1 stimulates neutrophil thromboxane release,[34] activated neutrophils adhering to endothelial cells may increase platelet aggregation. Finally, IL-1 has angiogenic properties in the rabbit eye anterior chamber model[264] and following brain injury;[84] this may be related to the fact that IL-1 and the related fibroblast growth factors share significant amino acid homologies. In general, the effects of IL-1 on endothelial cells represent a well-coordinated effort to localize tissue inflammation and contribute to the initiation of pathological lesions leading to vasculitic-like changes. Figure 3 illustrates the activity of IL-1 (and TNF, see below) on vascular tissue.

The effects of IL-1 stimulation of endothelial cell functions should be considered in light of the fact that endothelial cells produce their own IL-1. Concentrations in the ng/ml range of bacterial endotoxins or TNF induce cultured endothelial cells to release IL-1.[126] In addition, thrombin stimulates endothelial cell IL-1 production. Northern hybridization of endothelial cell mRNA supports the close relationship between the predominant IL-1β and endothelial cell-derived IL-1. Thus, the induction of endothelial cell IL-1 by two clinically relevant stimulators (endotoxin and thrombin) may initiate a cascade of events leading to further development of vasculitic processes. Although immune complexes stimulate monocyte IL-1 production, there are no reported studies as yet demonstrating that immune complexes stimulate endothelial cell IL-1 synthesis. Recent studies demonstrated that arterial smooth muscle produces IL-1,[127] that IL-1 is a growth factor for smooth muscle cells, and IL-1 induces IL-1 in these cells.[253]

C. CATABOLIC EFFECTS OF IL-1

The catabolic properties of IL-1 are usually considered in terms of its local effects. For example, IL-1 produced locally acts in a paracrine-like fashion in destructive joint and bone disease and local tumor invasion. On the other hand, IL-1 in the systemic circulation exerts its catabolic effects indirectly by affecting the metabolism of lipoproteins by liver and fat. IL-1 is a potent inducer of collagenase production in synovial cells;[37,117] in addition, IL-1 induces release of metalloproteinases and proteoglycanases from chondrocytes.[212,224] In fact, because of its local catabolic biological activities, pig IL-1 was previously known as "catabolin". Recombinant IL-1 added to bone cultures *in vitro* induce dramatic resorptive processes and shrinkage of bone matrix. Just as pig IL-1 was known previously as catabolin, osteoclast activating factor (OAF) is now identified as having the same amino acid sequence as the human IL-1β.[41] Thus, it is presently considered that the catabolic properties of IL-1 in cartilage and bone contribute to the tissue destruction and matrix loss in a variety of joint diseases.[117,190] As discussed below, TNF can also act as an osteoclast activating factor. IL-1 and the related FGF synergize in the induction of proteases from chrondrocytes.[191]

D. EFFECTS OF IL-1 ON FIBROBLASTS AND FIBROSIS

In contrast to its catabolic activities, IL-1 increases fibroblast proliferation[223] and collagen synthesis.[27] IL-1 is mitogenic for fibroblasts and is thought to play a major role in pannus formation. In fact, cellular infiltration and early pannus formation have been observed in rabbit joints injected with recombinant IL-1.[190] *In vitro*, however, IL-1-induced fibroblast and smooth muscle cell proliferation is often difficult to observe unless cyclooxygenase inhibitors are present.[126,127] This seems to be related to the PGE_2 levels induced by IL-1. This is not the case with other fibroblast growth factors such as PDGF, epidermal growth factor, and TGF. In comparison to epidermal growth factor and TGFβ, numbers of receptors for IL-1 on fibroblasts are low (2000/cell),[23,30] but compared to IL-1 receptors on other cells, the fibroblast ranks as one of the tissues with high numbers of receptors. One mechanism for IL-1-induced fibroblast growth is via increased production of receptors for endogenous growth factors such as epidermal growth factor. In terms of the role of IL-1 in fibrosis, recombinant IL-1 directly increases the transcription of type I and type III collagen[27] and type IV (basement membrane) collagen.[154]

E. OTHER CYTOKINES AFFECTING FIBROBLASTS AND FIBROSIS

Other cytokines share with IL-1 the ability to stimulate fibroblast proliferation. These include TNF,[116] FGF,[82] PDGF,[225] and TGFβ. In addition, another growth factor from macrophages, macrophage-derived growth factor, seems to act as a competence factor for PDGF-induced fibroblast growth;[150] however, this factor now seems to be PDGF itself. The mechanism of action of PDGF on cell proliferation includes a requirement for insulin whereas IL-1 and TNF effects are seen in the absence of insulin. Despite the fact that these various cytokines have distinct receptors, their effects on cell growth appear similar. These cytokine growth factors also share other biological properties. For example, like IL-1, PDGF is chemotactic for neutrophils and monocytes *in vivo*, induces cell aggregation and adhesiveness, and induces degranulation.[58,246] IL-1, TNF, TGF, and PDGF induce the synthesis of collagen and collagenases. At present, the multiple biological properties of IL-1 are clearly shared, to some extent, with these growth factors, raising issues such as synergism and antagonism between the cytokines on mesenchymal tissue. Recent data demonstrate that considerable synergism between IL-1 and TNF exist in a variety of biological effects; little is known about the synergism or antagonism between the non-IL-1 growth factors, except that TGFβ is immunosuppressive.[107]

V. SYSTEMIC VS. LOCAL EFFECTS OF IL-1

Table 1 lists the systemic effects of recombinant IL-1. These studies were carried out by injecting IL-1 into experimental animals either intravenously or intraperitoneally. In many cases, the IL-1 induced changes mimic the animal's responses to an injection of microbial toxins or antigen-antibody complexes. When administered intravenously into rabbits at 200 ng/kg, human recombinant IL-1 results in a fall in circulating neutrophils within 5 min and this is due to rapid margination on the endothelial surfaces; approximately 10 min after an intravenous injection, rectal temperature begins to rise and reaches peak elevation between 45 and 55 min after the injection.[54] Increases in slow wave sleep parallel the fever course but the sleep-inducing property of IL-1 is not linked to its ability to increase body temperature. After 4 to 6 h, temperature and sleep patterns return to preinjection levels, but there is an increase in circulating neutrophils, particularly new forms released from the marrow. After 12 h, serum alumin, iron, zinc, and cytochrome P-450 enzyme activity are decreased.[80] When approximately 10 times the amount of IL-1 is injected, a decrease in systemic arterial pressure, systemic vascular resistance, and central venous pressure can be observed within 10 min.[182] Although these hemodynamic changes are similar to the changes observed in

TABLE 1
Systemic Effects of Recombinant IL-1[a]

Central nervous system
Fever
Brain PGE_2 synthesis
Increased ACTH
Decreased REM sleep
Increased slow wave sleep
Decreased appetite

Hematologic
Neutrophilia
Nonspecific resistance
Increased GM-CSF
Radioprotection
Bone marrow stimulation
Tumor necrosis

Metabolic
Hypozincemia, hypoferremia
Decreased cytochrome P450 enzyme
Increased acute phase proteins
Decreased albumin synthesis
Increased insulin production
Inhibition of lipoprotein lipase
Increased sodium excretion
Increased corticosteroid synthesis

Vascular wall
Hypotension
Increased leukocyte adherence
Increased PGE synthesis
Decreased systemic vascular resistance
Decreased central venous pressure
Increased cardiac output
Increased heart rate
Decreased blood pH
Lactic acidosis
Chemoattractant

[a] These effects have been demonstrated by administration of recombinant IL-1 to animals.

animals given TNF, tissue damage is not characteristic of IL-1, at least at doses less than 5 μg/kg, whereas TNF is associated with necrosis in some organs.[244] Large doses of recombinant IL-1 injected into mice have been given without death or tissue damage unless the mice have been previously adrenalectomized.[265]

Information derived from the *in vitro* effects of IL-1 may relate to some of the biological properties of IL-1 observed *in vivo*. For example, IL-1 stimulates somatostatin release from cultured pituitary cells[220] and also increases steroid synthesis[206] from perfused adrenal glands. Therefore, it is not surprising that other neuropeptides are stimulated when IL-1 is given systemically. The effects of IL-1 on endothelial cell arachidonic acid metabolism, platelet activating factor generation, and procoagulant activity *in vitro* likely explain the shock-like state that IL-1 produces *in vivo*.[182] In addition, the ability of IL-1 to induce various lymphokines *in vitro*, for example, IFN-β1, IFN-γ, IL-2, IL-3, and IL-6, likely occurs *in vivo*, but it is difficult to demonstrate circulating levels of interferons and interleukins unless large doses of IL-1 are administered. One approach to interpreting the large body of evidence for

TABLE 2
Local Effects of Recombinant IL-1[a]

Nonimmunological
Chemoattractant (*in vivo*)
Basophil histamine release
Eosinophil degranulation
Increased collagenase production (*in vivo*)
Chondrocyte protease release
Bone resorption
Induction of fibroblast and endothelial CSF activity
Production of PGE_2 in dermal and synovial fibroblasts
Increased neutrophil and monocyte thromboxane synthesis
Cytotoxic for human melanoma cells
Cytotoxic for human β-islet cells
Suppression of thyroid function
Keratinocyte proliferation
Proliferation of dermal fibroblasts
Increased collagen synthesis
Mesangial cell proliferation
Gliosis

Immunological
T-cell activation
IL-2 production
Increased IL-2 receptors
B-cell activation
Synergism with IL-4
Induction and synergism with IL-6
Activation of NK cells
Synergism with IL-2 and interferons NK cells
Increased lymphokine production (IL-3, IL-6, IFN-γ)
Macrophage cytotoxicity
Growth factor for B-cells
Increased IL-1 production

[a]   These effects are derived from *in vitro* studies.

the multiple biological effects of IL-1 is to view local production and action as the "autocrine/paracrine" action of IL-1. These are listed in Table 2. By contrast, the systemic effects of IL-1 can be viewed as the "hormonal" property such as fever and decreased appetite.[160] At present, it seems that autocrine/paracrine effects of IL-1 predominate in some diseases such a type I diabetes mellitus,[15] whereas systemic effects are characteristic of IL-1 produced as a result of toxemia, septicemia, widespread tissue damage, or intravenous antigen challenge.

It is increasingly clear that tissues producing IL-1 are either themselves targets of IL-1 or are capable of acting on adjacent tissues. For example, IL-1 produced by macrophages in a lymph node acts on macrophages as well as on lymphocytes inducing IL-2, IL-2 receptors, IL-3, IL-6, and IFN-γ. IL-1 produced by microglia and astrocytes in the brain has its effect on local gliosis,[83] but may induce no systemic responses. A similar case can be made for the ability of IL-1 to stimulate production of granulocyte-macrophage colony stimulating factor,[11,262] IFN-β1,[248] and IL-6[249,250] in bone marrow. The local production and biological activity of IL-1 in the joint space has attracted considerable attention because of a potential role for IL-1 in the pathogenesis of various joint diseases. However, in the joint space, IL-1 likely exerts its autocrine/paracrine effects in the absence of major systemic responses. A similar case can be made for IL-1 which is found in the nerve fibers of the human hypothalamus.[26] Locally produced IL-1 in the brain may exert various neuroendocrinologic changes with no detectable systemic changes other than what is detected as normal physiologic changes. The ability of membrane or cell-associated IL-1 to be biologically active underscores the importance of local effects of IL-1 in the absence of systemic signs and symptoms.

VI. EFFECT OF IL-1 ON IMMUNOCOMPETENT CELLS

A. IS IL-1 REQUIRED FOR T CELL ACTIVATION?

Recombinant IL-1 has been used to confirm a role for IL-1 in the mechanism of T and B cell activation, eliminating previous doubts about the purity of natural IL-1 preparations and whether these were capable of participating in immune responses. This is a particularly important issue because recent data on the ability of IL-6, IL-4,[95] and granulocyte macrophage-colony stimulating factor (GM-CSF) to act as "lymphocyte activating factors" have been used to cast doubt on the role of IL-1 as an activator of lymphocytes. Clearly, some preparations of natural IL-1 could have been contaminated with other lymphokines and clouded the issue. However, recombinant IL-1 and antibodies to recombinant IL-1 or antibodies to synthetic IL-1 peptides have clarified the presence of IL-1 receptors on lymphocytes and that IL-1 acts as an activator of lymphocytes. Recombinant IL-1 has not, however, helped settle the issue of whether IL-1 is an absolute requirement for a primary immune response. Certain aspects of the biology of IL-1 have confounded the issue of whether soluble IL-1, like IL-2 and other T cell growth factors, is required for T cell activation. For example:

1. Some T cells synthesize IL-1[240]
2. IL-1 induces other cytokines, such as IL-6 and IFN-γ
3. IL-1 is biologically active as a cell-associated protein, presumably as a cell membrane surface protein[121]

There is little question that in many models of T and B cell activation, IL-1 amplifies the response to antigens or mitogens. This is particularly the case when suboptimal concentrations (concentrations that actually may be close to the *in vivo* situation) are used and when some attempt at macrophage depletion has been employed. In fact, the original immunologic effect of IL-1 was its ability to act in a costimulator assay, the so-called "lymphocyte activating factor" assay using murine thymocytes and suboptimal amounts of mitogens. It soon became clear that given the proper conditions, IL-1 would amplify the activation and induce IL-2 gene expression and IL-2 receptors.[235] What remains to be resolved since those initial observations is whether mature, resting T cells have an absolute requirement for IL-1 during primary activation. The present data suggest that in the strict absence of macrophage membranes, soluble, recombinant IL-1 does not restore the macrophage requirement for activation leading to proliferation. In examining the role for IL-1 in T cell activation, it appears best to divide the discussion into three areas: (1) the effect of IL-1 on thymocytes, (2) the effect of IL-1 on T cell cell lines, and (3) the ability of IL-1 to activate mature, resting T-cells.

B. EFFECT OF IL-1 ON THYMOCYTE RESPONSES TO MITOGENS

From the initial experiments of Gery and Waksman,[79] IL-1 had been "defined" as a co-mitogen for murine thymocytes. Further work demonstrated that when depleted of macrophages, rat thymocytes (or lymph node cells) will not proliferate when incubated with Concanavalin A (Con A) and are unresponsive to IL-2 but require IL-1. Although IL-1 treatment does not affect the ability of thymocytes to bind Con A, the addition of soluble, recombinant IL-1 renders the thymocytes and lymph node cells capable of responding to Con A by producing both IL-2 and IL-2 receptors.[229] In a similar fashion, peanut agglutinin-negative murine thymocytes proliferated when IL-1 was added to suboptimal concentrations of IL-2. The combination of IL-1 and IL-2 induces the IL-2 receptors.[147] The monoclonal antibody directed against the thymocyte receptor L3T4 blocks the ability of IL-1 to act as a co-mitogen and it has been speculated that the L3T4 molecule is functionally involved with IL-1-induced thymocyte proliferation.[135] Other data show that the Ly-1 antigen may serve as an IL-1 receptor.[134]

C. EFFECT OF IL-1 ON IL-2 PRODUCTION FROM T CELL LINES

The D10.G4.1 murine T helper cell line[106] responds to IL-1 in the femtomolar range and may be an ideal cell for studying the T cell response to IL-1. Initially this cell line enters a proliferative phase when IL-1 is added to mitogen-primed cells; in the absence of IL-1, there was no proliferative signal. Subsequently, it was shown that the effect of IL-1 on these cells was not through increased production of IL-2, but rather that IL-4 was providing the proliferative signal. Several laboratories have now demonstrated the exquisite sensitivity of these cells to IL-1 (subfemtomolar concentrations) and that these cells will proliferate to IL-1 in the absence of mitogens and antigens.[122] The IL-1 receptors for these cells have been demonstrated to be comprised of both a high and a low affinity class and the numbers of high affinity receptors are in excess of 20,000/cell.[216] At present it remains unclear whether these cells are inducing a secondary cytokine which provide the proliferative signal, such as IL-4[119] or CSFs.[120]

There is a growing body of evidence that the largest number of high affinity receptors for IL-1 exists on T cell lines. These include the EL4 mouse thymoma cell line, the LBRM33 mouse thymoma cell line, the NOB-1 line (a subclone of the EL4 cell), and the D10S subclone of the murine T helper cell line, D10.G4.1. With the exception of the NOB-1 and the D10S cells, cell lines produce little or no IL-2 in response to IL-1. However, when costimulated with mitogens, antibodies to the CD3 complex, ionophores, or phorbol esters, the cells produce large amounts of IL-2. For example, the human Jurkat cell line produces no Il-2 in response to IL-1, but in the presence of mitogens and phorbol esters, there is increased transcription of IL-2 mRNA.[6] Similar observations have been established in the EL4 and LBRM33 cell lines, i.e., IL-1 itself does not induce IL-2 secretion but requires a second signal, usually one which increases cytosolic calcium.[1,139,141,230]

These data are consistent with the well-established synergistic effect of IL-1 with antigens, mitogens, ionophores, or activators of protein kinase C and support the existence of a two-signal hypothesis for the induction of IL-2 in T cells and T cell lines.[1] The first signal is provided by agents which increase cytosolic calcium, whereas increases in protein kinase C are a signal 2 event. Thus, IL-2 synthesis takes place when cells are stimulated with ionophore and phorbol esters comparable to mitogen and IL-1, respectively. Examining the events in the LBRM33 cell line, mitogen induces rapid hydrolysis of phosphatidylinositol-4,5-bisphosphate (PI), and increased cytosolic calcium. Phorbol esters induced a protracted association of cellular protein kinase C with the plasma membrane. IL-1, however, although providing the signal which leads to increased IL-2 production when cells are stimulated with mitogen, did not activate protein kinase C nor mobilize calcium. Clearly, IL-1 in combination with mitogen-induced intracellular events was able to trigger IL-2 production by a non-phosphotidylinositol, noncalcium mechanism.

D. IL-1 INDUCED DIACYLGLYCEROL IN T CELLS THROUGH
PHOSPHATIDYLCHOLINE TURNOVER

In recent studies by Rosoff and co-workers,[209] similar findings were reported using the Jurkat cell line. As noted above, IL-1 amplifies the gene expression for mitogen or ionophore primed Jurkat cells.[6] These cells produce increased IL-2 when stimulated by a combination of phorbol esters and IL-1 or anti-CD3 and IL-1; however, despite this activation, IL-1 does not increase cytosolic calcium in these cells or in neutrophils.[78] On the other hand, IL-1 causes a rapid rise in diacylglycerol (DG) production. If this were due to hydrolysis of PI, generation of inositol triphosphate would have occurred, but similar to the results of others,[1] this did not occur. These results suggest that IL-1 induces phospholipid hydrolysis through a nonphosphatidylinositol turnover pathway, for example, phosphatidylcholine (PC).

When the Jurkat cells were labeled with ^{3}H-choline and then stimulated with IL-1, phosphorylcholine increased dramatically (within 5 s) in the supernatant, whereas the concentration of PC decreased in the organic phase of the cells. The increase in supernatant phosphorylcholine was not due to PC turnover via protein kinase C-stimulated diacylglycerol PI turnover because that pathway leads to increased cytosolic PC hydrolysis and the IL-1-stimulated PC turnover is primarily observed in the extracellular compartment. The concentration of IL-1 which induced the PC turnover was 30 fmol, reaching a maximum at 100 fmol, the concentration of IL-1 that stimulates T cell proliferation and other biological effects *in vitro*. The IL-1-induced PC turnover was also observed in the D10.G4.1 T helper cell line, the EL4 cell line, and in nylon wool purified human peripheral blood T cells.

When the Jurkat, EL4 and D10.G4.1 cells were examined for IL-1 receptor affinity and numbers, we observed that Jurkat cells have no high affinity (see below) IL-1 receptors whereas the EL4 and D10.G4.1 cells studied with the same labeled IL-1α and under the same equilibrium conditions clearly contained the typical 80 kDa IL-1 receptor. These studies suggest that the high affinity receptors for IL-1 are probably unrelated to the initiation of PC turnover and that this may be due to activation of a second, very low affinity receptor. This may explain the discrepancies in the biological response of many cells to IL-1 and the number of high affinity receptors.

Regardless of the proposed existence of a very low IL-1 receptor-IL-1 binding being the mechanism by which IL-1 stimulates PC turnover, the fact that there are at least two pathways by which DG becomes elevated in T cells may explain the co-mitogen effect of IL-1 in a variety of immunocompetent cells (and even some nonimmunocompetent cells). T cells are rich in protein kinases and several isoenzymes with different tissue distribution exist. It has been proposed that the different protein kinases differ in the binding sites of the DG and that this may be determined by the type of fatty acid side chain. For example, mitogens which stimulate DG through a PI turnover pathway result in activation of one type of protein kinase C, whereas IL-1 which stimulates DG through PC turnover stimulates another isoenzyme. In some cells like the Jurkat, there is a requirement for both (?synergism) protein kinases before IL-2 gene expression is initiated. The mitogen (in this case anti-CD3) is not sufficient without phorbol esters or IL-1 to provide the second signal, in this case another protein kinase, through a PC-specific DG. This may be one explanation for the ampliyfing effect of IL-1 in a variety of immunocompetent cells. In comparing the response of EL4 cells to IL-1, ionophore, and phorbol esters, Truneh et al.[245] concluded that IL-1 and TPA induce protein kinase C activation by two different mechanisms. It is thus probable that these two mechanisms reflect the two different pathways by which IL-1 and mitogens stimulate DG.

E. EFFECT OF IL-1 ON PERIPHERAL BLOOD T CELLS

Employing human peripheral blood T cells activated by immobilized antibodies directed against the CD3 cell surface protein complex, soluble IL-1 serves a cofactor for activation in the absence of macrophages.[257] Under these conditions, the addition of soluble recombinant IL-1 partially restores the role of the macrophage and one observes increased synthesis of IL-2 and expression of the IL-2 receptor. Increased DNA synthesis followed these events as an indicator of cell proliferation. When they are diluted, however, the ability of soluble IL-1 to replace the macrophage function is lost, suggesting that total macrophage depletion was not accomplished. IL-2 will, on the other hand, drive these cells to proliferate.

F. EFFECT OF IL-1 ON B CELL ACTIVATION

Many investigators have shown that B cells and other cells serve as accessory cells in antigen recognition, but have failed to demonstrate a role for IL-1 because IL-1 cannot be detected in B cell supernatants. This issue may have been resolved by studies which demonstrate that B cells produce IL-1[159,217] and that B cells express membrane-bound IL-1.[121] In fact, nearly all cells which can act as accessory cells produce IL-1. These include astrocytes, mesangial cells, keratinocytes, and endothelial cells. Effects of IL-1 on B cells and immunoglobulin production continue to occur.[131,171] The function of IL-1 in B cell activation seems to be similar to that shown in T cells, that is, IL-1 acts as a helper or cofactor during the activation process, particularly together with IL-4, also known as B cell stimulating factor-1. IL-1 activates B cells and contributes to the formation of antibody. The first experiments to show the critical role for IL-1 in B cell activation were performed with anti-IL-1.[132] Adding antibody early to human peripheral blood mononuclear cells stimulated with pokeweed mitogen completely prevented B cell activation and subsequent antibody formation. Other studies demonstrated that IL-1 synergized with various B cell growth and differentiation factors leading to increased proliferation and antibody formation.[67,68] Some of the biological activity of the natural B cell growth and differentiation factors may have been due to the presence of IL-6 (see below). The ability of IL-1 to synergize with IL-6 on T cell activation probably extends to B cell activation; its other ability to induce other B cell stimulating factors, including IL-6, IFN-γ, and IL-2 must also be considered since these substances activate B cells.

The recent evidence demonstrating that IL-1 induces the production of B cell stimulating factor-2/hybridoma growth factor should be considered as a role for IL-1 in B cell and immunoglobulin synthesis. The hybridoma growth factor protein also had the ability to stimulate plasmacytoma cell growth. The N-terminus of the palsmacytoma/hybridoma growth factor matches that of an IFN-β2.[249,250] Others have also reported a B cell stimulating factor,[94] which is the same sequence as the 26 kDa IFN-β2. IFN-β2 has also been identified as the factor previously known as hepatocyte stimulating factor, which caused an increase in C-reactive protein as well as other hepatic acute phase proteins.[77] IFN-β2 with its activity on B and liver cells is now termed IL-6. It seems that the role of IL-1 in augmenting B cell function and ultimately leading to the production of protective antibodies may be through its ability to induce the synthesis of B cell stimulating factors and/or upregulating their receptors.

G. IL-1 AND NK CELLS

IL-1 also plays a role in host defense against tumor cells. There is evidence that IL-1 increases the binding of NK cells to tumor targets and that tumor cells induce synthesis of IL-1 by NK cells.[92,93] In addition, NK cells from patients with large tumor burdens produce significantly less IL-1 and have decreased killing ability than cells from healthy individuals. When incubated with exogenous IL-1, impaired natural killer function is restored. IL-1 also augments the binding of NK cells from healthy donors to tumor targets. Since IL-1 induces IFN and since IFN synergizes with IL-1 with respect to its actions on NK cells,[40] one could view both mechanisms as an efficient aspect of host defense against tumors. Unlike augmentation of T and B cell responses by IL-1 which are enhanced at febrile temperatures,[59,89] however, the effect of IL-1 on NK cells is reduced by febrile temperatures.[51]

NK cells also produce IL-1.[218] Recent studies suggest that in addition to endotoxin, high dose IL-2 is a stimulant for IL-1 and TNF production by NK cells.[180] The ability of IL-2 to induce IL-1 and TNF production appears to be due to the CD4 receptor on monocytes. This is up-regulated by IFN-γ which also increases the responsiveness of NK cells to IL-1-induced cytokine production.

VII. THE IL-1 RECEPTOR

The initial studies on the binding of radiolabeled IL-1 were carried out using a variety of cells;[56] nearly all subsequent studies have focused on two cell types: murine thymoma cells and fibroblasts.[215] From these early studies, there appeared to be a single class of intermediate affinity receptor (K_d ranged from 400 pmol to 1 nM) and relatively few receptors (200/cell). Subsequent studies showed that the receptor number and affinity could be higher on thymoma cell lines and fibroblasts. Although the IL-1 receptor was specific in that it did not recognize other cytokines, the IL-1 receptor did not distinguish between IL-1α or IL-1β.[30,110,139,141,155,156] In general, the binding correlated with the capacity of the cells to respond to IL-1, however, it soon became clear that there were two classes of IL-1 receptors.[23,139] There is little question that an IL-1 receptor has been recognized by all groups and has a variable dissociation constant of 200 to 600 pmol. From cross-linking experiments, this binding protein is probably what is often called the IL-1 receptor — an 80 kDa glycosylated peptide whose unglycosylated form is approximately 55 kDa. This molecule has been solubilized[184] and cloned; the sequence reveals that the IL-1 receptor belongs to the immunoglobulin superfamily.[231]

The cloned molecule likely represents the high affinity receptor described by Lowenthal and MacDonald[139] and Bird and Saklatvala.[23] These groups described binding sites with an affinity of 5 to 10 pmol, considerably higher affinity than that previously reported. Furthermore, it has also been reported that both high and low affinity receptors exist on a wide variety of T cell lines and normal cells. We have also observed two classes of IL-1 receptors on the D10.G4.1 murine T helper cell line. In the case of our own studies,[216] receptors of both high and low affinity were detected simultaneously on a subclone (D10S) of these cells. The failure to detect both classes of receptors in some studies may be due to the low specific activity of the radiolabeled IL-1 or that the low affinity receptor is not easily detectable.

In addition to the conflicting data on the IL-1 receptor affinity, there are also low numbers of receptors. However, Lowenthal and MacDonald[139] and Savage et al.[216] have reported much higher numbers of IL-1 receptors on murine EL4 cells and murine T helper cells, respectively. The high numbers (about 20,000/cell) are not in the same range as those observed for other growth factor receptors which can be of the order of 100,000 to 200,000/cell.

A. COMPARISON OF THE IL-1 AND IL-2 RECEPTOR

In evaluating the significance of high and low affinity receptors for IL-1 on different cells, some investigators have compared the situation with that of the receptors for IL-2. IL-2 receptors also exhibit two classes distinguished by their ligand binding affinities.[142,204] The IL-2 receptor is made up of two distinct polypeptide chains (the so-called "TAC" 55 kDa antigen and a lower affinity polypeptide chain of 75 kDa) each of which may bind to IL-2. One of the components binds with a lower affinity than the other; the two may both interact and combine with IL-2 to produce the high affinity receptor. The binding of the IL-2 to its 75 kDa intermediate affinity receptor is sufficient to activate Na^+/H^+ exchange in YT 202,[162] a cell line expressing only the 75 kDa IL-2 binding component. The same situation has been proposed for the IL-2 receptor.[24] Our own studies on D10S cells suggests that the IL-1 receptor comprises more than one polypeptide chain[216] and others have also observed the existence of a second chain.[24]

Studies on the IL-2 receptor have revealed that high and low affinity receptors differ functionally and that a similar case can be made for the two classes of IL-1 receptors.[139] It has been proposed that the high affinity IL-1 receptor is incorporated into the cell and the number of IL-1 molecules endocytosed by various T-cell lines correlates with the number of high affinity IL-1 receptors expressed by these cells. This has been demonstrated for IL-2, where ligand internalization is believed to be mediated only by high affinity receptors.[255] In contrast, the internalization of IL-1 appears to be via a receptor with an intermediate affinity of 150 pmol.[23] Internalization of IL-1 by a large granular lymphocyte cell line was demonstrated by receptors with a K_d of about 100 pmol,[155,156] which is higher than the high affinity receptors of 5 to 10 pmol. One explanation for this discrepancy is that two different cell types have been studied, the fibroblast and the T cell, respectively.

B. BOTH IL-1α AND IL-1β BIND TO THE SAME RECEPTOR

Most studies have demonstrated that in using either form of IL-1 in receptor binding experiments, the one IL-1 form effectively competes with the binding of the other form. However, some studies suggest that although human and murine IL-1α may bind to human endothelial cells with an equal affinity, there is an unequal ability to induce a biological response.[241] Recombinant murine IL-1α was found to be 250- to 1250-fold less active than recombinant human IL-1α in inducing endothelial cell adherence of human lymphocytes. Furthermore, Bird et al.[24] have shown that the concentration of porcine IL-1β required to elicit half maximal IL-2 production from NOB-1, a subline of murine thymoma IL-4, was 100-fold greater than that for porcine IL-1α. However, both forms of IL-1 were equally active at similar doses when acting on BALB/c 3T3 fibroblasts to increase lactate production.

These results and those of other investigators suggest that contrary to what was first believed, the receptor binding site on IL-1α and IL-1β may not be recognizing the same receptor loci in the different cells. Some attempts have been made to localize the receptor binding site or specific recognition peptides on IL-1. MacDonald et al.[144] produced various mutations of the histidine residue at position 147 in IL-1β and showed that this resulted in up to 100-fold reduction in receptor-binding affinity. Short synthetic peptide fragments of human IL-1β with immunostimulatory activity[4,208] have been produced. These peptides code for hydrophobic regions of the IL-1β molecule which share significant amino acid homologies to those regions in the IL-1α molecule. Although they are biologically active, large amounts are required. Furthermore, there are no data suggesting that these peptides block the binding of full-length IL-1β to cells. Recently, attention has focused on the carboxyl terminal of the IL-1β structure. X-ray crystallographic studies of IL-1β have revealed that the histidine at position 147 as well as the N-terminus and carboxyl terminus are exposed and available for membrane interaction.[198] In one study, antibodies produced to the C-terminal (amino acids 247-269) blocked IL-1 biological activities whereas antibodies produced to the N-terminal amino acids (117-134) had no effect.[203] On the other hand, mutations in the IL-1β N-terminus have dramatically affected IL-1 binding.[97] It appears that both the N- and C-termini interact with the receptor.

C. REGULATION OF IL-1 RECEPTOR EXPRESSION

Both up-regulation and down-regulation of the IL-1 receptor may occur. Up-regulation of the IL-1 receptor on T cells has been reported on human peripheral T cells or murine splenic T cells stimulated with Con A[57,226] and human mononuclear cells treated with corticosteroids increase receptor number. EL4 cells treated with *trans*-retinoic acid increase their binding of IL-1.[110] Down-regulation of the IL-1 receptor has been reported by IL-1 itself.[155,164,216]

D. PHYSICAL STRUCTURE OF THE IL-1 RECEPTOR

Cross-linking experiments in a variety of cells identify a major binding protein of 80 kDa on sodium dodecylsulfate-polyacrylamide gel electrophoresis (SDS-PAGE). A second cross-linked species has been observed at 116 kDa. It has been suggested that the higher molecular mass species could either represent a protein of 116 kDa or a tertiary complex of the 80 kDa receptor, a 30 kDa binding protein, and IL-1. Cross-linking studies in rat brain indicate that the rat brain IL-1 receptor also has a molecular mass of 80 kDa.[69] It may be significant that these authors also found a second IL-1 binding protein in rat brain at 68 kDa. The homogeneous IL-1 receptor, purified from EL4 6.1 cells has been found to be a protein of 80 kDa which correlates with the results found for the affinity cross-linking experiments.

Most experimental evidence to date has confirmed the existence of a plasma membrane protein of molecular size ranging from 70 to 80 kDa for the IL-1 receptor. The Raji B-lymphoma cells have a lower binding affinity but much higher receptor density ($K_d = 2.1$ nM, 7709 sites/cell)[97] than the murine T cells ($K_d = 400$ pmol, 241 sites/cell). Cross-linking studies showed that the IL-1 receptor in the B cells had a lower molecular mass than that in the T cells (68 compared to 80 kDa). We, however, have found that the D10S subclone of the murine T helper cell D10.G4.1 possesses a high number of IL-1 receptors which would imply that the cells do not differ from the B cells in this regard.[216] It is likely that variations in the size of the IL-1 binding components in the different cells are caused by glycosylation. In fact, treatment of EL4 as well as fibroblast-derived IL-1 receptors with glycanases reduces the molecule size to about 50 kDa.[266]

In our laboratory we have digested radioactive IL-1 cross-linked proteins from EL4 and D10S cells with glycanase and generated bands 10 to 15 kDa lower in mass.[267] Most authors have also reported on the presence of minor radioactive bands either of higher or lower molecular mass than the major species. We have observed a 30 kDa IL-1-binding protein on D10S cells which was not observed with EL4 cells. It is possible that the 116 kDa protein is a combination of the 80 and 30 kDa proteins. The significance of these lower molecular weight IL-1-binding components is not clear; however, a recent report on the structure of the IL-1 receptor may explain the molecular weight differences (see below).

E. POSTRECEPTOR BINDING EVENTS

Information concerning the intracellular events following the IL-1-1/IL-1 receptor complex has only recently been studied. No clear picture has emerged. Of importance when considering the postreceptor events of IL-1 action is the fact that in addition to the growth promoting properties of IL-1, the cytokine has a wide variety of other biologic activities. These properties can only be explained if there are different receptors on the various cells, or alternatively, the receptors are identical but the postreceptor machinery differ in the various cells in which the biological events occur. When considering the cellular proliferating effects, some evidence suggests that like other growth factors such as EGF and insulin, IL-1 may activate a tyrosine kinase, although it is not known whether the kinase is part of the IL-1 receptor. However, the same authors have also observed plasma membrane protein phosphorylation as a result of IL-1 action on membranes from K562 cells. Surprisingly the K562 cells have been shown to possess very small numbers of receptors (<10 molecules bound/cell) and the effect of IL-1 in these cells is not to produce proliferation, but rather induce killing mechanisms. Do the two phosphorylation events induced by IL-1 differ? Results from our laboratory[268] show that recombinant IL-1 acting on the plasma membrane isolated from EL4 cells can also induce the phosphorylation of certain membrane proteins, although the site of phosphorylation is unknown at present. On the other hand, Matsushima et al.[158] have observed the phosphorylation of a cytosolic 65 kDa protein when IL-1 acts on normal human peripheral blood mononuclear leukocytes pretreated with glucocorticoids. Phosphorylation was observed in serine residues of the protein and not on tyrosine residue, as described by Martin et al.[149] for K-562 cells.

In addition to the phosphorylation effects of IL-1, internalization of the ligand occurs. Internalization of IL-1 has been shown by several groups.[23,155,156,164] Some studies show subsequent lysosomal trafficking of ligand and reutilization of receptors. After 3 h at 37°C, the ligand was located in the lysosomal fraction and there was an increase in the TCA soluble fraction at 6 h. In addition, some studies show electron microscopic evidence, using auto-radiographic detection techniques, for the appearance of radioactive IL-1 within the nucleus of the cells. There was little evidence for the degradation of IL-1 by the cells, at least up to 4 to 6 h. Lowenthal and MacDonald[140] have also observed the uptake of IL-1 in EL4 cells and that a significant fraction internalized IL-1 was found in the nucleus.

Another postreceptor event that has been described for IL-1 is on the ion flux of both Na^+ and Ca^{2+} across the plasma membrane of a murine pre-B cell line.[237] Major questions require clarification of the nature of the signal initiated by the formation of the cell surface IL-1 complex and the role of internalization of the IL-1 ligand in the transfer of information. The finding that IL-1 will rapidly increase PC turnover in Jurkat cells which do not manifest a detectable IL-1 receptor underscores the complexity of IL-1 effects on cells and the postexposure events. It is possible that there are both receptor (high affinity) events leading to PI turnover and the generation of DG in some cells and low affinity receptor interaction resulting in the generation of another DG from PC turnover. Moreover, both systems may work in some cells. The end result would perhaps provide a number of activated protein kinases.

VIII. COMPARISON OF IL-1, TNF AND IL-6

A. IL-1 AND TNF

TNF was initially identified in the circulation of animals following the injection of endotoxin. It was also discovered in the supernates from stimulated macrophage cell lines where its property as an inhibitor of lipoprotein lipase led to its being named "cachectin", since it produced a wasting syndrome when chronically administered to mice. The amino acid sequences of TNF[186] are identical to cachectin.[19] TNF, a product of stimulated monocytes and macrophages, is also produced by lymphocytes,[35] endothelial cells, and keratinocytes. A structurally related polypeptide, initially isolated from activated T cells, is lymphotoxin. Lymphotoxin and TNF produce similar biological changes in a variety of cells. The amino sequence of TNF and lymphotoxin are closely related[186] and both molecules are recognized by the same cell membrane receptor. Like IL-1β and -α, TNF and lymphotoxin are sufficiently structurally distinct molecules that antibodies produced to each cytokine do not cross-react with the other cytokine. Although originally studied for its ability to kill tumor cells *in vitro* as well as when injected into tumor bearing mice, the widespread biological effects of TNF on mesenchymal and other cells have been the focus of studies related to its inflammatory properties, particularly in mediating synovial cell activity and cartilage and bone degradation. Moreover, recombinant human TNF has been injected into human subjects and many of its systemic effects such as fever, leukopenia, and hypotension, which were studied in animals, have now been observed in humans.[29]

The biological properties of TNF share remarkable similarities to those of IL-1, particularly the nonimmunological effects of IL-1. Some lymphocyte-activating properties of IL-1 or IL-6 are shared with TNF but these require considerably higher concentrations of TNF than IL-1. There are recent reports on the ability of TNF to activate T cells,[200] including the expression of IL-2 receptors.[195] B cells are also stimulated by TNF.[102,107] Compared to IL-1, the molar concentration of TNF required to stimulate immunocompetent cells is one or two orders of magnitude greater than IL-1.[107,200] Since TNF induces the synthesis and release of immunostimulatory polypeptides such as IL-1 and IL-6 from monocytes, fibroblasts, and endothelial cells, it is possible that these cytokines augment the action of TNF on lymphocytes. Some investigators have attempted to separate a direct action of TNF on lymphocytes from that secondary to the induction of IL-1 or IL-6.[200] It also appears that unlike IL-1, the immunostimulatory effects of TNF are species-specific.

Nearly every nonimmunological biological property of IL-1 has also been observed with TNF. These include fever,[53] the induction of PGE_2 and collagenase synthesis in a variety of tissues,[37] bone and cartilage resorption,[211] inhibition of lipoprotein lipase,[18] increases in hepatic acute phase proteins, complement components, and a decrease in albumin synthe-

TABLE 3
Comparison of Biological Properties of IL-1 and TNF

Biological property	IL-1	TNF
Endogenous pyrogen fever	+	+
Slow wave sleep	+	+
Hemodynamic shock	+	+
Increased hepatic acute phase protein synthesis	+	+
Decreased albumin synthesis	+	+
Activation of endothelium	+	+
Decreased lipoprotein lipase	+	+
Decreased cytochrome P450	+	+
Decreased plasma Fe/Zn	+	+
Increased fibroblast proliferation	+	+
Increased synovial cell collagenase and PGE_2	+	+
Induction of IL-1	+	+
T/B cell activation	+	±
Hemopoietin-1 activity	−	+

sis.[188] Slow wave sleep and appetite suppression are also observed following the injection of TNF.[227] As discussed above, both molecules induce fibroblast proliferation collagen synthesis.[116] The cytotoxic activity of TNF differs from that of IL-1 in that IL-1 is inactive on a variety of tumor targets for which TNF is a potent cytotoxin. However, IL-1 exhibits cytotoxic effects on melanoma cells which are unaffected by TNF.[183] Another difference between IL-1 and TNF is that IL-1 can function as cofactor for stem cell activation (hemopoietin-1 activity),[165,167,236] whereas TNF suppresses bone marrow colony formation.[263] Both IL-1 and TNF induce the synthesis of CSFs.[11,262]

Similar to IL-1, TNF induces fever by its direct ability to stimulate hypothalamic PGE_2 synthesis.[53] Levels of circulating TNF rise rapidly in human subjects injected with endotoxin[91,161] and are associated with the symptoms of the prodrome and chill period of the fever. In addition to fever, TNF produces hypotension, leukopenia, and local tissue necrosis.[244] On a weight basis in rabbits, TNF is more potent than IL-1 in producing a shock.[182] Administration of anti-TNF antibodies to rabbits prevents the shock induced by endotoxin.[152] The shock-like responses to TNF likely reflect the effects on the vascular endothelium. TNF stimulates PGI_2, PGE_2, and platelet activating factor production by cultured endothelium. In addition, like IL-1, TNF stimulates procoagulant activity, leukocyte adherence, and plasminogen activator inhibitor on these cells. TNF also induces a capillary-leak syndrome. Despite the similarities, receptors for TNF and IL-1 are distinct and specific and receptor binding to the respective ligand is only displaced by the specific cytokine. Furthermore, IL-1 down-regulates its own receptor as well as that of TNF. The most likely explanation is that TNF and IL-1 stimulate similar intracellular messages by different pathways and alter the same cascade of intracellular metabolites. Table 3 lists the biological similarities between IL-1 and TNF. Of note is the fact that TNF stimulates human neutrophil oxidative metabolism,[112] whereas IL-1 does not;[78] on the other hand, IL-1 induces histamine and arylsulfatase release from human basophils[238] and eosinophils, respectively,[194] and TNF does not. There is another macrophage product with a molecular weight of 8 kDa which is chemotactic for neutrophils and is clearly not IL-1 nor TNF.[258,261] This factor may have been present in some preparations of natural IL-1 and TNF and could have accounted for their effects on neutrophils. The biological properties of this macrophage product in comparison to IL-1 and TNF remain to be ascertained.

B. SYNERGISM BETWEEN IL-1 AND TNF

The effects of IL-1 or TNF on a variety of cells *in vitro* as well as systemic effects *in vivo* are often biologically indistinguishable. When the two cytokines are used together in experimental studies, the net effect often exceeds the additive effect of each cytokine. Potentiation or frank synergism between these two molecules has been demonstrated in several studies. On fibroblasts, IL-1 and TNF act synergistically in the production of PGE_2.[63] The cytotoxic effect of TNF and IL-1 on certain tumor cells is also synergistic *in vitro*, and when administered to tumor-bearing mice *in vivo*, both molecules act synergistically to eliminate the tumor.[269] IL-1 combined with TNF protects rats exposed to lethal hyperoxia.[256] IL-1 and TNF act synergistically in the induction of radioprotection.[175,176] IL-1 induces cytotoxic effects on the insulin producing β cells of the islets of Langerhans; this effect is dramatically augmented by TNF.[145,146] IL-1 and TNF induce neutrophilic infiltration when injected intradermally into experimental animals; when injected together, these cytokines act synergistically and can replace endotoxin in the generation of the local Swartzman reaction.[169] Rats receiving intravenous infusions of IL-1 or TNF manifest metabolic changes reflected in plasma amino acid levels, but when given together, negative nitrogen balance and muscle proteolysis can be demonstrated.[197] Although high doses (10 to 20 μg/kg) of TNF produce a shock-like state with tissue damage,[244] IL-1 and TNF act synergistically to produce hemodynamic shock and pulmonary hemorrhage at doses of only 1 μg/kg when given together.[182] The two cytokines also act synergistically in the aggregation of neutrophils and the synthesis of thromboxanes.[34] Considering the fact that IL-1 and TNF are often present together in human body fluids, including inflammatory joint fluid, the synergism between the two cytokines cannot be considered a laboratory observation. The synergism between these two cytokines seems to be due to second message molecules rather than up-regulation of cell receptors; in fact, IL-1 reduces TNF receptors.[96]

C. IL-1 AND IL-6

The recent cloning and expression of B cell stimulating factor-2 (B cell growth factor-2)[94] and hybridoma growth factor[25] has supported the observation that these molecules are identical to IFN-β-2.[249,250] FN-β2 was cloned and expressed before its identification as B cell stimulating factor-2. In addition, IFN-β2 appears to be the same molecule previously termed "hepatocyte stimulating factor",[77] inducing a variety of hepatic acute phase proteins in cultured liver cells. The molecule IFN-β2, otherwise known as hybridoma growth factor, plasmacytoma growth factor, B cell stimulating factor-2, and hepatocyte stimulating factor is now termed IL-6. Like IL-1 and TNF, IL-6 is an endogenous pyrogen and an inducer of acute phase responses. In a clinical study, serum levels of IL-6 correlated with the amount of fever present in patients with burn injuries.[177] IL-6 levels have also been reported to be elevated in patients undergoing renal rejection[252] and in the cerebrospinal fluid of patients with CNS infections.[99] Although IL-6 is an inducer of fibrinogen synthesis in hepatic cell lines, these cultured cells require the presence of corticosteroids to observe a response.[3] In mice and rats, IL-6 does not induce fibrinogen unless corticosteroids are administered at the same time;[148] IL-1, on the other hand, induces large amounts of fibrinogen without the requirements of such cofactors.[16]

The effects of IL-6 on lymphocytes and bone marrow stem cells are broadly based. Attention has focused on the ability of natural or recombinant IL-6 to act as a lymphocyte activating factor in the typical murine thymocyte co-mitogenesis assay. Similar to recombinant IL-1α or IL-1β, recombinant IL-6, in the presence of Con A, induces the production of IL-2 from cytotoxic T cell lines (CTLL).[76] A similar response was observed when recombinant IL-6 was added with mitogen or antibody to the T cell antigen receptor-stimulated peripheral blood CD4+ T cell depleted of accessory cells. IL-2 was released and acted as the proliferative signal for these cells. Using high concentrations (100 U) of recombinant IL-1, production of IL-2 was not observed,[76] leading these authors to the conclusion that IL-6 rather than IL-1 was providing the "first signal" along with mitogen or anti-T cell receptor activation in mature circulating T cells. The molar concentration of the recombinant IL-6 used in these studies is difficult to ascertain and limiting dilutions of the purified T cell targets was not carried out. Therefore, like IL-1, it is difficult to ascertain whether IL-6 activates lymphocytes in the absence of macrophages, particularly since IL-6 is a product of activated macrophages; moreover, hemopoietic growth factors[260] as well as IL-6 are inducible by IL-1.[222,249,250]

IL-6 will act as a co-mitogen for human thymocytes and macrophage-depleted human T cells;[138] however, unlike IL-1, the co-mitogenesis effect of IL-6 was not inhibited by antibodies to the IL-2 receptor.[138] Similar studies have been reported for thymic and peripheral blood T cells of the L3T4+ and Lyt-2+ subsets.[247] Recombinant IL-6 acts as an autocrine growth factor for human myeloma cells *in vitro*,[105] and IL-1 has also been shown to act as an autocrine growth factor for EBV-transformed human B cells.[219] In addition, recombinant IL-6 induces the production of immunoglobulin from activated B cells in the absence of growth.[172]

We have compared recombinant IL-1 and IL-6 in a variety of assays. In the murine thymocyte co-mitogenesis assay, human recombinant IL-1 stimulates proliferation at 1 to 10 pg/ml, whereas 1 to 10 ng/ml of recombinant IL-6 is required for the same amount of proliferation. This may be due to the species specificity of IL-6. Using a highly IL-1-sensitive murine T helper cell line (D10.G4.1), 5 to 6 orders of magnitude greater concentrations of IL-6 compared to IL-1 are required for a proliferative signal. In rabbits, IL-6 behaves as an endogenous pyrogen, producing a rapid onset monophasic fever; however, 20- to 50-fold greater amounts of IL-6 are required to produce the same elevation in body temperature as that following IL-1.[55] Once again, this may be due to species specificity. However, when recombinant human IL-1 was compared to recombinant human IL-6 on human monocyte PGE_2 production, 50- to 100-fold more IL-6 than IL-1 was required. Similar dose-response differences have been observed using human synovial cell or fibroblasts as targets.[270] Unlike IL-1 and TNF, IL-6 does not induce IL-1 or TNF; in fact, IL-6 suppresses endotoxin- and TNF-induced IL-1 production.[55] IL-6 does not activate endothelial cells *in vitro*.[123,233] In general, IL-6 appears to be a weak inflammatory peptide. Of considerable importance is the observation that IL-1 and IL-6 both act as hemopoietin-1 on bone marrow cultures.[100,165,167] In addition, IL-6 protects granulocytopenic mice against lethal Gram-negative infection[271] similar to the protection afforded by IL-1.[251] IL-1 and IL-6 act synergistically in protecting mice given lethal irradiation.[272] The lack of inflammatory properties and postivie effects on B and T cell functions as well as bone marrow and nonspecific host defense mechanisms make IL-6 potentially useful in treating some diseases, especially bone marrow transplantation. Table 4 lists the biological activities of IL-1, TNF, and IL-6.

IX. IL-1 AND RELATED CYTOKINES IN HUMAN DISEASE

A. IL-1 and TNF IN HUMAN JOINT FLUID

IL-1 and TNF have been detected in human joint fluids from patients with a variety of joint diseases, including rheumatoid, traumatic, psoriatic, and osteoarthritis.[42,73,178] Recently, IL-6 has been detected in the fluid from patients with rheumatoid arthritis.[273] Although substances that inhibit the bioassays for IL-1, TNF, and IL-6 have made detection difficult, specific assays to detect immunoreactive levels of the cytokines are presently available.[133] Because of joint fluid proteases, it is not surprising to find IL-1 in small molecular weight fragments in the 10 and 4000 Da range. These fragments exhibit biological activity for T and B lymphocytes.[163] It is unclear whether TNF has biological activity after limited proteolysis. The sources of the IL-1, TNF, and IL-6 in human joint fluid includes the joint

TABLE 4
Comparison of IL-1, TNF, and IL-6

Biological property	IL-1	TNF	IL-6
Endogenous pyrogen fever	+	+	+
Hepatic acute phase proteins	+	+	+
T-cell activation	+	±	+
B-cell activation	+	±	+
B-cell Ig synthesis	±	−	+
Fibroblast proliferation	+	+	+
Stem cell activation (hemopoietin-1)	+	−	+
Nonspecific resistance to infection	+	+	+
Radioprotection	+	+	+
Synovial cell activation	+	+	−
Endothelial cell activation	+	+	−
Induction of IL-1 and TNF from monocytes	+	+	−
Induction of IL-6	+	+	−

macrophage and other cells such as B cells and the synovial dendritic cells.[60] Large granular lymphocytes (also known as NK cells) release IL-1 and TNF upon stimulation with endotoxin[218] or high dose IL-2.[180] The two major blood vessel cells, endothelium and smooth muscle, both produce IL-1 and may be a source of cytokines.[126,127] In disease processes in which antigen-antibody complexes mediate tissue injury and vessel disruption, endothelial and/or smooth muscle IL-1 likely acts as an autocoid and contributes to the progression of the lesion. In addition to the fixed cell pool in the synovium, IL-1 production may also take place in the joint space from B lymphocytes[159] and neutrophils.[243] Of importance is the finding that Epstein-Barr virus infection in B cells leads to IL-1 production;[217] some recent studies suggest that T cells may also be a source of IL-1, but these studies have been carried out only in transformed T cell lines.[61] On the other hand, human blood T cells stimulated with mitogens produce TNF.[35]

B. CIRCULATING IL-1, TNF AND IL-6 IN HUMAN DISEASE STATES

In general, the levels of these cytokines are low and most studies to date are based on bioassays. These include elevated IL-1 levels in humans following strenuous exercise, ultraviolet light for the treatment of psoriasis, in women following ovulation,[28] and in patients with renal allograft rejection. IL-6 levels have been reported to be elevated in patients with burn injuries[177] and those undergoing organ transplant rejection. TNF levels are elevated in patients with acute meningitis due to *Neisseria*. Recently, TNF levels, as measured by specific enzyme-linked immunoassay, were elevated in the plasma of human volunteers injected with endotoxin.[161] There are several unresolved issues of measuring cytokines in the circulation during various disease states; these include technical aspects of extracting cytokines that may bind to plasma proteins, specific plasma protein that inhibit the assays, rapid degradation by plasma proteases, rapid clearance of the cytokines by cell receptors or excretion into the urine, and transiently elevated cytokine levels. There has been considerable research effort focused on measuring circulating cytokine in various disease states but few convincing reports.

C. PRODUCTION OF IL-1 *IN VITRO* BY BLOOD MONOCYTES OF PATIENTS WITH DISEASES

The amount of IL-1 products from human blood monocytes *in vitro* has been examined in the setting of various disease states. There have been consistent results which indicate that IL-1 production is decreased in monocytes from patients with large tumor burdens[92] or metastatic disease.[196,214] It is unclear, however, whether this decreased production of IL-1 represents a mechanism relevant to cancer or reflects the state of nutrition of the individual. Malnourishment itself seems to reduce IL-1 production and this has been shown in experimental animal models[104] as well as in human studies.[22,90] On the other hand, there are several studies which suggest that blood monocytes from patients with active rheumatoid arthritis produce more IL-1 than blood monocytes from normal individuals.[151,179,228] Patients with ankylosing spondylitis produce the same amount of IL-1 as that produced by monocytes from healthy control subjects,[109] whereas decreased IL-1 production has been consistently demonstrated from monocytes of patients with scleroderma[213] or systemic lupus erythematosus.[2,98,130]

These and other data on IL-1 levels are based upon bioassays which are affected by a variety of substances present in the supernatant medium of cultured mononuclear cells. It is, however, unlikely that the "increase" in IL-1 production observed from monocytes of patients with rheumatoid arthritis is due to IL-2 since the amount of IL-2 produced from the cells of these patients is, in fact, decreased. On the other hand, the demonstration that IL-1 production by monocytes of patients with lupus erythematosus or scleroderma is decreased may be due to the presence of inhibitory factors which suppress the IL-1 bioassay. These inhibitory substances include prostaglandins as well as polypeptides. In one study, the decreased production of IL-1 from monocytes *in vitro* from patients with lupus erythematosus was only partially reversed by the addition of indomethacin.[98]

In general, the supernatant media of cultured human mononuclear cells contain polypeptides that specifically suppress T cell bioassays for IL-1 but not IL-2. These nondialyzable suppressor factors have been demonstrated in the supernatant media of stimulated human mononuclear cells from apparently healthy individuals under a variety of conditions including incubation with immune complexes and viruses.[5,205] There has been partial characterization of the IL-1 inhibitory protein found in the supernates of cytomegalovirus infected human mononuclear cells.[205] Cultured human mononuclear cells from the joint fluid of patients with rheumatoid arthritis produce an IL-1-specific inhibitor[137] which has been implicated as the cause of the depressed response of these cells to mitogens.[137] There is evidence that the IL-1 inhibitory protein produced by a human glioma cell line is TGFβ.[74] Clearly, these IL-1 inhibitory molecules are biologically functional molecules but their presence obscures the bioassays for IL-1. Hence, the data demonstrating decreased IL-1 production from the mononuclear cells of patients with autoimmune diseases may reflect excess production of inhibitory substances. Measurement of immunoreactive IL-1 will clarify whether a production defect for IL-1 (either increased or decreased amounts) exists in autoimmune diseases.

D. NATURAL INHIBITORS OF IL-1 ACTIVITY

Polypeptides which specifically inhibit IL-1 biological activity have also been detected in the serum of human volunteers injected with bacterial endotoxin[48] and isolated from the urine of febrile patients,[125] patients with myelomonocytic leukemia,[14] and in the urine of pregnant women. The urinary inhibitor isolated from pregnant women has been identified as uromodulin[170] which is a glycosylated form of the Tamm-Horstfal protein.[187] The carbohydrate portion of the uromodulin molecule binds IL-1 and TNF and this binding accounts for the inhibition of IL-1 activity in bioassays. In addition, the binding of IL-1 and TNF to uromodulin may be one mechanism in which biologically potent molecules are removed from the glomerular filtrate. An inhibitory molecule isolated from the urine of patients with myelomonocytic leukemia has been shown to block the binding of IL-1 to its receptor on thymoma cells.[14] In general, the urinary inhibitors from febrile patients are biochemically different from uromodulin.

E. CYTOKINE SELF-AUGMENTATION NETWORK

IL-1 and TNF participate in self-augmentation induction mechanisms. Recombinant human IL-1 and TNF are each capable of inducing the production of their respective molecules as well as each other.[52,53,101] IL-1 and TNF both induce IL-6. The target cells include monocytes, endothelial cells, smooth muscle cells, and B cells. The concentrations of IL-1 and TNF which stimulate their own production in this self-amplification cycle are within the range (1 to 10 ng/ml) of what has been measured in the supernatant media of cultured cells stimulated with viruses, bacterial toxins and active complement components, and immune complex.[181] In addition, the induction of circulating IL-1 by either TNF or by IL-1 itself can be demonstrated in experimental animals. In tissues such as joint spaces or lymph nodes, this self-amplification network may play an important role in sustaining a pathological process. As a result of exogenous activators or IL-1 itself, increased PGE_2 occurs in macrophages and endothelial cells which serves to suppress further production of IL-1. The suppressive effect of PGE_2 on IL-1 production is, however, not at the transcriptional level but rather at the translation of new IL-1 and this seems to be via PGE_2-induced cAMP.[113] B cell-derived IL-1 also has an autocrine effect for B cell functions involved in antibody formation.[219]

Besides PGE_2 providing a negative feedback signal for IL-1-induced IL-1 production, IFN-γ also suppresses IL-1-induced IL-1 production.[81] This effect of IFN-γ on IL-1 action has also been observed for IL-1 effects on osteoclasts and fibroblasts.[86,87] The ability of IFN-γ to reduce fibroblast collagen synthesis and IL-1-induced osteoclast activation is in contrast to the well-established ability of IFN-γ to augment IL-1 production by a variety of cell activators, including endotoxins, staphylococcal entertoxins, complement components, and synthetic adjuvants. The ability of IFN-γ to suppress IL-1-induced IL-1 production takes place in the presence of cyclooxygenase inhibition. Similarly, the ability of corticosteroids to reduce the transcription of IL-1 mRNA also takes place in the presence of cyclooxygenase inhibition. One possible explanation for the clinical efficacy of disease-modifying drugs on the progression of rheumatoid arthritis may relate to the ability of these drugs to reduce IL-1 and related cytokine production and arrest the self-amplication interactions.

ACKNOWLEDGMENTS

These studies are supported by NIH Grant AI15614. The author thanks Professor Nerina Savage for her contribution to the section on IL-1 receptors. The author also acknowledges the suggestions and help of the following persons: J. G. Cannon, B. Clark, S. Endres, P. Ghezzi, R. Ghorbani, T. Ikejima, G. Lonnemann, J. W. Mier, L. Miller, R. Numerof, S. F. Orencole, R. Schindler, S. D. Sisson, J. W. M. van der Meer, A. Vanstory, S. J. C. Warner, and S. M. Wolff.

REFERENCES

1. **Abraham, R. T., Ho, S. N., Barna, T. J., and McKean, D. J.,** *J. Biol. Chem.,* 262, 2719, 1987.
2. **Alcocer-Varela, J., Laffon, A., and Alarcon-Segovia, D.,** *Clin. Exp. Immunol.,* 55, 125, 1984.
3. **Andus, T., Geiger, T., Hirano, T., Northoff, H., Ganter, U., Bauer, J., Kishimoto, T., and Heinrich, P. C.,** *FEBS Lett.,* 221, 18, 1987.
4. **Antoni, G., Presentini, R., Perin, F., Tagliabue, A., Ghiara, P., Censini, S., Volpini, G., Villa, L., and Boraschi, D.,** *J. Immunol.,* 137, 3201, 1986.
5. **Arend, W. P., Joslin, F. G., and Massoni, R. J.,** *J. Immunol.,* 134, 3868, 1985.
6. **Arya, S. K. and Gallo, R. C.,** *Biochemistry,* 23, 6685, 1984.
7. **Atkins, E.,** *Physiol. Rev.,* 40, 580, 1960.
8. **Auron, P. E., Webb, A. C., Rosenwasser, L. J., Mucci, S. F., Rich, A., Wolff, S. M., and Dinarello, C. A.,** *Proc. Natl. Acad. Sci. U.S.A.,* 81, 7907, 1984.

9. Auron, P. E., Rosenwasser, L. J., Matsushima, K., Copeland, T., Dinarello, C. A., Oppenheim, J. J., and Webb, A. C., *J. Mol. Immunol.*, 2, 169, 1985.

10. Auron, P. E., Warner, S. J. C., Webb, A. C., Cannon, J. G., Bernheim, H. A., McAdam, K. J. P. W., Rosenwasser, L. J., LoPreste, G., Mucci, S. F., and Dinarello, C. A., *J. Immunol.*, 138, 1447, 1987.

11. Bagby, G. C., Jr., Dinarello, C. A., Wallace, P., Wagner, P., Hefeneider, S., and McCall, E., *J. Clin. Invest.*, 78, 1316, 1986.

12. Bakouche, O., Brown, D. C., and Lachman, L. B., *J. Immunol.*, 138, 4249, 1987.

13. Balavoine, J. F., deRochemonteix, B., Cruchaud, A., and Dayer, J. M., in *The Physiologic, Metabolic and Immunologic Actions of Interleukin-1*, Kluger, M. J., Powanda, M. C., and Oppenheim, J. J., Eds., Alan R. Liss, New York, 1985, 429.

14. Balavoine, J. F., deRochemonteix, B., Williamson, K., Seckinger, P., Cruchaud, A., and Dayer, J. M., *J. Clin. Invest.*, 78, 1120, 1986.

15. Bendtzen, K., Mandrup-Poulsen, T., Nerup, J., Nielson, J. H., Dinarello, C. A., and Svenson, M., *Science*, 232, 1545, 1986.

16. Bertini, R., Bianchi, M., Villa, P., and Ghezzi, P., *Int. J. Immunopharmacol.*, in press.

17. Beuscher, H. U., Fallon, R. J., and Colten, H. R., *J. Immunol.*, 139, 1896, 1987.

18. Beutler, B. and Cerami, A., *J. Immunol.*, 135, 3969, 1985.

19. Beutler, B. and Cerami, A., *Nature*, 320, 584, 1986.

20. Bevilacqua, M. P., Pober, J. S., Majeau, G. R., Cotran, R. S., and Gimbrone, M. A., Jr., *J. Exp. Med.*, 160, 618, 1984.

21. Bevilacqua, M. P., Pober, J. S., Wheeler, M. E., Mendrick, D., Cotran, R. S., and Gimbrone, M. A., Jr., *J. Clin. Invest.*, 76, 2003, 1985.

22. Bhaskaram, P. and Sivakumar, B., *Arch. Dis. Child.*, 61, 182, 1986.

23. Bird, T. A. and Saklatvala, J., *Nature*, 324, 263, 1986.

24. Bird, T. A., Gearing, A. J. H., and Saklatvala, J., *FEBS Lett.*, 225, 21, 1987.

25. Brakenhoff, J. P. J., de Groot, E. R., Evers, R. F., Pannekoek, H., and Aarden, L. A., *J. Immunol.*, 139, 4116, 1987.

26. Breder, C. D., Dinarello, C. A., and Saper, C. B., *Science*, 240, 321, 1988.

27. Canalis, E., *Endocrinology*, 118, 74, 1986.

28. Cannon, J. G. and Dinarello, C. A., *Science*, 227, 1247, 1985.

29. Chapman, P. B., Lester, T. J., Casper, E. S., Gabrilove, J. L., Wong, G. Y., Kempin, S. J., Gold, P. J., Welt, S., Warren, R. S., Starnes, H. F., Sherwin, S. A., Old, L. J., Oettgen, H. F., *J. Clin. Oncol.*, 5, 1942, 1987.

30. Chin, J., Cameron, P. M., Rupp, E., and Schmidt, J. A., *J. Exp. Med.*, 165, 70, 1987.

31. Clark, B. D., Collins, K. L., Gandy, M. S., Webb, A. C., and Auron, P. E., *Nucl. Acids Res.*, 14, 7897, 1986.

32. Clowes, G. H. A., Jr., George, B. C., Bosari, S., and Love, W., *J. Leuk. Biol.*, 42, 547, 1987.

33. Cohen, F. E. and Dinarello, C. A., *J. Leuk. Biol.*, 42, 548, 1987.

34. Conti, P., Cifone, M. G., Alesse, E., Reale, M., Fieschi, C., and Dinarello, C. A., *Prostaglandins*, 32, 111, 1986.

35. Cuturi, M. C., Murphy, M., Costa-Gomi, M. P., Weinmann, R., Perussia, B., and Trinchieri, G., *J. Exp. Med.*, 165, 1581, 1987.

36. Dayer, J.-M., Beutler, B., and Cerami, A., *J. Exp. Med.*, 162, 2163, 1985.

37. Dayer, J.-M., de Rochemonteix, B., Burrus, B., Demczuk, S., and Dinarello, C. A., *J. Clin. Invest.*, 77, 645, 1986.

38. Dejana, E., Brevario, F., Erroi, A., Bussolino, F., Mussoni, L., Gramse, M., Pintucci, G., Casali, B., Dinarello, C. A., VanDamme, J., and Mantovani, A., *Blood*, 69, 695, 1987.

39. Demczuk, S., Baumberger, C., Mach, D., and Dayer, J. M., *J. Mol. Cell. Immunol.*, 3, 255, 1987.

40. Dempsey, R. A., Dinarello, C. A., Mier, J. W., Rosenwasser, L. J., Allegretta, M., Brown, T. E., and Parkinson, D. R., *J. Immunol.*, 129, 2504, 1982.

41. Dewhirst, F. E., Stashenko, P. P., Mole, J. E., and Tsuramachi, T., *J. Immunol.*, 135, 2562, 1985.

42. DiGiovine, F. S., Nuki, G., and Duff, G. W., *Lancet*, in press.

43. Dinarello, C. A., *Rev. Infect. Dis.*, 6, 51, 1984.

44. Dinarello, C. A., *Year Immunol.*, 2, 68, 1986.

45. Dinarello, C. A., *FASEB J.*, 2, 108, 1988.

46. Dinarello, C. A. and Krueger, J. M., *Fed. Proc.*, 45, 2545, 1986.

47. Dinarello, C. A., Renfer, L., and Wolff, S. M. *Proc. Natl. Acad. Sci. U.S.A.*, 74, 4624, 1977.

48. Dinarello, C. A., Rosenwasser, L. J., and Wolff, S. M., *J. Immunol.*, 127, 2517, 1982.

49. Dinarello, C. A., Bishai, I., Rosenwasser, L. J., Coceani, F., *Int. J. Immunopharmacol.*, 6, 43, 1984.

50. Dinarello, C. A., Clowes, G. H. A., Jr., Gordon, A. H., Saravis, C. A., and Wolff, S. M., *J. Immunol.*, 133, 1332, 1984.

51. Dinarello, C. A., Dempsey, R. A., Allegretta, M., LoPreste, G., Dainiak, N., Parkinson, D. R., and Mier, J. W., *Cancer Res.*, 46, 6235, 1986.
52. Dinarello, C. A., Ikejima, T., Warner, S. J. C., Orencole, S. F., Lonnemann, G., Cannon, J. G., and Libby, P., *J. Immunol.*, 139, 1902, 1987.
53. Dinarello, C. A., Cannon, J. G., Wolff, S. M., Bernheim, H. A., Beutler, B., Cerami, A., Figari, I. S., Palladino, M. A., Jr., and O'Connor, J. V., *J. Exp. Med.*, 163, 1433, 1986.
54. Dinarello, C. A., Cannon, J. G., Mier, J. W., Bernheim, H. A., LoPreste, G., Lynn, D. L., Love, R. N., Webb, A. C., Auron, P. E., Reuben, R. C., Rich, A., Wolff, S. M., and Putney, S. D., *J. Clin. Invest.*, 77, 1734, 1986.
55. Dinarello, C. A., Cannon, J. G., Endres, S., Ghezzi, P., Ghorbani, R., Ikejuma, T., Miller, L., Orencole, S., and Schindler, R., *Lymphokine Res.*, in press.
56. Dower, S. K., Kronheim, S. R., March, C. J., Conlon, P. J., Hopp, T. P., Gillis, S., and Urdal, D. L., *J. Exp. Med.*, 162, 501, 1985.
57. Dower, S. K. and Urdal, D. L., *Immunol. Today*, 8, 46, 1987.
58. Duel, T. F., Senior, R. M., Huang, J. S., and Griffin, G. L., *J. Clin. Invest.*, 69, 1056, 1982.
59. Duff, G. W. and Durum, S. K., *Yale J. Biol. Med.*, 55, 437, 1982.
60. Duff, G. W., Forre, O., Waalen, K., Dickens, E., and Nuki, G., *Br. J. Rheumatol.*, 24(Suppl.), 94, 1985.
61. Durum, S. K., Finnegan, A., Brody, D. T., Kovacs, E. J., Smith, M. R., Berzofsky, J. A., Young, H. A., and Tartakovksy, B., *Lymphokine Res.*, 6, 1124, 1987.
62. Dustin, M. L., Rothelin, R., Bhan, A. K., Dinarello, C. A., and Springer, T. A., *J. Immunol.*, 137, 245, 1986.
63. Elias, J. A., Gustilo, K., Baeder, W., and Freundlich, B., *J. Immunol.*, 138, 3812, 1987.
64. Endres, S., Ghorbani, R., Lonnemann, G., van der Meer, J. W. M., and Dinarello, C. A.,,, *Clin. Immunol. Immunopathol.*, in press.
65. Endres, S., Cannon, J. G., Ghorbani, R., Dempsey, R. A., Lonnemann, G., van der Meer, J. W. M., and Dinarello, C. A., *J. Immunol.*, in press.
66. Endres, S., Ghorbani, R., Kelley, V. E., Georgilis, K., Lonnemann, G., van der Meer, J. W. M., Cannon, J. G., Klempner, M. S., Schaefer, E. J., Wolff, S. M., and Dinarello, C. A., *N. Engl. J. Med.*, in press.
67. Falkoff, R. J. M., Muraguchi, A., Hong, J. X., Butler, J. L., Dinarello, C. A., and Fauci, A. S., *J. Immunol.*, 131, 801, 1983.
68. Falkoff, R. J. M., Butler, J. L., Dinarello, C. A., and Fauci, A. S., *J. Immunol.*, 133, 692, 1984.
69. Farrar, W. L., Kilian, P. L., Ruff, M. R., Hill, J. M., and Pert, C. B., *J. Immunol.*, 139, 459, 1987.
70. Fenton, M. J., Clark, B. D., Collins, K. L., Webb, A. C., Rich, A., and Auron, P. E., *J. Immunol.*, 138, 3972, 1987.
71. Fenton, M. J., Vermeulen, M. W., Clark, B. D., Webb, A. C., and Auron, P. E., *J. Immunol.*, 140, 2267, 1988.
72. Folks, T. M., Justement, J., Kinter, A., Dinarello, C. A., and Fauci, A. S., *Science*, 238, 800, 1987.
73. Fontana, A., Hengarrtner, H., Weber, E., Fehr, K., Grob, P. J., and Cohen, G., *Rheumatol. Int.*, 2, 49, 1982.
74. Fontana, A., Bodmer, S., Siepi, C., Wrann, M., Martin, R., Hofer-Warbinek, R., and Hofer, E., *J. Leukotriene Biol.*, 42, 543, 1987.
75. Furutani, Y., Notake, M., Fuki, T., Ohue, M., Nomura, H., Yamada, M., and Nakamura, S., *Nucl. Acids Res.*, 14, 3167, 1986.
76. Garman, R. D., Jacobs, K. A., Clark, S. C., and Raulet, D. H., *Proc. Natl. Acad. Sci. U.S.A.*, 84, 7629, 1987.
77. Gauldie, J., Richards, C., Harnish, D., Lansdorp, P., and Baumann, H., *Proc. Natl. Acad. Sci. U.S.A.*, 84, 7251, 1987.
78. Georgilis, K., Schaefer, C., Dinarello, C. A., and Klempner, M. S., *J. Immunol.*, 138, 3403, 1987.
79. Gery, I. and Waksman, B. H., *J. Exp. Med.*, 136, 143, 1972.
80. Ghezzi, P., Saccardo, B., Villa, P., Rossi, V., Bianchi, M., and Dinarello, C. A., *Infect. Immunol.*, 54, 837, 1986.
81. Ghezzi, P. and Dinarello, C. A., *J. Immunol.*, in press.
82. Gimenez-Gallego, G., Rodkey, J., Bennett, C., Rios-Candelore, M., DiSalvo, J., and Thomas, K., *Science*, 230, 1385, 1985.
83. Giulian, D. and Lachman, L. B., *Science*, 228, 497, 1985.
84. Giulian, D., Woodward, J., Young, D. G., and Krebs, J. F., *J. Neurosci.*, in press.
85. Goldberg, A. L., Kettelhut, I. C., Furuno, K., Fagan, J. M., and Baracos, V., *J. Clin. Invest.*, 81, 1378, 1988.
86. Gowen, M., Wood, D. D., Mundy, G. R., and Russell, R. G. G., *Br. J. Rheumatol.*, 24(Suppl.), 147, 1985.

87. Granstein, R. D., Murphy, G. F., Margolis, R. J., Byrne, M. H., and Amento, E. P., *J. Clin. Invest.*, 79, 1254, 1987.
88. Haak-Frendscho, M., Dinarello, C. A., and Kaplan, A. P., *J. Allergy Clin. Immunol.*, in press.
89. Hanson, D. F. and Murphy, P. A., *J. Immunol.*, 135, 3011, 1985.
90. Helyar, L. and Sherman, A. R., *Am. J. Clin. Nutr.*, 46, 346, 1987.
91. Hesse, D. G., Tracey, K. J., Fong, Y., Manogue, K. R., Palladino, M. A., Jr., Cerami, A., Shires, G. T., and Lowry, S. F., *Surg. Gynecol. Obstet.*, 166, 147, 1988.
92. Herman, J., Kew, M. C., and Rabson, A. R., *Cancer Immunol. Immunother.*, 16, 182, 1985.
93. Herman, J., Dinarello, C. A., Kew, M. C., and Rabson, A. R., *J. Immunol.*, 135, 2882, 1985.
94. Hirano, T., Yasukawa, K., Harada, H., Taga, T., Wantanabe, Y., Matsuda, T., Kashiwamura, S., Nakajima, K., Koyama, K., Iwasmatsu, A., Tsunasawa, S., Sakiyama, F., Matsui, H., Takahara, Y., Taniguchi, T., and Kishimoto, T., *Nature*, 324, 73, 1986.
95. Ho, S., Abraham, R. T., Nilson, A., Handwerger, B. S., and McKean, D. J., *J. Immunol.*, 139, 1532, 1987.
96. Holtmann, H. and Wallach, D., *J. Immunol.*, 139, 1161, 1987.
97. Horuk, R., Huang, J. J., Covington, M., and Newton, R. C., *J. Biol. Chem.*, 262, 16275, 1987.
98. Horwitz, D. A., Linger-Israeli, M., and Gray, J. D., *J. Immunol. Immunopharmacol.*, 7, 43, 1987.
99. Houssiau, F. A., Bukasa, K., Sindic, C. J. M., van Damme, J., van Snick, J., *Clin. Exp. Immunol.*, 71, 320, 1988.
100. Ikebuchi, K., Wong, G. G., Clark, S. C., Ihle, J. N., Hirai, Y., and Ogawa, M., *Proc. Natl. Acad. Sci. U.S.A.*, 84, 9035, 1987.
101. Ikejima, T., van der Meer, J. W. M., Endres, S., and Dinarello, C. A., *J. Leukotriene Biol.*, 42, 552, 1987.
102. Jelinek, D. F. and Lipsky, P. E., *J. Immunol.*, 139, 2970, 1987.
103. Kampschmidt, R. F., in *Physiologic and Metabolic Responses of the Host*, Powanda, M. D. and Canonico, P. G., Eds., Elsevier/North Holland, Amsterdam, 1981, 55.
104. Kauffman, C. A., Jones, P. G., and Kluger, M. J., *Am. J. Clin. Nutr.*, 44, 449, 1986.
105. Kawano, M., Hirano, T., Matsuda, T., Taga, T., Horii, Y., Iwato, K., Asaoku, H., Tang, B., Tanabe, O., and Tanaka, H., *Nature*, 332, 83, 1988.
106. Kaye, J., Gillis, S., Mizel, S. B., Shevach, E. M., Malek, T. R., Dinarello, C. A., Lachman, L. B., and Janeway, C. A., Jr. *J. Immunol.*, 133, 1339, 1984.
107. Kehrl, J. H., Miller, A., and Fauci, A. S., *J. Exp. Med.*, 166, 786, 1987.
108. Kern, J. A., Lamb, R. J., Reed, J. C., Daniels, R. P., and Nowell, P. C., *J. Clin. Invest.*, 81, 237, 1988.
109. Keystone, E. C., Jagial, S., and Shore, A., *J. Rheumatol.*, 13, 944, 1986.
110. Kilian, P. L., Kaffka, K. L., Stern, A. S., Woehle, D., Benjamin, W. R., DeChiara, T. M., Gubler, U., Farrar, J. J., Mizel, S. B., and Lomedico, P. T., *J. Immunol.*, 136, 4509, 1986.
111. Kimball, E. S., Pickerall, S. F., Oppenheim, J. J., and Rossio, J. L., *J. Immunol.*, 133, 256, 1984.
112. Klebanoff, S. J., Vadas, M. A., Harlan, J. M., Sparks, L. H., Gamble, J. R., Agosti, J. M., and Waltersdorph, A. M., *J. Immunol.*, 137, 2695, 1986.
113. Knudsen, P. J., Dinarello, C. A., and Strom, T. B., *J. Immunol.*, 137, 3189, 1986.
114. Knudsen, P. J., Dinarello, C. A., and Strom, T. B., *J. Immunol.*, 139, 4129, 1987.
115. Kobayashi, Y., Appella, E., Yamada, M., Copeland, T. D., Oppenheim, J. J., and Matsushima, K., *J. Immunol.*, 140, 2279, 1988.
116. Kohase, M., May, L. T., Tamm, I., Vilcek, J., and Sehgal, P. B., *Mol. Cell. Biol.*, 7, 273, 1987.
117. Krane, S. M., Dayer, J.-M., Simon, L. S., and Byrne, S., *Collagen Rel. Res.*, 5, 99, 1985.
118. Kunkel, S. L. and Chensue, S. W., *Biochem. Biophys. Res. Commun.*, 128, 892, 1985.
119. Kupper, T., Horowitz, M., Lee, F., Robb, R., and Flood, P. M., *J. Immunol.*, 138, 4280, 1987.
120. Kupper, T., Flood, P., Coleman, D., and Horowitz, M., *J. Immunol.*, 138, 4288, 1987.
121. Kurt-Jones, E. A., Kiely, J. M., and Unanue, E. R., *J. Immunol.*, 135, 1548, 1985.
122. Lacey, D. L., Chappel, J. C., and Teitelbaum, S. L., *J. Immunol.*, 139, 2649, 1987.
123. Lapierre, L. A., Fiers, W., and Pober, J. S., *J. Exp. Med.*, 167, 794, 1988.
124. Lepe-Zuniga, B. and Gery, I., *Clin. Immunol. Immunopathol.*, 31, 222, 1984.
125. Liao, Z., Grimshaw, R. S., and Rosenstreich, D. L., *J. Exp. Med.*, 159, 126, 1984.
126. Libby, P., Ordovas, J. M., Auger, K. R., Robbins, A. H., Birinyi, L. K., and Dinarello, C. A., *Am. J. Pathol.*, 124, 179, 1986.
127. Libby, P., Ordovas, J. M., Auger, K. R., Robbins, A. H., Birinyi, L. K., and Dinarello, C. A., *J. Clin. Invest.*, 78, 1432, 1986.
128. Lichtman, A. H., Kurt-Jones, E. A., and Abbas, A. K., *Proc. Natl. Acad. Sci. U.S.A.*, 84, 824, 1987.
129. Lichtman, A. H., Williams, M. E., Ohara, J., Paul, W. E., Faller, D. V., and Abbas, A. K., *J. Immunol.*, 138, 3276, 1987.

130. **Linker-Israeli, M., Bakke, A. C., Kitridou, R. C., Gendler, S., Gillis, S., and Horwitz, D. A.,** *J. Immunol.,* 130, 2651, 1983.
131. **Lipsky, P. E.,** *Contemp. Topics Mol. Immunol.,* 10, 195, 1985.
132. **Lipsky, P. E., Thompson, P. A., Rosenwasser, L. J., and Dinarello, C. A.,** *J. Immunol.,* 130, 2708, 1983.
133. **Lisi, P. J., Chu, C.-W., Koch, G. A., Endres, S., Lonnemann, G., and Dinarello, C. A.,** *Lymphokine Res.,* 6, 229, 1987.
134. **Loegdberg, L. and Shevach, E. M.,** *Eur. J. Immunol.,* 15, 1007, 1985.
135. **Loegdberg, L., Wassmer, P., and Shevach, E. M.,** *Cell. Immunol.,* 94, 299, 1985.
136. **Lomedico, P. T., Gubler, U., Hellman, C. P., Dukovich, M., Giri, J. G., Pan, Y. E., Collier, K., Semionow, R., Chua, A. O., and Mizel, S. B.,** *Nature,* 312, 458, 1984.
137. **Lotz, M., Tsoukas, C. D., Robinson, C. A., Dinarello, C. A., Carson, D. A., and Baughan, J. H.,** *J. Clin. Invest.,* 78, 713, 1986.
138. **Lotz, M., Jirik, F., Kobouridis, P., Tsoukas, C., Hirano, T., Kishimoto, T., and Carson, D. A.,** *J. Exp. Med.,* 167, 1253, 1988.
139. **Lowenthal, J. W. and MacDonald, H. R.,** *J. Exp. Med.,* 164, 1060, 1986.
140. **Lowenthal, J. W. and MacDonald, H. R.,** *J. Immunol.,* 138, 1, 1987.
141. **Lowenthal, J. W., Cerottini, J. C., and MacDonald, H. R.,** *J. Immunol.,* 137, 1226, 1986.
142. **Lowenthal, J. W., Zubler, R. H., Nabholz, M., and MacDonald, H. R.,** *Nature,* 315, 675, 1985.
143. **MacDonald, H. R. and Lowenthal, J. W.,** *Ann. Inst. Pasteur Immunol.,* 138, 482, 1987.
144. **MacDonald, H. R., Wingfield, P., Schmeissner, U., Shaw, A., Clore, G. M., and Gronenborn, A. M.,** *FEBS Lett.,* 209, 295, 1986.
145. **Mandrup-Poulsen, T., Bendtzen, K., Dinarello, C. A., and Nerup, J.,** *J. Immunol.,* 139, 4077, 1987.
146. **Mandrup-Poulsen, T., Bendtzen, K., Nerup, J., Dinarello, C. A., Svenson, M., and Nielson, J. H.,** *Diabetologia,* 29, 63, 1986.
147. **Maennel, D. N., Mizel, S. B., Diamantstcin, T., and Falk, W.,** *J. Immunol.,* 134, 3108, 1985
148. **Marinkovic, S., Jahreis, J. P., Wang, G. G., and Baumann, H.,** *Science,* in press.
149. **Martin, M., Lovett, D. H., and Resch, K.,** *Immunobiology,* 171, 145, 1986.
150. **Martinet, Y., Rom, W. N., Grotendorst, G. R., Martin, G. R., and Crystal, R. G.,** *N. Engl. J. Med.,* 317, 202, 1987.
151. **Martini, A., Ravello, A., Notarangelo, L. D., Maccario, R., Lanfranchi, A., Rondena, D., Ugazio, A. G., and Burgio, R.,** *J. Rheumatol.,* 13, 3, 1986.
152. **Mathison, J. C., Wolfson, E., and Ulevitch, R. J.,** *J. Clin. Invest.,* 81, 1925, 1988.
153. **Massone, A., Baldari, C., Censini, S., Bartalini, M., Nucci, D., Boraschi, D., and Telford, J. L.,** *J. Immunol.,* 140, 3812, 1988.
154. **Matsushima, K., Bano, M., Kidwell, W. R., and Oppenheim, J. J.,** *J. Immunol.,* 134, 904, 1985.
155. **Matsushima, K., Yodoi, J., Tagaya, Y., and Oppenheim, J. J.,** *J. Immunol.,* 137, 3183, 1986.
156. **Matsushima, K., Akahoshi, T., Yamada, M., Furutani, Y., and Oppenheim, J. J.,** *J. Immunol.,* 136, 4496, 1986.
157. **Matshushima, K., Taguchi, M., Kovacs, E. J., Young, H. A., and Oppenheim, J. J.,** *J. Immunol.,* 136, 2883, 1986.
158. **Matsushima, K., Kobayashi, Y., Copeland, T. D., Akahoshi, T., and Oppenheim, J. J.,** *J. Immunol.,* 139, 3367, 1987.
159. **Matsushima, K., Procopio, A., Abe, H., Scala, G., Ortaldo, J. R., and Oppenheim, J. J.,** *J. Immunol.,* 135, 1132, 1985.
160. **McCarthy, D. O., Kluger, M. J., and Vander, A. J.,** *Am. J. Clin. Nutr.,* 42, 1179, 1987.
161. **Michie, H. R., Manogue, K. R., Spriggs, D. R., Revhaug, A., O'Dwyer, S., Dinarello, C. A., Cerami, A., Wolff, S. M., and Wilmore, D. W.,** *N. Engl. J. Med.,* 318, 1481, 1988.
162. **Mills, G. B. and May, C.,** *J. Immunol.,* 139, 4083, 1987.
163. **Miossec, P., Dinarello, C. A., and Ziff, M.,** *Arthritis Rheum.,* 29, 461, 1986.
164. **Mizel, S. B., Kilian, P. L., Lewis, J. C., Paganelli, K. A., and Chizzonite, R. A.,** *J. Immunol.,* 138, 2906, 1987.
165. **Mochizuki, D. Y., Eisenman, J. R., Conlon, P. J., Larsen, A. D., and Tushinski, R. J.,** *Proc. Natl. Acad. Sci. U.S.A.,* 84, 5267, 1987.
166. **Moldawer, L. L., Svaninger, G., Gelin, J., and Lundholm, K. G.,** *Am. J. Physiol.,* 253, C773, 1987.
167. **Moore, M. A. and Warren, D. J.,** *Proc. Natl. Acad. Sci. U.S.A.,* 84, 7134, 1987.
168. **Mosley, B., Urdal, D. L., Prickett, K. S., Larsen, A., Cosman, D. L., Conlon, P. J., Gillis, S., and Dower, S. K.,** *J. Biol. Chem.,* 262, 2941, 1986.
169. **Movat, H. Z., Burrowes, C. E., Cybulsky, M. I., and Dinarello, C. A.,** *Am. J. Pathol.,* 129, 463, 1987.
170. **Muchmore, A., Shifrin, S., and Decker, J. M.,** *J. Immunol.,* 138, 2547, 1987.

171. Muraguchi, A., Kehrl, J. H., Butler, J. L., and Fauci, A. S., *J. Clin. Immunol.*, 4, 337, 1984.
172. Muraguchi, A., Hirano, T., Tang, B., Matsuda, T., Horii, Y., Nakajima, K., and Kishimoto, T., *J. Exp. Med.*, 167, 332, 1988.
173. Murphy, P. A., Chesney, J., and Wood, W. B., Jr., *J. Lab. Clin. Med.*, 83, 310, 1974.
174. Nachman, R. L., Hajjar, K. A., Silverstein, R. L., and Dinarello, C. A., *J. Exp. Med.*, 163, 1545, 1986.
175. Neta, R., Douches, S., and Oppenheim, J. J., *J. Immunol.*, 136, 2483, 1987.
176. Neta, R., Oppenheim, J. J., and Douches, S. D., *J. Immunol.*, 140, 108, 1988.
177. Nijsten, M. W. N., De Groot, E. R., Ten Duis, H. J., Klasen, H. J., Hack, C. E., and Aarden, L. A., *Lancet*, 2, 921, 1987.
178. Nouri, A. M. E., Panayi, G. S., and Goodman, S. M., *Clin. Exp. Immunol.*, 55, 295, 1984.
179. Nouri, A. M. E., Panayi, G. S., Goodman, S. M., and Waugh, A. P. W., *Br. J. Rheumatol.*, 24(Suppl.), 191, 1985.
180. Numerof, R. P., Dinarello, C. A., Endres, S., Lonnemann, G., van der Meer, J. W. M., and Mier, J. W., *J. Immunol.*, in press.
181. Okusawa, S., Dinarello, C. A., Yancey, K. B., Endres, S., Lawley, T. J., Frank, M. M., Burke, J. F., and Gelfand, J. A., *J. Immunol.*, 139, 2635, 1987.
182. Okusawa, S., Gelfand, J. A., Ikejima, T., Connolly, R. A., and Dinarello, C. A., *J. Clin. Invest.*, 81, 1162, 1988.
183. Onozaki, K., Matsushima, K., Aggarwal, B. B., and Oppenheim, J. J., *J. Immunol.*, 135, 3962, 1985.
184. Paganelli, K. A., Stern, A. S., and Kilian, P. L., *J. Immunol.*, 138, 2249, 1987.
185. Palaszynski, E. W., *Biochem. Biophys. Res. Commun.*, 147, 204, 1987.
186. Pennica, D., Nedwin, G. E., Hayflick, J. S., Seeburg, P. H., Derynck, R., Palladino, M. A., Kohr, W. J., Aggarwal, B. B., and Goeddel, D. V., *Nature*, 312, 724, 1984.
187. Pennica, D., Kohr, W. J., Kuang, W. J., Glaister, D., Aggarwal, B. B., Chen, E. Y., and Goeddel, D. V., *Science*, 236, 83, 1987.
188. Perlmutter, D. H., Dinarello, C. A., Punsal, P., and Colten, H. R., *J. Clin. Invest.*, 78, 1349, 1986.
189. Perlmutter, D., Goldberger, G., Dinarello, C. A., Mizel, S. B., and Colten, H. R., *Science*, 232, 850, 1986.
190. Pettipher, E. R., Higgs, G. A., and Henderson, B., *Proc. Natl. Acad. Sci. U.S.A.*, 83, 8749, 1986.
191. Phadke, K., *Biochem. Biophys. Res. Commun.*, 142, 448, 1987.
192. Philip, R. and Epstein, L. B., *Nature*, 323, 86, 1986.
193. Pierart, M. E., Tome, N., Appelboom, T. E., and Deschodt-Lanckman, M. M., *J. Immunol.*, 140, 3808, 1988.
194. Pincus, S. H., Whitcomb, E. A., and Dinarello, C. A., *J. Immunol.*, 137, 3509, 1986.
195. Plaetinck, G., Declercq, W., Tavernier, J., Nabholz, M., and Fiers, W., *Eur. J. Immunol.*, 17, 1835, 1987.
196. Pollack, S., Micali, A., Kinne, D. W., Enker, W. E., Geller, N., Oettgen, H. F., and Hoffman, M. K., *Int. J. Cancer*, 32, 733, 1983.
197. Pomoselli, J. J., Flores, E. A., Bistrian, B. R., Zeisel, S., Dinarello, C. A., Drabik, M., and Blackburn, G. L., *Clin. Res.*, 35, 514A, 1987.
198. Priestle, J. P., Schaer, H.-P., and Gruetter, M. G., *EMBO J.*, in press.
199. Ramadori, G., Sipe, J. D., Dinarello, C. A., Mizel, S. B., and Colten, H. R., *J. Exp. Med.*, 162, 930, 1985.
200. Ranges, G. E., Zlotnik, A., Espevik, T., Dinarello, C. A., Cerami, A., and Palladino, M. A., Jr., *J. Exp. Med.*, 167, 1472, 1988.
201. Rhyne, J. A., Mizel, S. B., Wheeler, J. G., and McCall, C. E., *J. Immunol.*, in press.
202. Rimsky, L., Wakasugi, H., Ferrara, P., Robin, P., Capdevielle, J., Tursz, T., Fradelizi, D., and Bertoglio, J., *J. Immunol.*, 136, 3304, 1986.
203. Riveau, G., Dinarello, C. A., and Chedid, L., *Int. J. Immunopharm.*, in press.
204. Robb, R. J., Greene, W. C., and Rusk, C. M., *J. Exp. Med.*, 160, 1126, 1986.
205. Rogers, B. C., Scott, D. M., Mundin, J., and Sissons, J. G. P., *J. Virol.*, 55, 527, 1987.
206. Roh, M. S., Drazenovich, K. A., Jeffrey, B. S., Barbose, J. J., Dinarello, C. A., and Cobb, C. F., *Surgery*, 102, 140, 1987.
207. Rola-Pleszczynski, M. and Lemaire, I., *J. Immunol.*, 135, 3958, 1985.
208. Rosenwasser, L. J., Webb, A. C., Clark, B. D., Irie, S., Chang, L., Dinarello, C. A., Gehrke, L., Wolff, S. M., Rich, A., and Auron, P. E., *Proc. Natl. Acad. Sci. U.S.A.*, 83, 1, 1986.
209. Rosoff, P. M., Savage, N., and Dinarello, C. A., *Cell*, in press.
210. Rossi, V., Breviario, F., Ghezzi, P., Dejana, E., and Mantovani, A., *Science*, 229, 1174, 1985.
211. Saklatvala, J., *Nature*, 322, 547, 1986.
212. Saklatvala, J., Sarsfield, S. J., and Townsend, Y., *J. Exp. Med.*, 162, 1208, 1985.

213. **Sandborg, C. I., Berman, M. A., Andrews, B. S., and Friou, G. J.,** *Clin. Exp. Immunol.,* 59, 332, 1985.
214. **Santos, L. B., Yamada, F. T., and Steinberg, M. A.,** *Cancer,* 56, 1553, 1985.
215. **Savage, N. and Dinarello, C. A.,** *Crit. Rev. Immunol.,* in press.
216. **Savage, N., Orencole, S. F., and Dinarello, C. A.,** *J. Immunol.,* in press.
217. **Scala, G., Kuang, Y. D., Hall, R. E., Muhmore, A. V., and Oppenheim, J. J.,** *J. Exp. Med.,* 159, 1637, 1984.
218. **Scala, G., Allaven, P., Djew, J. X., Kasahara, T., Ortaldo, J. R., Herberman, R. B., and Oppenheim, J. J.,** *Nature,* 309, 56, 1984.
219. **Scala, G., Morrone, G., Tamburrini, M., Alfinito, F., Pastore, C. I., D'Alessio, G., and Venuto, S.,** *J. Immunol.,* 138, 2527, 1987.
220. **Scarborough, D. E., Dinarello, C. A., and Reichlin, S.,** *J. Leukotriene Biol.,* 42, 560, 1987.
221. **Schindler, R. and Dinarello, C. A.,** *Lymphokine Res.,* in press.
222. **Schindler, R., Endres, S., Ghorbani, R., Wu, A., and Dinarello, C. A.,** *Lymphokine Res.,* in press.,
223. **Schmidt, J. A., Oliver, C. N., Lepe-Zuniga, J. L., Green, I., and Gery, I.,** *J. Clin. Invest.,* 73, 1462, 1984.
224. **Schnyder, J., Payne, T., and Dinarello, C. A.,** *J. Immunol.,* 138, 496, 1987.
225. **Shimokado, K., Raines, E. W., Madtes, D. K., Barrett, T. B., Benditt, E. P., and Ross, R.,** *Cell,* 43, 277, 1985.
226. **Shirakawa, F., Tanaka, Y., Ota, T., Suzuki, H., Eto, S., and Yamashita, U.,** *J. Immunol.,* 138, 4243, 1987.
227. **Shoham, S., Davenne, D., Cady, A. B., Dinarello, C. A., and Krueger, J. M.,** *Am. J. Physiol.,* 253, R142, 1987.
228. **Shore, A., Jagial, S., and Keystone, E. C.,** *Clin. Exp. Immunol.,* 65, 298, 1986.
229. **Simic, M. M. and Stosic-Grujicic, S.,** *Folia Biol.,* 31, 410, 1985.
230. **Simon, P. L.,** *Cell Immunol.,* 87, 720, 1984.
231. **Sims, J. E., March, C. T., Cosman, D. J., Widmer, M. B., MacDonald, H. R., MacMahan, C. J., Gruben, C. E., Wignall, J. M., Jackson, J. L., Call, S. M., Friend, D., Albert, A. A., Gillis, S., Urdal, D. L., and Dower, S. K.,** *Science,* in press.
232. **Singer, I. I., Scott, S., Hall, G. L., Limjuco, G., Chin, J., and Schmidt, J. A.,** *J. Exp. Med.,* 167, 389,
223. **Sironi, M., Breviario, F., Biondi, A., Dejana, E., and Mantovani, A.,** *J. Immunol.,* in press.
234. **Sisson, S. D. and Dinarello, C. A.,** *Blood,* in press.
235. **Smith, K. A., Lachman, L. B., Oppenheim, J. J., and Favata, M. F.,** *J. Exp. Med.,* 151, 1551, 1980.
236. **Stanley, E. R., Bartocci, A., Patinkin, D., Rosendall, M., and Bradley, T. R.,** *Cell,* 45, 667, 1986.
237. **Stanton, T. H., Maynard, M., and Bomsztyk, K.,** *J. Biol. Chem.,* 2, 701, 1986.
238. **Subramanian, N. and Bray, M. A.,** *J. Immunol.,* 138, 271, 1987.
239. **Tagaya, Y., Okada, M., Sugie, K., Kasahara, T., Kondo, N., Hamuro, J., Matsushima, K., Dinarello, C. A., and Yodoi, J.,** *J. Immunol.,* 140, 1, 1988.
240. **Tartakovsky, B., Kovacs, E. J., Takacs, L., and Durum, S. K.,** *J. Immunol.,* 137, 160, 1986.
241. **Thieme, T. R., Hefeneider, S. H., Wagner, C. R., and Bach, D. R.,** *J. Immunol.,* 139, 1173, 1987.
242. **Thomas, K. A., Rios-Candelore, M., Gimez-Gallego, G., Di Salvo, J., Bennett, C., Rodkey, J., and Fitzpatrick, S.,** *Proc. Natl. Acad. Sci. U.S.A.,* 82, 6409, 1985.
243. **Tiku, K., Tiku, M. L., and Skosey, J. L.,** *J. Immunol.,* 136, 3677, 1986.
244. **Tracey, K. J., Beutler, B., Lowry, S. F., Merryweather, J., Wolpe, S., Milsark, I. W., Hairi, R. J., Fahey, T. J., Zentella, A., Albert, J. D., and Cerami, A.,** *Science,* 234, 470, 1986.
245. **Truneh, A., Simon, P., and Schmitt-Verhulst, A. M.,** *Cell Immunol.,* 103, 365, 1986.
246. **Tzeng, D. Y., Duel, T. F., Huang, J. S., Senior, R. M., Boxer, L. A., and Baehner, R. L.,** *Blood,* 64, 123, 1984.
247. **Uyttenhove, C., Coulie, P. G., and Van Snick, J.,** *J. Exp. Med.,* 167, 1417, 1988.
248. **Van Damme, J., De Ley, M., Opdenakker, G., Billiau, A., and De Somer, P.,** *Nature,* 314, 266, 1985.
249. **Van Damme, J., De Ley, M., Van Snick, J., Dinarello, C. A., and Billiau, A.,** *J. Immunol.,* 139, 1867, 1987.
250. **Van Damme, J., Opdenakker, G., Simpson, R. J., Rubira, M. R., Cayphas, S., Vink, A., Billiau, A., and Van Snick, J.,** *J. Exp. Med.,* 165, 914, 1987.
251. **van der Meer, J. W. M., Barza, M., Wolff, S. M., and Dinarello, C. A.,** *Proc. Natl. Acad. Sci. U.S.A.,* 85, 1620, 1988.
252. **van Oers, M. H., van der Heyden, A. A., and Aarden, L. A.,** *Clin. Exp. Immunol.,* 71, 314, 1988.
253. **Warner, S. J. C., Auger, K. R., and Libby, P.,** *J. Exp. Med.,* 165, 1316, 1987.
254. **Webb, A. C., Collins, K. L., Auron, P. E., Eddy, R. L., Nakai, H., Byers, M. G., Haley, L. L., Henry, W. M., and Shows, T. B.,** *Lymphokine Res.,* 5, 77, 1986.

255. **Weissman, A. M., Hartford, J. B., Svetlik, P. B., Depper, J. M., Waldmann, T. A., Greene, W., and Klausner, R. D.**, *Proc. Natl. Acad. Sci. U.S.A.*, 83, 1463, 1986.

256. **White, C. W., Ghezzi, P., Dinarello, C. A., Caldwell, S. A., McMurtry, I. J., and Repine, J. E.**, *J. Clin. Invest.*, 79, 1863, 1987.

257. **Williams, J. M., DeLoria, D., Hansen, J. A., Dinarello, C. A., Loertscher, R., Shapiro, H. M., and Strom, T. B.**, *J. Immunol.*, 135, 2249, 1985.

258. **Wolpe, S. D., Davatelis, G., Sherry, B., Beutler, B., Hesse, D. G., Nguyen, H. T., Moldawer, L. L., Nathan, C. F., Lowry, S. F., and Cerami, A.**, *J. Exp. Med.*, 167, 570, 1988.

259. **Wood, D. D., Ihrie, E. J., Dinarello, C. A., and Cohen, P. L.**, *Arthritis Rheum.*, 26, 975, 1983.

260. **Yang, Y. C., Tsai, S., Wong, G. G., and Clark, S. C.**, *J. Cell. Physiol.*, 134, 292, 1988.

261. **Yoshimura, T., Matsushima, K., Tanaka, S., Robinson, E. A., Appella, E., Oppenheim, J. J., and Leonard, E. J.**, *Proc. Natl. Acad. Sci. U.S.A.*, 84, 9233, 1987.

262. **Zucali, J. R., Dinarello, C. A., Gross, M. A., Anderson, L., Oblon, D., and Weiner, R. S.**, *J. Clin. Invest.*, 77, 1857, 1986.

263. **Zucali, J. R., Broxmeyer, H. E., Gross, M. A., and Dinarello, C. A.**, *J. Immunol.*, 140, 840, 1988.

264. **Prendergast, N. and Dinarello, C. A.**, unpublished observations.

265. **Ghezzi, P.**, personal communication.

266. **Bird, T. A., Saklatvala, J., and MacDonald, H. R.**, personal communication.

267. **Savage, N., et al.**, unpublished observations.

268. **Von Bulow, G., Savage, N., Dinarello, C. A.**, unpublished data.

269. **Palladino, M.**, personal communication.

270. **Dayer, J.-M.**, personal communication.

271. **van der Meer, J. W. M.**, personal communication.

272. **Neta, R.**, personal communication.

273. **Kishimoto, T.**, personal communication.

Chapter 9

THE MOLECULAR BASIS OF INTERLEUKIN-2 ACTION

Daniel E. Sabath and Michael B. Prystowsky

TABLE OF CONTENTS

I. INTRODUCTION

Interleukin-2 (IL-2) is an important regulatory hormone of the immune system. As the major T cell growth hormone, it is responsible for amplification of antigen-specific T lymphocytes, and it may regulate the function of B cells, monocytes, and other cells which participate in immune responses. It acts through a specific membrane receptor which is fairly well characterized, although the mechanism of signal transduction is not known. When T cells are stimulated by IL-2, the result is DNA synthesis and cell division, preceded by the synthesis of new RNA and protein. In this review, we focus on the actions of IL-2 at the molecular level. The structure of IL-2 and its gene is discussed, as well as the mechanisms responsible for regulation of IL-2 gene expression. We then summarize what is known about the IL-2 receptor (IL-2R) structure, consider the available data regarding possible second signals, and discuss the implications for possible transmembrane signaling. How these signals ultimately result in new gene expression is not known, but by studying genes induced by IL-2 this connection can be explored. Changes in gene expression after IL-2 stimulation is an area of active study in our laboratory as well as many others, and the current progress in this area is reviewed. Finally, because of the powerful effects of IL-2 on the immune system, including the stimulation of lymphokine-activated killer cells which may have potent antitumor activity, the potential therapeutic uses for IL-2 are summarized.

IL-2 was originally isolated from the supernatants of concanavalin A (Con A) stimulated murine spleen cells[1] or PHA stimulated human peripheral blood or tonsil cells.[2,3] It has been purified to homogeneity,[4,5] and has been cloned by several different laboratories.[6-10] Recombinant IL-2 has been produced in both prokaryotic[9,10] and eukaryotic systems.[6,8] IL-2 is a polypeptide hormone of 15,500 kDa and its structure has been solved to 3.0 Å.[11] Results from structure-function studies suggest that the N-terminal portion of the molecule is important for receptor binding and biological function.[12,13] The molecule has three cysteine residues at positions 58, 105, and 125 (in human IL-2); site-directed mutagenesis experiments show that changing the cysteines at positions 58 or 105 to serine essentially abolishes biological activity, while mutations at position 125 have no effect on activity.[14-16] This suggests that cysteines 58 and 105 may be involved in a disulfide linkage, which is consistent with the X-ray crystallographic data.[11]

IL-2 is produced by T helper lymphocytes upon stimulation with antigen, and as its original name would suggest, this molecule is a growth factor for activated T lymphocytes. Traditionally, it was thought that all T helper (T_H) cells produced IL-2 in response to antigen and then proliferated in response to IL-2. Now there is evidence that there may be at least two distinct subsets of T_H cells, each of which produces a different set of lymphokines upon stimulation.[12-17] $T_H 1$ cells produce IL-2 in response to antigenic stimulation and use IL-2 as an autocrine growth factor. $T_H 2$ cells, on the other hand, make and respond to IL-4 in an analogous fashion, and while they can proliferate in response to IL-2, they do not secrete it. The physiological significance of these two subsets of T_H cells is unclear. In this review, we concentrate primarily on the actions of the T_H cells, and they are referred to simply as T_H cells.

II. T CELL ACTIVATION

T cells bear on their surface an antigen-specific receptor capable of recognizing antigen when presented in association with products of the major histocompatability complex (MHC). The receptor consists of a disulfide-linked heterodimer associated with the CD3 complex. T_H cells bearing the CD4 molecule are stimulated by antigen in the context of class II MHC products, which are found primarily on the surfaces of macrophages and B cells, although many other cell types can be induced to express class II MHC by γ-interferon. It is likely that any cell bearing class II MHC molecules can function as an antigen-presenting cell (APC).[22] T cells can also be stimulated *in vitro* by antibodies to the CD3 complex alone or in combination with antibodies to other cell surface proteins. Stimulation by antigen leads to an increase in cytosolic free calcium concentration, and is associated with the breakdown of phosphatidyl-inositol bisphosphate into diacylglycerol and inositol trisphosphate. Diacylglycerol in combination with calcium is thought to be the physiologic activator of protein kinase C and inositol trisphosphate may contribute to the rise in intracellular calcium concentration. It is also known that calcium ionophores in combination with phorbol esters can activate resting T cells. These two sets of data suggest that a combination of protein kinase C activation and a rise in intracellular calcium concentration may be sufficient signals for T cell activation, IL-2R expression, and lymphokine production.[23] The various factors required for T cell activation and the molecular events following T cell activation have been studied extensively,[24,25] but are beyond the scope of this review.

When a T_H cell encounters antigen on the surface of an APC, it is stimulated to produce lymphokines, notably IL-2. In addition, it expresses receptors for IL-2 on its surface.[26] While IL-2 has no intrinsic antigen specificity, it is functionally antigen specific, since only T cells which have encountered antigen express IL-2R, and therefore only antigen-specific cells can respond to IL-2. In this manner, clones of antigen-specific T cells are expanded while unstimulated T cells are not. Thus, IL-2 serves to amplify the immune response to antigen.

III. REGULATION OF EXPRESSION OF IL-2

The regulation of expression of the IL-2 gene is mediated at the transcriptional level by sequences in the 5′ flanking region of the gene. These sequences share homology with the 5′ sequences of the IL-2 receptor and several other lymphokine genes that are coordinately expressed with IL-2, implying a common mechanism of expression.[27-29] When T cells are stimulated, there are changes in the DNA structure in this region, rendering it more sensitive to DNAase I digestion.[30-31] A nuclear factor has been identified that is present in activated T cells, along with other T cell-specific factors that are present in unstimulated cells.[32] Interestingly, these 5′ sequences of the IL-2 gene are similar to sequences in the long terminal repeats of the adult T-cell leukemia virus (ATLV),[33] and of the human immunodeficiency virus (HIV),[27] which are thought to regulate viral gene expression. This suggests that ATLV may take advantage of T cell-specific transcription factors for its own expression.

In addition to sequences in the 5′ region of the IL-2 gene that positively regulate IL-2 expression, there may also be sequences that regulate inhibition of IL-2 production. A region has been identified that may regulate the inhibition of IL-2 expression in unstimulated cells.[34] Sequences have also been identified that may be important for the inhibitory effects exerted by the immunosuppressive agent cyclosporine A on the production of IL-2 and other lymphokines following antigen or lectin stimulation.[35] These two regions actually overlap in a region about 70 bp upstream from the transcription start site, raising the possibility that cyclosporine may interact with the sequences of the IL-2 gene that normally are responsible for preventing expression in unstimulated T cells.

The expression of IL-2 is also regulated at the post-transcriptional level. When T cells are activated *in vitro* by mitogenic lectins, IL-2 mRNA is induced transiently. When the cells are activated in the presence of cycloheximide, IL-2 mRNA is "superinduced".[36] A possible explanation for this phenomenon is that in the absence of cycloheximide a protein is produced that either shuts off IL-2 transcription or increases the rate of IL-2 mRNA degradation. In the presence of cycloheximide, this protein is not synthesized, resulting in an increase in the steady-state level of IL-2 mRNA. A similar phenomenon has been noted for other genes that are induced in many different cell types following a proliferation signal, including c-*myc,* c-*fos,* the IL-2 receptor, γ-interferon, and others.[37-40] A common feature of these genes is an AU-rich region in the 3' untranslated region of their mRNAs, which have been shown to confer RNA instability in unstimulated cells.[41]

IV. THE INTERLEUKIN-2 RECEPTOR

A. HIGH AND LOW AFFINITY FORMS

The nature of the IL-2 receptor remained somewhat enigmatic for many years, due to an apparent discrepancy between the number of receptors determined by IL-2 binding and the number determined by anti-IL-2R antibody binding.[42,43] The IL-2 receptor exists in both a high and low affinity form, with K_D's of approximately 10 pM and 10 nM, respectively,[44] on both T and B cells.[45] In addition an intermediate affinity IL-2 receptor has recently been described which is found primarily on natural killer (NK) cells.[46-48] It has been generally felt that the high-affinity receptor is responsible for transducing the IL-2 signal for proliferation.[42,49] The first antibodies to the IL-2R precipitated a 55-kDa protein (p55)[43,50] that was present on activated, but not resting T cells, the same cells that proliferated in response to IL-2. However, when cDNAs corresponding to the IL-2 receptor were isolated, it was discovered that the intracellular domain was very small,[51-53] consisting of only 13 amino acids, and not likely to be adequate for signal transduction. This was especially true when compared to other growth factor receptors such as the EGF,[54] platelet-derived growth factor (PDGF),[55] insulin,[56] and CSF-1[57,58] receptors, all of which have large cytoplasmic domains with tyrosine kinase activity. Furthermore, transfection of IL-2R cDNA into nonlymphoid cell lines yielded only low-affinity receptors,[59-61] implying that native p55 was not the functional high-affinity receptor. In addition, a secreted form of the IL-2R has been identified,[62] and IL-2R lacking the transmembrane and intracytoplasmic tail have been created.[63,64] Both of these soluble forms of IL-2R bind IL-2 with low affinity.[63-66] Interestingly, when the extracellular portion of p55 was fused to the intracellular domain of the EGF receptor, high affinity IL-2 receptors were generated which seemed to produce an EGF-like signal, resulting in oncogenic transformation of two fibroblast lines.[67] This suggested that there was another component of the wild-type IL-2 receptor that cooperated with the p55 molecule to generate the functional high-affinity IL-2 receptor.

B. A SECOND RECEPTOR MOLECULE

A clue that the p55 molecule could be modified to form the high affinity receptor came from an experiment where L cell membranes bearing low-affinity p55 molecules were fused to T cell membranes, generating high-affinity receptors,[68] suggesting that there is a second protein present in T cell membranes capable of converting p55 from a low affinity to a high affinity form. To characterize this "converter" protein, a number of laboratories have done experiments in which radiolabeled IL-2 is cross-linked to its receptor and the complex is immunoprecipitated with anti-p55 antibodies, dissociated, and analyzed by gel electrophoresis. This approach has demonstrated a second protein of 75 kDa that binds IL-2 in association with the p55 molecule.[46,69-71] This protein can be expressed in the absence of p55, as demonstrated on the cell line YT, which has receptors which bind IL-2 with intermediate affinity (K_D of about 1 nM), and are not immunoprecipitated by anti-p55 antibodies.[46] Additionally, the p55 molecule can be induced on YT cells by adult T cell conditioned medium,[72] TNF-α,[73] or IL-1-β,[74] and the induction of p55 correlates with the induction of high-affinity IL-2 binding sites, implying that the interaction of p55 with this intermediate affinity protein produces the classical high affinity IL-2 receptor. Similarly, p75 molecules have been found on large granular lymphocytes (LGL), which proliferate in response to high concentrations of IL-2 and upon which the p55 molecule and high affinity receptors can be induced by IL-2.[47] Kinetic analysis of the two chains suggest that the rates of IL-2 association and dissociation with the p55 molecule are fast ($t_{1/2}$ of 2 to 6 s at 37°C), while the rates of association and dissociation for the p75 molecule are much slower ($t_{1/2}$ of 46 min at 37°C).[48,75] The high-affinity receptor combines the fast kinetics of association of the p55 molecule ($t_{1/2}$ of 16 s) with the slow kinetics of dissociation of the p75 molecule ($t_{1/2}$ of 37 to 50 min), generating the observed low K_D. The way the high affinity receptor may function is that the p55 molecule rapidly associates with IL-2, bringing it into close proximity to the p75 molecule, which then would hold the IL-2 firmly to the receptor. Alternatively, the p75 molecule might undergo a conformational change causing IL-2 to associate with faster kinetics. Antibodies to the p75 molecule should soon be available, which will facilitate the further characterization and cloning of the p75 molecule and permit the investigation of its function.

C. REGULATION OF IL-2 RECEPTOR EXPRESSION

The IL-2 receptor is induced under those conditions that activate T cells, as discussed above. IL-2 itself can also induce IL-2R expression,[76,77] when measured by anti-p55 antibodies, but the receptors induced are of the low affinity variety.[42] The IL-2R, as well as IL-2, can also be induced by the product of the *tat* genes of HTLV-I[78] and HTLV-II,[79] which may be responsible for creating T cells that are neoplastic based on their ability to synthesize their own growth factor and its receptor.

V. SIGNAL TRANSDUCTION

In order for IL-2 to exert its effect on its target cells, it must, through the interaction with its receptor, generate intracellular signals that cause new genes to be expressed and ultimately cause DNA synthesis and cell division. As mentioned above, while many growth factor receptors have obvious tyrosine kinase activity which is probably important for signal transduction, the p55 molecule of the IL-2 receptor does not seem capable of generating such a second signal. The newly described p75 molecule is an attractive candidate for being a signal-generating protein, but there are currently no data to support this hypothesis, and it is entirely possible that there may be as-yet undiscovered proteins associated with the IL-2R that perform the signal transduction function. It has been shown by a number of laboratories that high-affinity IL-2 receptors are internalized by IL-2 binding,[80-83] but whether this endocytosis has any role in signal transduction is unknown. Since there is no direct evidence for the nature of the signal generated by the IL-2R, the mechanism by which the IL-2 signal gets from the cell surface to the interior of the cell must be deduced from changes in phosphorylation, ion concentrations, and second messengers which occur following IL-2 stimulation of T cells.

A. PROTEIN PHOSPHORYLATION

Alterations in protein phosphorylation are commonly seen in many inducible cell systems. Activation of protein kinases is associated with changes is levels of cyclic nucleotides, calcium, phospholipids, and hormones binding their receptors. It is no surprise then that there are changes in protein phosphorylation following IL-2 stimulation, although it is not clear whether these changes are necessary or sufficient for DNA synthesis and cell division.

IL-2 stimulation of either Con A-activated spleen cells or IL-2-dependent cell lines results in phosphorylation of many membrane proteins, including the IL-2R[84] the the γ-chain of the T cell receptor.[85] Phosphorylation of specific proteins of 67,[86,87] 63,[87] 85,[88] 26, and 27 kDa[89] has been documented, and all are phosphorylated on serine or threonine residues. Similar proteins are phosphorylated when cells are treated with phorbol esters,[86,87] although there exist proteins that are phosphorylated with IL-2 stimulation that are not phosphorylated upon exposure to phorbol esters.[90] Similarly, it has been shown that although protein kinase C phosphorylates the ribosomal S6 protein, this protein is a substrate for another protein kinase.[91] While these data suggest that protein kinase C may be involved in IL-2-mediated cell activation, it is likely that other protein kinases will be important for IL-2 signal transduction as well. Recently, it has been shown that a protein kinase activity coprecipitates with the IL-2 receptor, and that the p75 molecule is phosphorylated *in vitro* upon stimulation with IL-2.[92] This raises the attractive possibility that the IL-2 receptor might be associated with a protein kinase and is autophosphorylated like other growth factor receptors.

Evidence that protein kinase C is activated by IL-2 is indirect. This is in contrast to antigen stimulation of T cells, where phoshatidylinositol turnover has been well documented, implying that protein kinase C is at least in part responsible for transducing the antigen signal.[25] IL-2 has been shown to cause translocation of protein kinase C from the cytosolic to the membrane fraction of CT6 cells,[93] implying but not proving that protein kinase C is activated by IL-2. The p55 molecule of the IL-2 receptor and other molecules become phosphorylated upon stimulation with IL-2 or phorbol ester,[90] and have been shown to be substrates for protein kinase C *in vitro*,[94,95] again suggesting indirectly that protein kinase C may be activated by IL-2 under physiologic conditions. Despite this evidence, however, no one has demonstrated conclusively that there is production of diacylglycerol upon IL-2 stimulation,[96,97] which would be necessary for protein kinase C activation *in vivo*. A possible explanation for these apparent discrepancies is that different cell systems have been used for different experiments, and that results obtained may depend upon the state of activation of the cells used.[98] That is, a cell in G_0 of the cell cycle may have different activation requirements than cells that are in G_1 or continuously cycling when stimulated by IL-2.

B. THE ROLE OF CALCIUM

While it is clear that calcium is important in the activation of T cells via the antigen receptor,[99] its role, if any, in the stimulation of T cells by IL-2 is unclear. In the CT6 IL-2-dependent T cell line, IL-2 causes a transient increase in the uptake of ^{45}Ca from the medium.[100] In another study, again using IL-2-dependent T cell lines, a rise in cytosolic free calcium was observed, both from intracellular and extracellular sources.[101] These findings may be unrelated to proliferation, as it has been shown that PHA-stimulated human peripheral blood lymphocytes can proliferate in response to IL-2, even in the absence of calcium in the medium (although if calcium is present it is taken up by the cells).[102] Yet another report shows no effect of IL-2 on intracellular calcium concentration, this time using activated human peripheral blood lymphocytes, murine thymus, spleen, and IL-2-dependent T cell lines, none of which had an increase in cytoplasmic free calcium.[103] Again, the most likely cause for these conflicting results is the differences in cell systems used in the experiments. In addition, it is possible to have an influx in calcium without a rise in cytosolic calcium, either due to an absolute increase in cell volume or to calcium becoming associated with the membranes. More work needs to be done in this area before any conclusions can be drawn regarding calcium and IL-2 stimulation.

C. THE ROLE OF CYCLIC NUCLEOTIDES

In many systems, transmembrane signaling is accomplished by activation of adenylate or guanylate cyclase through a G protein coupled to a hormone receptor. For some time it has been known that an increase in cyclic adenosine monophosphate (cAMP) exerts an antiproliferative response on mitogen-stimulated T cells,[104,105] perhaps by inhibiting phosphatidylinositide turnover,[106] and that an increase in cyclic guanosine monophosphate (cGMP) may provide a positive signal for proliferation.[107] In the IL-2 system, agents that increase cAMP, such as prostaglandin E_2 (PGE_2)[108,109] and theophylline,[110] are inhibitory to IL-2-induced proliferation. Similarly, the cAMP analog, 8-Br-cAMP, inhibits IL-2-induced protein phosphorylation, albeit by a relatively small amount.[84] As far as cGMP is concerned, one report shows IL-2-stimulated guanosine triphosphatase (GTPase) activity in isolated cell membranes of an IL-2-dependent cell line,[111] but no one has demonstrated an increase in cGMP levels following IL-2 stimulation, nor a stimulatory effect of cGMP analogs on IL-2 induced T cell proliferation.

D. OTHER SECOND MESSENGERS

While there is conflicting evidence about the role of "traditional" second messengers in IL-2 signal transduction, some information is available about biochemical changes which occur following IL-2 stimulation of T cells. One change that has been found is cytoplasmic alkalinization that occurs following IL-2 stimulation sensitive to amiloride, implying that the N^+/H^+ antiport is responsible.[112] It is not clear, however, that alkalinization is required for proliferation.

The importance of potassium in T cell activation and proliferation has been demonstrated in a number of laboratories. In collaboration with Dr. C. Deutsch, we have shown that IL-2 causes an increase in whole-cell potassium conductance in a cloned T lymphocyte, and that quinine, a K^+ channel blocker, inhibits IL-2 induced proliferation.[113,114] Similar results have been obtained with lectin-stimulated cells and other potassium channel blockers.[115-119] As with phosphorylation, calcium, or other second messengers, no direct connection has been made between these early biochemical events and later changes in gene expression or the induction of DNA synthesis. Presumably there are DNA-binding proteins that are modified either by phosphorylation or directly by second messengers, which then exert effects on DNA structure and RNA transcription.

Recently, a novel second messenger system has been described in T cells which may be important in T cell activation. Human T cells stimulation with lectin were shown to increase their synthesis of a glycosyl-phosphatidylinositol molecule. When subsequently stimulated with insulin, a specific phospholipase was activated causing the generation of an inositol phosphate-glycan which inhibited a cAMP-dependent protein kinase.[120] It is possible that this represents a second messenger system that opposes the cAMP system in T cells, which is known to be growth inhibitory. While no data are available yet showing the importance of this system in IL-2-stimulated T cell proliferation, it may be involved in IL-2 signal transduction, which might explain the difficulty in finding "standard" second messengers in IL-2-stimulated cells.

VI. IL-2-INDUCED GENE EXPRESSION

Following an IL-2 signal, T cells bearing high-affinity IL-2 receptors are stimulated to enter the cell cycle, with DNA synthesis and cell division as the ultimate result. DNA synthesis has traditionally been the assay for T cell activation, and G_1 has been poorly characterized in terms of the sequence of molecular events occurring prior to the onset of DNA synthesis. During G_1, significant changes in gene expression take place. In addition to the synthesis of structural proteins and metabolic enzymes, which must increase in quantity before a cell can divide, a variety of regulatory proteins and synthetic machinery for DNA, RNA, and protein must be synthesized. Presumably, the second signal(s) generated by IL-2 binding its receptor results in the direct activation of a number of genes. The protein products of these genes may in turn regulate the expression of genes needed later in the cell cycle. Therefore, genes induced by IL-2 can be grouped into two large sets. The first set is expressed independently of prior protein synthesis, and therefore protein synthesis inhibitors such as cycloheximide do not inhibit the accumulation of these mRNAs. The second set of genes requires the expression of some of the first set genes, and therefore the expression of second set genes is sensitive to protein synthesis inhibitors.

In PDGF-stimulated fibroblasts, the oncogenes c-*fos* and c-*myc* are among the earliest genes to be induced following growth factor stimulation, and both genes are induced by lectin stimulation of resting T cells.[38,39] In IL-2-stimulated lymphocytes, c-*myc* mRNA has been shown to be at maximal steady-state levels 1 to 2 h after IL-2 stimulation.[37,40,109,121-123] In addition, c-*fos* has been shown to be induced by IL-2, but only in one system,[109,121] suggesting that this is probably an unusual cell type. Another oncogene associated with IL-2 stimulation is c-*myb*, which is induced by IL-2 in PHA-stimulated human peripheral blood lymphocytes[124,125] and is regulated at least in part at the transcriptional level.[125] It is not clear how IL-2 causes increased transcription of these genes, nor is the function of these genes in the cell cycle understood. Since c-*fos* is expressed only rarely after IL-2 stimulation, it may be that this gene is needed for the G_0 to G_1 transition, and that IL-2-responsive cells are already beyond this stage of activation. On the other hand, c-*myc* may be induced as part of general cell activation, regardless of the prestimulation state of the cell.

Later in G_1, transferrin receptors appear on the T cell surface, and there are data to suggest that transferrin must bind its receptor for successful transit through G_1 into S phase.[126] It has also been shown that T cells can be stimulated to produce transferrin,[127] raising the possibility of another autocrine growth factor system in addition to the IL-2/IL-2R system. Other genes induced during G_1 include the p55 molecule of the IL-2R, as mentioned above, resulting in an increased number of low-affinity IL-2R,[42,76,77,128] and γ-interferon.[128-130] Both p55 and γ-interferon appear to be regulated in part at the transcriptional level.[77,129,130]

In our laboratory we have been interested in regulation of gene expression during the G_1 to S phase transition of the cell cycle. This interest stems from experiments in which the cloned antigen-dependent T cell line, L2, was stimulated with IL-2, and protein synthesis was examined by two-dimensional gel electrophoresis.[114] We demonstrated that while some proteins were synthesized at gradually increasing rates throughout G_1 and others were synthesized at high rates early in G_1 and then had decreased rates of synthesis, a third group had greatly increased rates of synthesis late in G_1, close to the onset of DNA synthesis. It was felt that the regulation of expression of some of these proteins might be tied to the regulation of DNA synthesis. Support for this idea came from the identification of one of these proteins as proliferating cell nuclear antigen (PCNA) or cyclin.[131,132] PCNA/cyclin has been shown to be a cofactor for DNA polymerase δ,[133,134] which is required for SV40 DNA replication,[135] and probably functions by coordinating leading and lagging strand DNA synthesis at the replication fork.[136] PCNA expression follows that of transferrin receptors, identifying yet another stage of G_1 progression.[137]

Because there were a large number of unidentified IL-2 induced proteins seen on two-dimensional gels, we attempted to isolate cDNA clones corresponding to these proteins. A cDNA library was constructed from L2 cells that were in late G_1 of the cell cycle, and was screened by differential hybridization to isolate those cDNAs that had higher RNA levels in IL-2-stimulated cells than in unstimulated cells. Of 40,000 clones screened, a total of 90 IL-2-induced clones were obtained. There were 21 different cDNAs represented among the 90. One cDNA cross-hybridized to 53 of the 90 original clones, making it the most commonly isolated IL-2-induced clone. When used to probe the entire cDNA library, this clone hybridized to 0.7% of the clones, and it hybridized to an extremely abundant mRNA that was induced approximately 5-fold upon IL-2 stimulation. The cDNA was sequenced and found to be the murine homolog of glyceraldehyde 3-phosphate dehydrogenase. In addition, 5 other glycolytic enzymes were found among the 21 different clones obtained. It is not known why GAPDH should be such an abundant mRNA, although T cells have been shown to be dependent upon glycolysis for energy production, rather than oxidative phosphorylation.[138,139] Similar findings were obtained when a library of serum-stimulated fibroblast RNA was screened by differential hybridization.[140] In this study, however, the primary library consisted of only 300 clones and may not have been representative of the total RNA pool in those cells.

Another set of genes that was isolated from the L2 cell library include the cytoskeletal proteins vimentin, α-tubulin, and γ-actin. Vimentin has also been shown to be induced by serum in cultured fibroblasts.[141] It is interesting to speculate that these two sets of genes might represent examples of coordinate regulation of gene expression during T cell proliferation. It is likely that the factors which regulate GAPDH gene expression are shared by all the glycolytic enzymes. Such a situation exists in yeast, where the GAPDH and enolase genes share 5′ flanking sequences that are probably acted on by common transcription factors.[142] There may be a mechanism for coordinate expression of the cytoskeletal genes as well.

In addition to the above-mentioned genes, we are in the process of identifying the other 12 genes which may belong to other families of coordinately regulated genes. Having isolated a large number of genes that are induced during T cell proliferation, we now will be able to analyze the mechanisms that are responsible for their expression. By understanding these mechanisms, we will come closer to understanding the molecular basis for cell proliferation in general.

VII. THE EFFECTS OF IL-2 ON OTHER CELLS

In addition to its effects on T cells, IL-2 has been shown to have effects on many different cell types important in the host response to infection. IL-2 acts as a B cell stimulatory factor by inducing growth and immunoglobulin secretion in activated human tonsillar B cells,[143] murine splenic cells,[45,144] as well as several B cell lines.[145,146] When B cells are stimulated with lipopolysaccharide (LPS), *Staphylococcus aureus,* anti-μ, or IL-5, they become responsive to IL-2 and respond by proliferating and/or secreting immunoglobulin. These agents have all been shown to induce expression of IL-2 receptors on B cells.[45,143-146] Similarly, IL-2 receptors can be induced by LPS in human peripheral blood monocytes, and IL-2 causes these activated monocytes to produce O_2^- and H_2O_2.[147,148] IL-2 can also increase NK cell killing[149] and can induce lymphokine-activated killer cells.[150] It has been reported that IL-2 can cause proliferation and synthesis of myelin basic protein in oligodendrocytes.[151] Finally, IL-3 has been shown to induce IL-2 receptors on nonlymphoid hematopoietic cells, suggesting a possible role for IL-2 in hematopoiesis.[152] It is likely that more effects of IL-2 on nonlymphoid cells will be discovered, which will further demonstrate the importance of IL-2 as a regulatory molecule in host defense and inflammation.

VIII. CLINICAL EXPERIENCE WITH IL-2

Because IL-2 is known to have powerful immunostimulatory effects, it is logical to consider it for use in disease states where immunologic function is compromised or insufficient, such as HIV infection or disseminated cancer. The discovery of lymphokine-activated killer (LAK) cells[150] which will lyse fresh human tumor cells *in vitro*, as well as the availability of large amounts of purified human IL-2 because of recombinant DNA technology, have made it possible to attempt immunotherapy of human tumors *in vivo*. It was first shown in a murine system that intravenous administration of IL-2 and LAK cells[153,154] or IL-2 alone[155] could cause regression of pulmonary metastases of murine sarcomas and melanomas. In the first report of using LAK cells and IL-2 for human malignancies, 25 patients were treated by removing lymphocytes by leukophoresis, treating them *in vitro* with IL-2 to stimulate LAK cells, and then reinfusing the cells into the patients along with additional IL-2. In this first trial there was 1 complete regression (disappearance of all measurable tumor) of pulmonary metastases from a melanoma, 10 partial regressions (at least 50% reduction in tumor size) from assorted tumors, and 14 cases with no response.[156] Toxicities associated with this therapy included malaise, fever, chills, and dyspnea associated with pulmonary edema, requiring intubation in two cases. In a second series involving 108 patients treated with IL-2 plus LAK cells and 49 treated with IL-2 alone, similar results were obtained, with 8 complete responses from assorted tumors, 15 partial responses, and 10 minor responses (between 25 and 50% reduction in tumor size) for those treated with IL-2 plus LAK cells, and less success with those patients treated with IL-2 alone.[157] While the majority of patients had no response to therapy, those who had a complete response remained in remission for a considerable length of time. The most encouraging results were obtained in two cases with non-Hodgkin's lymphoma. A complete response was obtained in both cases, demonstrating that IL-2 therapy may have efficacy in selected tumors. When examined histologically, a successful response correlated with an increase in HLA-DR expression on the tumor cells and an infiltrate of T cells into the tumor, where in nonresponders there was no T cell infiltrate or increased HLA-DR expression.[158]

IL-2 has also been used on a limited basis in attempts to reconstitute immune function in patients with acquired immune deficiency syndrome (AIDS). Since the primary defect in this disease is the destruction of CD4$^+$ lymphocytes, the primary source of IL-2, it was thought that exogenous administration of IL-2 would overcome some of the immunological defects in this disease. A number of phase I trials have been undertaken to assess the utility of IL-2 therapy in AIDS patients, but so far there has been no clear evidence that IL-2 can reverse the pathology seen in AIDS.[159-161] There is an indication that IL-2 may improve some of the immunological parameters in patients with AIDS-related complex (ARC), who may have enough remaining immune function to take advantage of the presence of exogenous IL-2.[161]

A limiting factor in IL-2 therapy has been its toxicity, which in some cases has been severe enough to be life-threatening. The side effects are generally reversible upon cessation of IL-2 administration,[156] however. The most common toxicities noted have been constitutional symptoms such as fever, chills, malaise, and weight gain.[156,162,163] Also common has been an increase in vascular permeability resulting in severe hypotension, pulmonary edema requiring mechanical ventilation in a number of cases,[156,157,162,164] and pleural effusions. The effective decrease in intravascular volume may also be responsible for the prerenal azotemia that has been observed.[157,164] Hematologic abnormalities have also been common, including anemia, thrombocytopenia, eosinophilia, and a decrease in erythroid and myeloid precursors in the peripheral blood.[163,165] A pruritic macular rash has been seen in many patients, along with a lymphoid infiltrate into the dermis.[166] Endocrine abnormalities have also been observed in patients treated with IL-2, with elevations in serum cortisol, ACTH, prolactin, growth hormone,[162] and the development of hypothyroidism.[167] Finally, neuropsychiatric changes have been noted in patients undergoing IL-2 therapy. Patients have experienced cognitive alterations, disorientation, and paranoid delusions that did not seem to correlate with known underlying psychiatric disorders.[168] Most IL-2-related side effects were reversible and remitted after IL-2 therapy was discontinued, and one study showed improvement in fever, pruritis, mental status, renal function, and pulmonary function when corticosteroids were administered concomitantly with the IL-2.[169] In addition to these symptomatic side effects, many patients develop anti-IL-2 antibodies, although these antibodies have never been shown to inhibit IL-2 function.[170,171] One possible reason that so many side effects have been seen is that massive doses of IL-2 must be administered because of the extremely short serum half-life of IL-2. It is also possible that some of the toxicities are not due to IL-2 itself, but to contaminants such as sodium dodecyl sulfate (SDS), which is present in small amounts in purified recombinant IL-2. SDS has not been shown to cause these effects *in vivo* by itself, however.[163,169] Perhaps improvements in methods of IL-2 dosing, formulation, or the generation of IL-2 analogs that are more stable in the serum will reduce the incidence and severity of side effects secondary to IL-2 administration.

IX. CONCLUSIONS

While the existence of a T cell growth factor has been known since the mid-1970s, it is only now that many of the details of IL-2 biology are beginning to be worked out. One reason has been the unavailability of pure IL-2, but this problem has been overcome by the production of recombinant IL-2. Another mystery has been the nature of the signal that IL-2 delivers. Unlike other growth factors, which have well-characterized receptors with clear signal-transducing functions, the IL-2 receptor has remained poorly characterized. Considerable information about the mechanism of signal transduction may be available soon, as the p75 molecule becomes better characterized. Finally, as these questions are answered, new discoveries will be made regarding the regulation of gene expression following IL-2 stimulation, including the identification of regulatory proteins that may both regulate gene expression and in turn be regulated by the signal delivered by the IL-2 receptor. As the molecular basis of IL-2 function becomes better understood, it will become possible to devise new therapies for clinical situations in which there is immune system dysfunction. IL-2 may prove useful in the therapy of both immunodeficiencies and cancer, as well as for autoimmune diseases where there is inappropriate immune system activation.

ACKNOWLEDGMENTS

We would like to thank Ms. Nancy Thornton for her invaluable assistance in assembling this manuscript. M. B. P. is a Hartford Fellowship recipient. D. E. S. was supported by MSTP training grant 5-T32-GM-07170.

REFERENCES

1. **Gillis, S. and Smith, K. A.**, Long term culture of tumour-specific cytotoxic T cells, *Nature,* 268, 154, 1977.
2. **Morgan, D. A., Ruscetti, F. W., and Gallo, R.**, Selective *in vitro* growth of T lymphocytes from normal human bone marrows, *Science,* 193, 1007, 1976.
3. **Gillis, S., Ferm, M. M., Ou, W., and Smith, K. A.**, T cell growth factor: parameters of production and quantitative microassay for activity, *J. Immunol.,* 120, 2027, 1978.
4. **Robb, R. J., Kutny, R. M., and Chowdry, V.**, Purification and partial sequence analysis of human T cell growth factor, *Proc. Natl. Acad. Sci. U.S.A.,* 80, 5990, 1983.
5. **Welte, K., Wang, C. Y., Mertelsmann, R., Venuta, S., Feldman, S. P., and Moore, M. A. S.**, Purification of human interleukin 2 to apparent homogeneity and its molecular heterogeneity, *J. Exp. Med.,* 156, 454, 1982.
6. **Yokota, T., Arai, N., Lee, F., Rennick, D., Mosmann, T., and Arai, K.-I.**, Use of a cDNA expression vector for isolation of mouse interleukin 2 cDNA clones: expression of T-cell growth-factor activity after transfection of monkey cells, *Proc. Natl. Acad. Sci. U.S.A.,* 82, 68, 1985.
7. **Holbrook, N. J., Smith, K. A., Fornace, A. J. J., Comeau, C. M., Wiskoch, R. L., and Crabtree, G. R.**, T-cell growth factor: complete nucleotide sequence and organization of the gene in normal and malignant cells, *Proc. Natl. Acad. Sci. U.S.A.,* 81, 1634, 1984.
8. **Taniguchi, T., Matsui, H., Fujita, T., Takaoka, C., Kashima, N., Yoshimoto, R., and Hamuro, J.**, Structure and expression of a cloned cDNA for human interleukin 2, *Nature,* 302, 305, 1983.
9. **Clark, S. C., Arya, S. K., Wong-Staal, F., Matsumoto-Kobayashi, M., Kay, R. M., Kaufman, R. J., Brown, E. L., Shoemaker, C., Copeland, T., Oroszlan, S., Smith, K., Sarngadharan, M. G., Lindner, S. G., and Gallo, R. C.**, Human T-cell growth factor: partial amino acid sequence, cDNA cloning, and organization and expression in normal and leukemic cells, *Proc. Natl. Acad. Sci. U.S.A.,* 81, 2543, 1984.
10. **Rosenberg, S. A., Grimm, E. A., McGrogan, M., Doyle, M., Kawasaki, E., Koths, K., and Mark, D. F.**, Biological activity of recombinant human interleukin-2 produced in *Escherichia coli, Science,* 223, 1412, 1984.

11. **Brandhuber, B. J., Boone, T., Kenney, W. C., and McKay, D. B.,** Three-dimensional structure of interleukin-2, *Science,* 238, 1707, 1987.

12. **Kuo, L.-M. and Robb, R. J.,** Structure-function relationships for the IL 2-receptor system. I. Localization of a receptor binding site on IL 2, *J. Immunol.,* 137, 1538, 1986.

13. **Zurawski, S. M., Mosmann, T. R., Benedik, M., and Zurawski, G.,** Alterations in the amino-terminal third of mouse interleukin 2: effects of biological activity and immunoreactivity, *J. Immunol.,* 137, 3354, 1986.

14. **Wang, A., Lu, S.-D., and Mark, D. F.,** Site-specific mutagenesis of the human interleukin-2 gene: structure-function analysis of the cysteine residues, *Science,* 224, 1431, 1984.

15. **Yamada, T., Fujishima, A., Kawahara, K., Kato, K., and Nishimura, O.,** Importance of disulfide linkage for constructing the biologically active human interleukin-2, *Arch. Biochem. Biophys.,* 257, 194, 1987.

16. **Arakawa, T., Boone, T., Davis, J. M., and Kenney, W. C.,** Structure of unfolded and refolded recombinant derived [Ala-125]interleukin 2, *Biochemistry,* 25, 8274, 1986.

17. **Mosmann, T. R., Cherwinski, H., Bond, M. W., Giedlin, M. A., and Coffman, R. L.,** Two types of murine helper T cell clone. I. Definition according to profiles of lymphokine activities and secreted proteins, *J. Immunol.,* 136, 2348, 1986.

18. **Cher, D. J. and Mosmann, T. R.,** Two types of murine helper cell clone. II. Delayed-type hypersensitivity is mediated by TH1 clones, *J. Immunol.,* 138, 3688, 1987.

19. **Reynolds, D. S., Boom, W. H., and Abbas, A. K.,** Inhibition of B lymphocyte activation by interferon-gamma, *J. Immunol.,* 139, 767, 1987.

20. **Cherwinski, H. M., Schumacher, J. H., Brown, K. D., and Mosmann, T. R.,** Two types of mouse helper T cell clone. III. Further differences in lymphokine synthesis between Th1 and Th2 clones revealed by RNA hybridization, functionally monospecific bioassays, and monoclonal antibodies, *J. Exp. Med.,* 166, 1229, 1987.

21. **Kurt-Jones, E. A., Hamberg, S., Ohara, J., Paul, W. E., and Abbas, A. K.,** Heterogeneity of helper/inducer T lymphocytes. I. Lymphokine production and lymphokine responsiveness, *J. Exp. Med.,* 166, 1774, 1987.

22. **Malissen, B., Price, M. P., Goverman, J. M., McMillan, M., White, J., Kappler, J., Marrack, P., Pierres, A., Pierres, M., and Hood, L.,** Gene transfer of H-2 class II genes: antigen presentation by mouse fibroblast and hamster B-cell lines, *Cell,* 36, 319, 1984.

23. **Weiss, A. and Imboden, J. B.,** Cell surface molecules and early events involved in human T lymphocyte activation, *Adv. Immunol.,* 41, 1, 1987.

24. **Alcover, A., Ramarli, D., Richardson, N. E., Chang, H.-C., and Reinherz, E. L.,** Functional and molecular aspects of human T lymphocyte activation via T3-Ti and T11 pathways, *Immunol. Rev.,* 95, 5, 1987.

25. **Isakov, N., Mally, M. I., Scholz, W., and Altman, A.,** T-lymphocyte activation: the role of protein kinase C and the bifurcating inositol phospholipid signal transduction pathway, *Immunol. Rev.,* 95, 89, 1987.

26. **Hemler, M. E., Brenner, M. B., McLean, J. M., and Strominger, J. L.,** Antigenic stimulation regulates the level of expression of interleukin 2 receptor on human T cells, *Proc. Natl. Acad. Sci. U.S.A.,* 81, 2172, 1984.

27. **Fujita, T., Shibuya, H., Ohashi, T., Yamanishi, K., and Taniguchi, T.,** Regulation of human interleukin-2 gene: functional DNA sequences in the 5' flanking region for the gene expression in activated T lymphocytes, *Cell,* 46, 401, 1986.

28. **Stanley, E., Metcalf, D., Sobieszczuk, P., Gough, N. M., and Dunn, A. R.,** The structure and expression of the murine gene encoding granulocyte-macrophage colony stimulating factor: evidence for utilisation of alternative promoters, *EMBO J.,* 4, 2569, 1985.

29. **Fujita, T., Takaoka, C., Matsui, H., and Taniguchi, T.,** Structure of the human interleukin 2 gene, *Proc. Natl. Acad. Sci. U.S.A.,* 80, 7437, 1983.

30. **Siebenlist, U., Durand, D. B., Bressler, P., Holbrook, N. J., Norris, C. A., Kamoun, M., Kant, J. A., and Crabtree, G. R.,** Promoter region of interleukin-2 gene undergoes chromatin structure changes and confers inducibility on chloramphenicol acetyltransferase gene during activation of T cells, *Mol. Cell. Biol.,* 6, 3042, 1986.

31. **Durand, D. B., Bush, M. R., Morgan, J. G., Weiss, A., and Crabtree, G. R.,** A 275 basepair fragment at the 5' end of the interleukin 2 gene enhances expression from a heterologous promoter in response to signals from the T cell antigen receptor, *J. Exp. Med.,* 165, 395, 1987.

32. **Durand, D. B., Shaw, J.-P., Bush, M. R., Replogle, R. E., Belagaje, R., and Crabtree, G. R.,** Characterization of antigen receptor response elements within the interleukin-2 enhancer, *Mol. Cell. Biol.,* 8, 1715, 1988.

33. **Holbrook, N. J., Lieber, M., and Crabtree, G. R.,** DNA sequence of the 5' flanking region of the human interleukin 2 gene: homologies with adult T-cell leukemia virus, *Nucl. Acids Res.,* 12, 5005, 1984.

34. **Nabel, G. J., Gorka, C., and Baltimore, D.,** T-cell-specific expression of interleukin 2: evidence for a negative regulatory site, *Proc. Natl. Acad. Sci. U.S.A.,* 85, 2934, 1988.
35. **Williams, T. M., Eisenberg, L., Burlein, J. E., Norris, C. A., Pancer, S., Yao, D., Burger, S., Kamoun, M., and Kant, J. A.,** Two regions within the human interleukin-2 (IL2) gene promoter are important for inducible IL2 expression, *J. Immunol.,* 123, 1068, 1988.
36. **Efrat, S. and Kaempfer, R.,** Control of biologically active interleukin 2 messenger RNA formation in induced human lymphocytes, *Proc. Natl. Acad. Sci. U.S.A.,* 81, 2601, 1984.
37. **Reed, J. C., Sabath, D. E., Hoover, R. G., and Prystowsky, M. B.,** Recombinant interleukin 2 regulates levels of c-*myc* mRNA in a cloned murine T lymphocyte, *Mol. Cell. Biol.,* 5, 3361, 1985.
38. **Kelly, K., Cochran, B. H., Stiles, C. D., and Leder, P.,** Cell-specific regulation of the c-*myc* gene by lymphocyte mitogens and platelet-derived growth factor, *Cell,* 35, 603, 1983.
39. **Muller, R., Bravo, R., Burckhardt, J., and Curran, T.,** Induction of c-*fos* gene and protein by growth factors precedes activation of c-*myc*, *Nature,* 312, 716, 1984.
40. **Kronke, M., Leonard, W. J., Depper, J. M., and Greene, W. C.,** Sequential expression of genes involved in human T lymphocyte growth and differentiation, *J. Exp. Med.,* 161, 1593, 1985.
41. **Shaw, G. and Kamen, R.,** A conserved AU sequence from the 3′ untranslated region of GM-CSF mRNA mediates selective mRNA degradation, *Cell,* 46, 659, 1986.
42. **Smith, K. A. and Cantrell, D. A.,** Interleukin 2 regulates its own receptors, *Proc. Natl. Acad. Sci. U.S.A.,* 82, 864, 1985.
43. **Robb, R. J. and Greene, W. C.,** Direct demonstration of the identity of T cell growth factor binding protein and the Tac antigen, *J. Exp. Med.,* 158, 1332, 1983.
44. **Robb, R. J., Greene, W. C., and Rusk, C. M.,** Low and high affinity cellular receptors for interleukin 2. Implications for the level of Tac antigen, *J. Exp. Med.,* 160, 1126, 1984.
45. **Lowenthal, J. W., Zubler, R. H., Nabholz, M., and MacDonald, H. R.,** Similarities between interleukin-2 receptor number and affinity on activated B and T lymphocytes, *Nature,* 315, 669, 1985.
46. **Teshigawara, K., Wang, H.-M., Kato, K., and Smith, K. A.,** Interleukin 2 high-affinity receptor expression requires two distinct binding proteins, *J. Exp. Med.,* 165, 223, 1987.
47. **Tsudo, M., Goldman, C. K., Bongiovanni, K. F., Chan, W. C., Winton, E. F., Yagita, M., Grimm, E. A., and Waldmann, T. A.,** The p75 peptide is the receptor for interleukin 2 expressed on large granular lymphocytes and is responsible for the interleukin 2 activation of these cells, *Proc. Natl. Acad. Sci. U.S.A.,* 84, 5394, 1987.
48. **Lowenthal, J. W. and Greene, W. C.,** Contrasting interleukin 2 binding properties of the alpha (p55) and beta (p70) protein subunits of the human high-affinity interleukin 2 receptor, *J. Exp. Med.,* 166, 1156, 1987.
49. **Robb, R. J., Munck, A., and Smith, K.,** T cell growth factor receptors: quantitation, specificity, and biological relevance, *J. Exp. Med.,* 154, 1455, 1981.
50. **Ortega, G. R., Robb, R. J., Shevach, E. M., and Malek, T. R.,** The murine IL 2 receptor. I. Monoclonal antibodies that define distinct functional epitopes on activated T cells and react with activated B cells, *J. Immunol.,* 133, 1970, 1984.
51. **Miller, J., Malek, T. R., Leonard, W. J., Greene, W. C., Shevach, E. M., and Germain, R. N.,** Nucleotide sequence and expression of a mouse interleukin 2 receptor cDNA, *J. Immunol.,* 134, 4212, 1985.
52. **Leonard, W. J., Depper, J. M., Crabtree, G. R., Rudikoff, S., Pumphrey, J., Robb, R. J., Kronke, M., Svetlik, P. B., Peffer, N. J., Waldmann, T. A., and Greene, W. C.,** Molecular cloning and expression of cDNAs for the human interleukin-2 receptor, *Nature,* 311, 626, 1984.
53. **Cosman, D., Cerretti, D. P., Larsen, A., Park, L., March, C., Dower, S., Gillis, S., and Urdal, D.,** Cloning, sequence and expression of human interleukin-2 receptor, *Nature,* 312, 768, 1984.
54. **Ullrich, A., Coussens, L., Hayflick, J. S., Dull, T. J., Gray, A., Tam, A. W., Lee, J., Yarden, Y., Libermann, T. A., Schlessinger, J., Downward, J., Mayes, E. L. V., Whittle, N., Waterfield, M. D., and Seeburg, P. H.,** Human epidermal growth factor receptor cDNA sequence and aberrant expression of the amplified gene in A431 epidermoid carcinoma cells, *Nature,* 309, 418, 1984.
55. **Yarden, Y., Escobedo, J. A., Kuang, W.-J., Yang-Feng, T. L., Daniel, T. O., Tremble, P. M., Chen, E. Y., Ando, M. E., Harkins, R. N., Francke, U., Fried, V. A., Ullrich, A., and Williams, L. T.,** Structure of the receptor for platelet-derived growth factor helps define a family of closely related growth factor receptors, *Nature,* 323, 226, 1986.
56. **Ebina, M., Ellis, L., Jarnagin, K., Edery, M., Graf, L., Clauser, E., Ou, J.-H., Masiarz, F., Kan, Y. W., Goldfine, C. D., Roth, R. A., and Rutter, W. J.,** The human insulin receptor cDNA: the structural basis for hormone-activated transmembrane signalling, *Cell,* 40, 747, 1985.
57. **Coussens, L., Van Beveren, C., Smith, D., Chen, E., Mitchell, R. L., Isacke, C. M., Verma, I. M., and Ullrich, A.,** Structural alteration of viral homologue of receptor proto-oncogene *fms* at carboxyl terminus, *Nature,* 320, 277, 1986.

58. **Sherr, C. J., Rettenmier, C. W., Sacca, R., Roussei, M. F., Look, A. T., and Stanley, E. R.,** The c-*fms* proto-oncogene product is related to the receptor for the mononuclear phagocyte growth factor, CSF-1, *Cell,* 41, 665, 1985.

59. **Hatakeyama, M., Minamoto, S., Uchiyama, T., Hardy, R. R., Yamada, G., and Taniguchi, T.,** Reconstitution of functional receptor for human interleukin-2 in mouse cells, *Nature,* 318, 467, 1985.

60. **Cosman, D., Wignall, J., Lewis, A., Alpert, A., Cerretti, D. P., Park, L., Dower, S. K., Gillis, S., and Urdal, D. L.,** High level stable expression of human interleukin-2 receptors in mouse cells generates only low affinity interleukin-2 binding sites, *Mol. Immunol.,* 23, 935, 1986.

61. **Greene, W. C., Robb, R. J., Svetlik, P. B., Rusk, C. M., Depper, J. M., and Leonard, W. J.,** Stable expression of cDNA encoding in the human interleukin 2 receptor in eukaryotic cells, *J. Exp. Med.,* 162, 363, 1985.

62. **Rubin, L. A., Kurman, C. C., Fritz, M. E., Biddison, W. E., Boutin, B., Yarchoan, R., and Nelson, D. L.,** Soluble interleukin 2 receptors are released from activated human lymphoid cells *in vitro, J. Immunol.,* 135, 3172, 1985.

63. **Shimizu, A., Kondo, N., Kondo, S., Hamuro, J., and Honjo, T.,** Production and characterization of the extracytoplasmic portion of the human interleukin-2 receptor, *Mol. Biol. Med.,* 3, 509, 1986.

64. **Treiger, B. F., Leonard, W. J., Svetlik, P., Rubin, L. A., Nelson, D. L., and Greene, W. C.,** A secreted form of the human interleukin 2 receptor encoded by an "anchor minus" cDNA, *J. Immunol.,* 136, 4099, 1986.

65. **Robb, R. J. and Kutny, R. M.,** Structure-function relationships for the IL2-receptor system. IV. Analysis of the sequence and ligand-binding properties of soluble Tac protein, *J. Immunol.,* 139, 855, 1987.

66. **Rubin, L. A., Jay, G., and Nelson, D. L.,** The released interleukin 2 receptor binds interleukin 2 efficiently, *J. Immunol.,* 137, 3841, 1986.

67. **Bernard, O., Fazekas de St. Groth, B., Ullrich, A., Green, W., and Schlessinger, J.,** High-affinity interleukin 2 binding by an oncogenic hybrid interleukin 2-epidermal growth factor receptor molecule, *Proc. Natl. Acad. Sci. U.S.A.,* 84, 2125, 1987.

68. **Robb, R. J.,** Conversion of low-affinity interleukin 2 receptors to a high-affinity state following fusion of cell membranes, *Proc. Natl. Acad. Sci. U.S.A.,* 83, 3992, 1986.

69. **Sharon, M., Klausner, R. D., Cullen, B., Chizzonite, R., and Leonard, W. J.,** Novel interleukin-2 receptor subunit detected by cross-linking under high-affinity conditions, *Science,* 234, 859, 1986.

70. **Tsudo, M., Kozak, R. W., Goldman, C. K., and Waldmann, T. A.,** Demonstration of a non-Tac peptide that binds interleukin 2: a potential participant in a multichain interleukin 2 receptor complex, *Proc. Natl. Acad. Sci. U.S.A.,* 83, 9694, 1986.

71. **Saragovi, H. and Malek, T. R.,** The murine interleukin 2 receptor. Irreversible cross-linking of radiolabeled interleukin 2 to high affinity interleukin 2 receptors reveals a noncovalently associated subunit, *J. Immunol.,* 139, 1918, 1987.

72. **Okada, M., Maeda, M., Tagaya, Y., Taniguchi, Y., Teshigawara, K., Yoshiki, T., Diamantstein, T., Smith, K. A., Uchiyama, T., Honjo, T., and Yodoi, J.,** TCGF (IL 2)-receptor inducing factor(s). II. Possible role of ATL-derived factor (ADF) on constitutive IL 2 receptor expression of HTLV-I(+) T cell lines, *J. Immunol.,* 135, 3995, 1985.

73. **Lee, J. C., Truneh, A., Smith, M. F. J., and Tsang, K. Y.,** Induction of interleukin 2 receptor (Tac) by tumor necrosis factor in YT cells, *J. Immunol.,* 139, 1935, 1987.

74. **Shirakawa, F., Tanaka, Y., Eto, S., Suzuki, H., Yodoi, J., and Yamashita, U.,** Effect of interleukin 1 on the expression of interleukin 2 receptor (Tac antigen) on human natural killer cells and natural killer-like cell line (YT cells), *J. Immunol.,* 137, 551, 1986.

75. **Wang, H.-M. and Smith, K. A.,** The interleukin 2 receptor. Functional consequences of its bimolecular structure, *J. Exp. Med.,* 166, 1055, 1987.

76. **Malek, T. R. and Ashwell, J. D.,** Interleukin 2 upregulates expression of its receptor on a T cell clone, *J. Exp. Med.,* 161, 1575, 1985.

77. **Depper, J. M., Leonard, W. J., Drogula, C., Kronke, M., Waldmann, T. A., and Greene, W. C.,** Interleukin 2 (IL-2) augments transcription of the IL-2 receptor gene, *Proc. Natl. Acad. Sci. U.S.A.,* 82, 4230, 1985.

78. **Inoue, J.-I., Seiki, M., Taniguchi, T., Tsuru, S., and Yoshida, M.,** Induction of interleukin 2 receptor gene expression by p40^x encoded by human T-cell leukemia virus type I, *EMBO J.,* 5, 2883, 1986.

79. **Greene, W. C., Leonard, W. J., Wano, Y., Svetlik, P. B., Peffer, N. J., Sodroski, J. G., Rosen, C. A., Goh, W. C., and Haseltine, W.A.,** Trans-activator gene of HTLV-II induces IL-2 receptor and IL-2 cellular gene expression, *Science,* 232, 877, 1986.

80. **Weissman, A. M., Harford, J. B., Svetlik, P. B., Leonard, W. L., Depper, J. M., Waldmann, T. A., Greene, W. C., and Klausner, R. D.,** Only high-affinity receptors for interleukin 2 mediate internalization of ligand, *Proc. Natl. Acad. Sci. U.S.A.,* 83, 1463, 1986.

81. **Fujii, M., Sugamura, K., Sano, K., Nakai, M., Sugita, K., and Yorio, H.,** High-affinity receptor-mediated internalization and degradation of interleukin 2 in human T cells, *J. Exp. Med.,* 163, 550, 1986.

82. **Lowenthal, J. W., MacDonald, H. R., and Iacopetta, B. J.,** Intracellular pathway of interleukin 2 following receptor-mediated endocytosis, *Eur. J. Immunol.,* 16, 1461, 1986.

83. **Duprez, V. and Dautry-Varsat, A.,** Receptor-mediated endocytosis of interleukin 2 in a human tumor T cell line. Degradation of interleukin 2 and evidence for the absence of recycling of interleukin receptors, *J. Biol. Chem.,* 261, 15450, 1986.

84. **Gaulton, G. N. and Eardley, D. D.,** Interleukin 2-dependent phosphorylation of interleukin 2 receptors and other T cell membrane proteins, *J. Immunol.,* 136, 2470, 1986.

85. **Lieberman, J., Verret, C. R., Kranz, D. M., Hubbard, S. C., Saito, H., Raulet, D. H., Tonegawa, S., and Eisen, H. N.,** A phosphorylated, disulfide-linked membrane protein in murine cytotoxic T lymphocytes, *Proc. Natl. Acad. Sci. U.S.A.,* 83, 7870, 1986.

86. **Ishii, T., Sugamura, K., Nakamura, M., and Hinuma, Y.,** Interleukin 2 (IL-2) rapidly induces phosphorylation of a cellular protein, pp67, in an IL-2 dependent murine CTLL line, *Biochem. Biophys. Res. Commun.,* 135, 487, 1986.

87. **Ishii, T., Kohno, M., Nakamura, M., Hinuma, Y., and Sugamura, K.,** Characterization of interleukin 2-stimulated phosphorylation of 67 and 63 kDa proteins in human T-cells, *Biochem. J.,* 242, 211, 1987.

88. **Mire, A. R., Wickremasinghe, R. G., Michalevicz, R., and Hoffbrand, A. V.,** Interleukin-2 induces rapid phosphorylation of an 85 kilodalton protein in permeabilized lymphocytes, *Biochim. Biophys. Acta,* 847, 159, 1985.

89. **Kohno, M., Kuwata, S., Namba, Y., and Hanaoka, M.,** Interleukin 2 induces rapid phosphorylation of cellular proteins in murine T lymphocytes, *FEBS Lett.,* 198, 33, 1986.

90. **Evans, S. W. and Farrar, W. L.,** Identity of common phosphoprotein substances stimulated by interleukin 2 and diacylglycerol suggests a role of protein kinase C for IL 2 signal transduction, *J. Cell. Biochem.,* 34, 47, 1987.

91. **Evans, S. W. and Farrar, W. L.,** Interleukin 2 and diacylglycerol stimulate phosphorylation of ribosomal S6 protein. Correlation with increased protein synthesis and S6 kinase activation, *J. Biol. Chem.,* 262, 4624, 1987.

92. **Benedict, S. H., Mills, G. B., and Gelfand, E. W.,** Interleukin 2 activates a receptor-associated protein kinase, *J. Immunol.,* 139, 1694, 1987.

93. **Farrar, W. L. and Anderson, W. B.,** Interleukin-2 stimulates association of protein kinase C with plasma membrane, *Nature,* 315, 233, 1985.

94. **Taguchi, M., Thomas, T. P., Anderson, W. B., and Farrar, W. L.,** Direct phosphorylation of the IL-2 receptor Tac antigen epitope by protein kinase C, *Biochem. Biophys. Res. Commun.,* 135, 239, 1986.

95. **Shackelford, D. A. and Trowbridge, I. S.,** Identification of lymphocyte integral membrane proteins as substrates for protein kinase C. Phosphorylation of the interleukin-2 receptor, Class I HLA antigens, and T200 glycoprotein, *J. Biol. Chem.,* 261, 8334, 1986.

96. **Mills, G. B., Stewart, D. J., Mellors, A., and Gelfand, E.,** Interleukin 2 does not induce phosphatidylinositol hydrolysis in activated T cells, *J. Immunol.,* 136, 3019, 1986.

97. **Kozumbo, W. J., Harris, D. T., Gromkowski, S., Cerottini, J.-C., and Cerutti, P. A.,** Molecular mechanisms involved in T cell activation. II. The phosphatidylinositol signal-transducing mechanism mediates antigen-induced lymphokine production but not interleukin 2-induced proliferation in cloned cytotoxic T lymphocytes, *J. Immunol.,* 138, 606, 1987.

98. **Heckford, S. E., Gelmann, E. P., Agnor, C. L., Jacobson, S., Zinn, S., and Matis, L. A.,** Distinct signals are required for proliferation and lymphokine gene expression in murine T cells, *J. Immunol.,* 137, 3652, 1986.

99. **Gelfand, E., Mills, G. B., Cheung, R. K., Lee, J. W. W., and Grinstein, S.,** Transmembrane ion fluxes during activation of human T lymphocytes: role of Ca^{2+}, Na^+/H^+ exchange and phospholipid turnover, *Immunol. Rev.,* 95, 59, 1987.

100. **Johnson, H. M., Vassalo, T., and Torres, B. A.,** Interleukin 2-mediated events in gamma-interferon production are calcium dependent at more than one site, *J. Immunol.,* 134, 967, 1985.

101. **Utsunomiya, N., Tsuboi, M., and Nakanishi, M.,** Interleukin 2 increases T lymphocyte membrane mobility before the rise in cytosolic calcium concentration, *Biochemistry,* 25, 2582, 1986.

102. **Larsen, C. S., Knudsen, T. E., and Johnson, H. E.,** The role of calcium in stimulation of activated T lymphocytes with interleukin 2, *Scand. J. Immunol.,* 24, 689, 1986.

103. **Mills, G. B., Cheung, R. K., Grinstein, S., and Gelfand, E. W.,** Interleukin 2-induced lymphocyte proliferation is independent of increases in cytosolic-free calcium concentrations, *J. Immunol.,* 134, 2431, 1985.

104. **Byus, C. V., Klimpel, G. R., Lucas, D. O., and Russel, D. H.,** Type I and type II cyclic AMP-dependent protein kinase as opposite effectors of lymphocyte mitogenesis, *Nature,* 268, 63, 1977.

105. **Wang, T., Sheppard, J. R., and Foker, J. E.,** Rise and fall of cyclic AMP required for onset of lymphocyte DNA synthesis, *Science,* 201, 155, 1978.

106. **Taylor, M. V., Metcalfe, J. C., Hesketh, T. R., Smith, G. A., and Moore, J. P.,** Mitogens increase phosphorylation of phosphoinositides in thymocytes, *Nature,* 312, 462, 1984.

107. **Hadden, J. W. and Coffey, R. G.,** Cyclic nucleotides in mitogen-induced lymphocyte proliferation, *Immunol. Today,* 3, 299, 1982.
108. **Beckner, S. K. and Farrar, W.,** Interleukin 2 modulation of adenylate cyclase. Potential role of protein kinase C, *J. Biol. Chem.,* 261, 3043, 1986.
109. **Farrar, W. L., Evans, S. W., Rapp, U. R., and Cleveland, J. L.,** Effects of anti-proliferative cyclic AMP on interleukin 2-stimulated gene expression, *J. Immunol.,* 139, 2075, 1987.
110. **Knudsen, T. E., Larsen, C. S., and Johnsen, H. E.,** A study of cyclic nucleotides as second messengers after interleukin 2 stimulation of human T lymphocytes, *Scand. J. Immunol.,* 25, 527, 1987.
111. **Evans, S. W., Becker, S. K., and Farrar, W. L.,** Stimulation of specific GTP binding and hydrolysis activities in lymphocyte membrane by interleukin-2, *Nature,* 325, 166, 1987.
112. **Mills, G. B., Cragoe, E. J. J., Gelfand, E. W., and Grinstein, S.,** Interleukin 2 induces a rapid increase in intracellular pH through activation of a Na^+/H^+ antiport. Cytoplasmic alkalinization is not required for lymphocyte proliferation, *J. Biol. Chem.,* 260, 12500, 1985.
113. **Lee, S. C., Sabath, D. E., Deutsch, C., and Prystowsky, M. B.,** Increased voltage-gated potassium conductance during interleukin 2-stimulated proliferation of a mouse helper T lymphocyte clone, *J. Cell Biol.,* 102, 1200, 1986.
114. **Sabath, D. E., Monos, D. M., Lee, S. C., Deutsch, C., and Prystowsky, M. B.,** Cloned T-cell proliferation and synthesis of specific proteins are inhibited by quinine, *Proc. Natl. Acad. Sci. U.S.A.,* 83, 4739, 1986.
115. **Matteson, D. R. and Deutsch, C.,** K channels in T lymphocytes: a patch clamp study using monoclonal antibody adhesion, *Nature,* 307, 468, 1984.
116. **Deutsch, C., Krause, D., and Lee, S. C.,** Voltage-gated potassium conductance in human T lymphocytes stimulated with phorbol ester, *J. Physiol.,* 372, 405, 1986.
117. **DeCoursey, T. E., Chandy, K. G., Gupta, S., and Cahalan, M. D.,** Voltage-gated K^+ channels in human T lymphocytes: a role in mitogenesis, *Nature,* 307, 465, 1984.
118. **Chandy, K. G., DeCoursey, T. E., Cahalan, M. D., and Gupta, S.,** Electroimmunology: the physiologic role of ion channels in the immune system, *J. Immunol.,* 135, 787s, 1985.
119. **Cahalan, M. D., Chandy, K. G., DeCoursey, T. E., and Gupta, S.,** A voltage-gated potassium channel in human T lymphocytes, *J. Physiol.,* 358, 197, 1985.
120. **Gaulton, G. N., Kelly, K. L., Pawlowski, J., Mato, J. M., and Jarett, L.,** Regulation and function of an insulin-sensitive glycosyl-phosphatidylinositol during T lymphocyte activation, *Cell,* 53, 963, 1988.
121. **Cleveland, J. L., Rapp, U. R., and Farrar, W. L.,** Role of c-*myc* and other genes in interleukin 2 regulated CT6 T lymphocytes and their malignant variants, *J. Immunol.,* 138, 3495, 1987.
122. **Kaczmarek, L., Calabretta, B., Elfenbein, I. B., and Mercer, W. E.,** Cell cycle analysis of human peripheral blood T lymphocytes in long-term culture, *Exp. Cell Res.,* 173, 70, 1987.
123. **Kaczmarek, L., Calabretta, B., and Baserga, R.,** Effect of interleukin-2 on the expression of cell cycle genes in human T lymphocytes, *Biochem. Biophys. Res. Commun.,* 133, 410, 1985.
124. **Stern, J. B. and Smith, K. A.,** Interleukin-2 induction of T-cell G_1 progression and c-*myb* expression, *Science,* 233, 203, 1986.
125. **Pauza, C. D.,** Regulation of human T-lymphocyte gene expression by interleukin 2: immediate-response genes include the proto-oncogene c-*myb,* *Mol. Cell. Biol.,* 7, 342, 1987.
126. **Neckers, L. M. and Cossman, J.,** Transferrin receptor induction in mitogen-stimulated human T lymphocytes is required for DNA synthesis and cell division and is regulated by interleukin 2, *Proc. Natl. Acad. Sci. U.S.A.,* 80, 3494, 1983.
127. **Lum, J. B., Infante, A. J., Makker, D. M., Yang, F., and Bowman, B. H.,** Transferrin synthesis by inducer T lymphocytes, *J. Clin. Invest.,* 77, 841, 1986.
128. **Reem, G. H. and Yeh, N.-H.,** Interleukin 2 regulates expression of its receptor and synthesis of gamma interferon by human T lymphocytes, *Science,* 225, 429, 1984.
129. **Farrar, W. L., Birchenall-Sparks, M. C., and Young, H. B.,** Interleukin 2 induction of interferon-gamma mRNA synthesis, *J. Immunol.,* 137, 3836, 1986.
130. **Young, H. A., Dray, J. F., and Farrar, W. L.,** Expression of transfected human interferon-gamma DNA: evidence for cell-specific regulation, *J. Immunol.,* 136, 4700, 1986.
131. **Moore, K. S., Sullivan, K., Tan, E. M., and Prystowsky, M. B.,** Proliferating cell nuclear antigen/ cyclin is an interleukin 2-responsive gene, *J. Biol. Chem.,* 262, 8447, 1987.
132. **Shipman, P. M., Sabath, D. E., Fischer, A. H., Comber, P. G., Sullivan, K., Tan, E. M., and Prystowsky, M. B.,** Cyclin mRNA and protein expression in recombinant interleukin 2-stimulated cloned murine T lymphocytes, *J. Cell. Biochem.,* 38, 189, 1988.
133. **Bravo, R., Frank, R., Blundell, P. A., and Macdonald-Bravo, H.,** Cyclin/PCNA is the auxiliary protein of DNA polymerase-delta, *Nature,* 326, 515, 1987.
134. **Prelich, G., Tan, C.-K., Kostura, M., Mathews, M. B., So, A. G., Downey, K. M., and Stillman, B.,** Functional identity of proliferating cell nuclear antigen and a DNA polymerase-delta auxiliary protein, *Nature,* 326, 517, 1987.

135. **Prelich, G., Kostura, M., Marshak, D. R., Mathews, M. B., and Stillman, B.,** The cell-cycle regulated proliferating cell nuclear antigen is required for SV40 DNA replication *in vitro, Nature,* 326, 471, 1987.

136. **Prelich, G. and Stillman, B.,** Coordinated leading and lagging strand synthesis during SV40 DNA replication *in vitro* requires PCNA, *Cell,* 53, 117, 1988.

137. **Kurki, P., Lotz, M., Ogata, K., and Tan, E. M.,** Proliferating cell nuclear antigen (PCNA)/cyclin in activated human T lymphocytes, *J. Immunol.,* 138, 4114, 1987.

138. **Wang, T., Marquardt, C., and Foker, J.,** Aerobic glycolysis during lymphocyte proliferation, *Nature,* 261, 702, 1976.

139. **Polgar, P. R., Foster, J. M., and Cooperbrand, S. R.,** Glycolysis as an energy source for stimulation of lymphocytes by phytohemagglutinin, *Exp. Cell Res.,* 49, 231, 1968.

140. **Matrisian, L. M., Rautmann, G., Magun, B. E., and Breathnach, R.,** Epidermal growth factor or serum stimulation of rat fibroblasts induces an elevation in mRNA levels for lactate dehydrogenase and other glycolytic enzymes, *Nucl. Acids Res.,* 13, 711, 1985.

141. **Ferrari, S., Battini, R., Kaczmarek, L., Rittling, S., Calabretta, B., De Riel, J. K., Philiponis, V., Wei, J.-F., and Baserga, R.,** Coding sequence and growth regulation of the human vimentin gene, *Mol. Cell. Biol.,* 6, 3614, 1986.

142. **Holland, J. P., Labieniec, L., Swimmer, C., and Holland, M. J.,** Homologous nucleotide sequences at the 5′ termini of messenger RNAs synthesized from the yeast enolase and glyceraldehyde-3-phosphate dehydrogenase gene families, *J. Biol. Chem.,* 258, 5291, 1983.

143. **Muraguchi, A., Kehrl, J. H., Longo, D. L., Volkman, D. J., Smith, K. A., and Fauci, A. S.,** Interleukin 2 receptors on human B cells. Implications for the role of interleukin 2 in human B cell function, *J. Exp. Med.,* 161, 181, 1985.

144. **Harada, N., Matsumoto, M., Koyama, N., Shimizu, A., Honjo, T., Tominaga, A., and Takatsu, K.,** T cell replacing factor/interleukin 5 induces not only B-cell growth and differentiation, but also increased expression of interleukin 2 receptor on activated B-cells, *Immunol. Lett.,* 15, 205, 1987.

145. **Nakanishi, K., Hashimoto, T., Hiroishi, K., Matsui, K., Yoshimoto, T., Morse, H. C. I., Furuyama, J.-I., Hamaoka, T., Higashino, K., and Paul, W. E.,** Demonstration of upregulated IL 2 receptor expression on an *in vitro* cloned BCL1 subline, *J. Immunol.,* 138, 1817, 1987.

146. **Bitoh, S., Yamamoto, H., Fujimoto, S., and Ohtsuki, Y.,** Long-term-cultured mouse B-lymphocyte line. I. Establishment and characterization of mouse B-lymphocyte line, *Cell. Immunol.,* 107, 138, 1987.

147. **Holter, W., Goldman, C. K., Casabo, L., Nelson, D. L., Greene, W. C., and Waldmann, T. A.,** Expression of functional IL 2 receptors by lipopolysaccharide and interferon-gamma stimulated human monocytes, *J. Immunol.,* 138, 2917, 1987.

148. **Wahl, S. M., McCartney-Francis, N., Hunt, D. A., Smith, P. D., Wahl, L. M., and Katona, I. M.,** Monocyte interleukin 2 receptor gene expression and interleukin 2 augmentation of microbicidal activity, *J. Immunol.,* 139, 1342, 1987.

149. **Zarcone, D., Prasthofer, E. F., Malavasi, F., Pistoia, V., LoBuglio, A. F., and Grossi, C. E.,** Ultrastructural analysis of human natural killer cell activation, *Blood,* 69, 1725, 1987.

150. **Grimm, E. A.,** Human lymphokine-activated killer cells (LAK cells) as a potential immunotherapeutic modality, *Biochim. Biophys. Acta,* 865, 267, 1986.

151. **Benveniste, E. N., Herman, P. K., and Whitaker, J. N.,** Myelin basic protein-specific RNA levels in interleukin-2-stimulated oligodendrocytes, *J. Neurochem.,* 49, 1274, 1987.

152. **Birchenall-Sparks, M. C., Farrar, W. L., Rennick, D., Kilian, P. L., and Ruscetti, F. W.,** Regulation of expression of the interleukin-2 receptor on hematopoietic cells by interleukin-3, *Science,* 233, 455, 1986.

153. **Mazumder, A. and Rosenberg, S. A.,** Successful immunotherapy of natural killer-resistant established pulmonary melanoma metastases by the intravenous adoptive transfer of syngeneic lymphocytes activated *in vitro* by interleukin 2, *J. Exp. Med.,* 159, 495, 1984.

154. **Mule, J. J., Shu, S., Schwarz, S. L., and Rosenberg, S. A.,** Adoptive immunotherapy of established pulmonary metastases with LAK cells and recombinant interleukin-2, *Science,* 225, 1487, 1984.

155. **Rosenberg, S. A., Mule, J. J., Spiess, P. J., Reichert, C. M., and Schwarz, S. L.,** Regression of established pulmonary metastases and subcutaneous tumor mediated by the systemic administration of high-dose recombinant interleukin 2, *J. Exp. Med.,* 161, 1169, 1985.

156. **Rosenberg, S. A., Lotze, M. T., Muul, L. M., Leitman, S., Chang, A. E., Ettinghausen, S. E., Matory, Y. L., Skibber, J. M., Shiloni, E., Vetto, J. T., Seipp, C. A., Simpson, C., and Reichert, C. M.,** Observations on the systemic administration of autologous lymphokine-activated killer cells and recombinant interleukin-2 to patients with metastatic cancer, *N. Engl. J. Med.,* 313, 1485, 1985.

157. **Rosenberg, S. A., Lotze, M. T., Muul, L. M., Chang, A. E., Avis, F. P., Leitman, S., Linehan, W. M., Robertson, C. N., Lee, R. E., Rubin, J. T., Seipp, C. A., Simpson, C. G., and White, D. E.,** A progress report on the treatment of 157 patients with advanced cancer using lymphokine-activated killer cells and interleukin-2 or high-dose interleukin-2 alone, *N. Engl. J. Med.,* 316, 889, 1987.

158. **Cohen, P. J., Lotze, M. T., Roberts, J. R., Rosenberg, S. A., and Jaffe, E. S.,** The immunopathology of sequential tumor biopsies in patients treated with interleukin-2, *Am. J. Pathol.,* 129, 208, 1987.

159. **Lane, H. C., Masur, H., Gelmann, E. P., and Fauci, A. S.,** Therapeutic approaches to patients with AIDS, *Cancer Res.,* 45(Suppl.), 4674s, 1985.
160. **Lane, H. C. and Fauci, A. S.,** Immunologic reconstitution in the acquired immunodeficiency syndrome, *Ann. Intern. Med.,* 103, 714, 1985.
161. **Ernst, M., Kern, P., Flad, H.-D., and Ulmer, A. J.,** Effects of systemic *in vivo* interleukin-2 (IL-2) reconstitution in patients with acquired immune deficiency syndrome (AIDS) and AIDS-related complex (ARC) on phenotypes and functions of peripheral blood mononuclear cells (PBMC), *J. Clin. Immunol.,* 6, 170, 1986.
162. **Atkins, M. B., Gould, J. A., Alegretta, M., Li, J. J., Dempsey, R. A., Rudders, R. A., Parkinson, D. R., Reichlin, S., and Mier, J. W.,** Phase I evaluation of recombinant interleukin-2 in patients with advanced malignant disease, *J. Clin. Oncol.,* 4, 1380, 1986.
163. **Lotze, M. T., Matory, Y. L., Rayner, A. A., Ettinghausen, S. E., Vetto, J. T., Seipp, C. A., and Rosenberg, S. A.,** Clinical effects and toxicity of interleukin-2 in patients with cancer, *Cancer,* 58, 2764, 1986.
164. **Belldegrun, A., Webb, D. E., Austin, H. A. I., Steinberg, S. M., White, D. E., Linehan, W. M., and Rosenberg, S. A.,** Effects of interleukin-2 on renal function in patients receiving immunotherapy for advanced cancer, *Ann. Intern. Med.,* 106, 817, 1987.
165. **Ettinghausen, S. E., Moore, J. G., White, D. E., Platanias, L., Young, N. S., and Rosenberg, S. A.,** Hematologic effects of immunotherapy with lymphokine-activated killer cells and recombinant interleukin-2 in cancer patients, *Blood,* 69, 1654, 1987.
166. **Gaspari, A. A., Lotze, M. T., Rosenberg, S. A., Stern, J. B., and Katz, S. I.,** Dermatologic changes associated with interleukin 2 administration, *JAMA,* 258, 1624, 1987.
167. **Atkins, M. B., Mier, J. W., Parkinson, D. R., Gould, J. A., Berkman, E. M., and Kaplan, M. M.,** Hypothyroidism after treatment with interleukin-2 and lymphokine-activated killer cells, *N. Engl. J. Med.,* 318, 1557, 1988.
168. **Denicoff, K. D., Rubinow, D. R., Papa, M. Z., Simpson, C., Seipp, C. A., Lotze, M. T., Chang, A. E., Rosenstein, D., and Rosenberg, S. A.,** The neuropsychiatric effects of treatment with interleukin-2 and lymphokine-activated killer cells, *Ann. Intern. Med.,* 107, 293, 1987.
169. **Vetto, J. T., Papa, M. Z., Lotze, M. T., Chang, A. E., and Rosenberg, S. A.,** Reduction of toxicity of interleukin-2 and lymphokine-activated killer cells in humans by the administration of corticosteroids, *J. Clin. Oncol.,* 5, 496, 1987.
170. **Thompson, J. A., Lee, D. J., Cox, W. W., Lindgren, C. G., Collins, C., Neraas, K., Dennin, R. A., and Fefer, A.,** Recombinant interleukin 2 toxicity, pharmacokinetics, and immunomodulatory effects in a phase I trial, *Cancer Res.,* 47, 4202, 1987.
171. **Allegretta, M., Atkins, M. B., Dempsey, R. A., Bradley, E. C., Konrad, M. W., Childs, A., Wolfe, S. N., and Mier, J. W.,** The development of anti-interleukin-2 antibodies in patients treated with recombinant human interleukin-2 (IL-2), *J. Clin. Immunol.,* 6, 481, 1986.

Chapter 10

CACHECTIN (TUMOR NECROSIS FACTOR) AND LYMPHOTOXIN AS PRIMARY MEDIATORS OF TISSUE CATABOLISM, INFLAMMATION, AND SHOCK

Bruce Beutler and Anthony Cerami

TABLE OF CONTENTS

I. INTRODUCTION

Among its many components, no aspect of the cellular immune response is more ancient nor more universal than inflammation. Inflammation is obviously intended to protect the host; anti-inflammatory drugs have been shown to foster the growth and spread of microbial infection. However, inflammation may also threaten host survival.

The participation of arachidonate metabolites in local inflammatory processes has become clear during the past 2 decades. Prostaglandins and leukotrienes appear to act as terminal mediators of the inflammatory response; however, their production and release are, at least in part, governed by primary mediators of inflammation, many of which are proteins of leukocyte origin.

At a systemic level, inflammation is accompanied by a variety of metabolic and physiologic changes.[1,2] Glucose intolerance, lipid and protein catabolism, fever, shock, and coagulopathy are among these. These derangements also appear to be mediated by specific cytokines. In recent years, techniques of genetic analysis have progressed to the point that individual agents responsible for initiating inflammatory changes can be studied in isolation.[3]

One of the most dramatic and most dangerous examples of host injury caused by inflammatory processes can be witnessed in the setting of Gram negative sepsis.[4-14] When infected by Gram negative organisms, mammals develop a "shock" state in which hypotension, hypoglycemia, metabolic acidosis, and ischemic injury of several end organs results. These events, once thought to be mediated by bacterial lipopolysaccharide (LPS), are in fact known to be attributable to endogenous mediators. The C3H/HeJ mouse, which is resistant to the lethal effect of LPS, can be rendered sensitive by transplantation of marrow from an LPS-sensitive, histocompatible donor.[15] This observation effectively proves that endotoxicity is dependent upon cell(s) of hematopoietic origin, or their products.

One of the most important of these mediators of endotoxicity is that molecule known as "cachectin", or "tumor necrosis factor" (TNF). The isolation of cachectin/TNF and the discovery of its role as a primary mediator of diverse inflammatory processes was accomplished through two separate lines of investigation.

II. HYPERTRIGLYCERIDEMIA IN WASTING DISEASES AND IN ENDOTOXIC SHOCK

In the late 1970s, Rouzer and Cerami observed that Trypanosome-infected rabbits developed a profound wasting syndrome despite the fact that they harbored a low parasite burden.[16,17] The cachexia displayed by these animals offered an excellent opportunity to analyze the hypercatabolic state that prevails in infection, since it could not be explained by a simple competitive mechanism. Oddly, these animals were also noted to be remarkably hypertriglyceridemic.[16] The hypertriglyceridemia was soon seen to result from a clearing defect; the animals displayed an acquired, systemic deficiency of the enzyme lipoprotein lipase (LPL),[16] which normally acts to cleave triglycerides, permitting their removal from the plasma. Thus, in these animals, hypertriglyceridemia was maintained at the expense of adipocyte stores. Systemic suppression of LPL activity was taken to represent a biochemical marker of the wasting diathesis that accompanied trypanosome infection.

A similar hypertriglyceridemia was found to occur in endotoxin-sensitive (C3H/HeN) mice following injection of LPS. LPL expression was entirely suppressed in the plasma and fatty tissues of these animals. Conversely, C3H/HeJ (endotoxin-resistant) mice did not exhibit this response to LPS.[18] However, adipocyte LPL expression could be suppressed in LPS-resistant mice by a serum factor obtained from endotoxin-treated C3H/HeN mice. Moreover, isolated macrophages obtained from endotoxin-sensitive animals and exposed to endotoxin *in vitro* produced a similar bioactivity.[18,19]

The LPL suppressing factor, termed "cachectin", was found to act upon isolated adipocytes in culture and was shown to be capable of suppressing LPL expression *in vitro*,[19] as well as stimulating lipolysis in these target cells.[20] Other enzymes, including fatty acid synthetase and acetyl CoA carboxylase, were also suppressed by the conditioned medium of LPS-activated macrophages.[21]

Cachectin was purified to homogeneity in four steps.[22] It was found to be a 17.5-kDa protein, secreted in copious quantities by LPS-activated macrophages. Mouse cachectin appeared to exist as a multimer of varying size when analyzed by gel filtration. It constituted approximately 1 to 2% of the total secretory protein produced by endotoxin-treated RAW 264.7 (mouse macrophage) cells, or by endotoxin-treated mouse peritoneal macrophages.

Highly purified preparations of mouse cachectin were radioiodinated with excellent preservation of biological activity. The radioiodinated protein was shown to bind with high affinity to cultured adipocytes (3T3-L1 cells), C2 myotubules, crude liver cell membrane preparations,[22] and subsequently to a variety of other tissues as well. The affinity constant (Ka) of the receptor was measured by Scatchard analysis and found to be approximately $3 \times 10^9 \ M^{-1}$. Approximately 10,000 receptor sites per cell were identified on each of the cultured cell lines mentioned above.

The receptor was immediately utilized as the basis of a sensitive and highly specific radioreceptor competition assay.[23] Rabbits were injected with LPS, and cachectin levels were assayed in serum samples obtained at frequent intervals over a 10-h period. Measurable quantities of the hormone were detected in the plasma within 15 min following LPS administration. Levels peaked at 2 h, and thereafter declined rapidly to approach baseline levels within 5 h. Direct measurements of the clearance of active radiolabeled cachectin in mice suggested that the hormone was eliminated with a half-life of approximately 6 min. Large quantities of the protein were recovered from the skin, liver, gastrointestinal tract, and kidneys. The principal means of clearance appeared to be receptor binding, endocytosis, and destruction. Very little of the hormone was cleared by a renal mechanism.

When the amino terminal sequence of mouse cachectin was determined,[24] it became apparent that the hormone was structurally homologous to human TNF, the sequence of which had also been determined recently.[25] It further became evident that the bioactivities of these two proteins were exactly concordant, e.g., cachectin was capable of lysing TNF-sensitive tumor cell lines *in vitro* and TNF was capable of eliciting LPL suppression. The discovery of identity between cachectin and TNF greatly expanded the set of biological functions that had previously been ascribed to each of these proteins.

III. THE HISTORY OF TUMOR NECROSIS FACTOR

Late in the 19th century, Dr. William Coley, an oncologic surgeon in New York City, made an intriguing observation.[26,30] He noted that a sarcoma-bearing patient exhibited marked clinical improvement following a streptococcal infection (erysipelas). The primary tumor became hemorrhagic and diminished in size. Coley attempted to reproduce the phenomenon by culturing *Streptococcus* and *Serratia* organisms *in vitro* and injecting filtrates of the bacterial broths into patients with a wide variety of neoplastic diseases. In some instances, he apparently succeeded in inducing remissions and even cures; however, the toxic effects associated with this early form of chemotherapy were severe and precluded its general use.

During the 1930s and 1940s Shear and his associates[31-36] attempted to isolate the bacterial principle bacterial that was responsible for the induction of hemorrhagic necrosis. Shear isolated a substance he termed the "bacterial polysaccharide" (now known as lipopolysaccharide or endotoxin). While Shear's objective had been the isolation of a factor with low toxicity, LPS, which induces hemorrhagic necrosis of tumors, also proved to be among the most toxic components of the culture filtrate.

Subsequently, however, O'Malley and Shear[37] and later Carswell et al.[38] demonstrated that LPS exerts its effect on tumor tissues by an indirect means. They found that LPS evokes the production of an endogenous mediator, subsequently dubbed "tumor necrosis factor" (TNF), a product of macrophages, which is in turn responsible for the destructive effects witnessed in the tumor. TNF, as well the related cytotoxin known as lymphotoxin, was purified to homogeneity from cultured cell lines by Aggarwal and colleagues.[25,39] Shortly thereafter, the cDNA and genes encoding these proteins in humans, mice, and rabbits were cloned.[40-49] It was observed that TNF (cachectin) and lymphotoxin are closely linked on chromosome 6 in man and on chromosome 17 in the mouse, and reside within the major histocompatibility complex. In the latter species, the genes lie approximately 70 kb proximal to the D locus.

TNF (cachectin) and lymphotoxin share a common receptor[50] and display a highly concordant spectrum of biological activities. Interestingly, however, lymphotoxin is secreted by T lymphocytes and B lymphoblastoid cells,[39,51,52] whereas cachectin/TNF is produced principally by macrophages.[53-58] Moreover, the stimuli required to elicit production of lymphotoxin[51] differ markedly from those required to elicit production of cachectin/TNF.[59]

Lymphotoxin was originally identified as a potential reactant in the delayed-type hypersensitivity reaction.[60-66] Its production occurs in response to certain mitogenic or specific antigenic stimuli. When animal tissues are used as an antigenic stimulus, lymphotoxin production is MHC restricted. On the other hand, macrophages are known to produce cachectin/TNF in response to the B cell mitogen LPS, and in response to certain viruses[67-69] and other invasive pathogens. Its production is augmented by "priming" with certain facultative intracellular pathogens,[55,70-74] but production in response to specific antigens is unknown.

The control of cachectin/TNF and lymphotoxin production is a subject of considerable importance and is discussed more fully below.

IV. THE ROLE OF CACHECTIN/TNF AS A MEDIATOR OF ENDOTOXICITY

The identity of cachectin and TNF immediately raised an interesting possibility. Since endotoxin was known to elicit a wide array of biological responses and since two disparate biological effects of endotoxin administration (e.g., hypertriglyceridemia and the hemorrhagic necrosis of tumors) appeared to be mediated by a single polypeptide hormone, it appeared possible that many or perhaps all of the physiologic derangements wrought by LPS might depend upon the production of this protein. This hypothesis seemed reasonable when viewed in the context of cachectin's highly catabolic character, its early production following LPS administration, and the enormous quantities expressed *in vivo*. Abe et al.[75] reported measurements suggesting that individual rabbits might produce TNF in quantities approximating milligrams per kilogram of body mass.

In an effort to determine whether cachectin/TNF was, in fact, an essential mediator of endotoxicity, mice were passively immunized against cachectin prior to challenge with LPS in various doses.[76] Such animals were shown to be rendered partially resistant to the lethal effect of LPS. In a series of related experiments, mice were injected with highly purified preparations of recombinant human cachectin, containing LPS in quantities that were not pharmacologically significant. These animals exhibited piloerection, diarrhea, weakness, anorexia, and weight loss. If sufficient quantities of cachectin were administered as a single bolus, or if mice were repeatedly challenged with sublethal quantities of the hormone, death would ensue.

In separate studies, rats were cannulated by arterial and venous routes and monitored before, during, and after infusion of active recombinant human cachectin.[77] Such animals became mildly hypotensive, mildly tachypneic, and would generally succumb to a sudden respiratory arrest. Well in advance of death, such animals were noted to be profoundly acidotic and were also shown to be markedly hemoconcentrated, suggesting that a loss of fluid from the intravascular compartment had occurred. A transient phase of hyperglycemia occurred shortly after cachectin infusion and was followed by a sharp decline in plasma glucose concentration shortly before death.

The histopathologic changes witnessed in rats following the administration of a lethal dose of cachectin were very striking. Pulmonary leukostasis was generally observed and was most likely a factor in ventillatory arrest. Acute renal tubular necrosis was also observed, together with an acute glomerulonephritis, which often led to gross hematuria. In addition, gastrointestinal ischemia was usually present and frequently led to the infarction of large portions of the digestive tract. Adrenal hemorrhage and pancreatic hemorrhage were also occasionally noted.

These changes, while in many instances more severe than lesions caused by administration of LPS alone, suggested that cachectin was indeed a major mediator of the host response to endotoxin. The mechanism by which cachectin evokes a shock state remains unclear, although several of the effects of this hormone on individual tissues (see below) may shed light upon its mode of action. It remains to be determined whether cachectin plays a direct role in eliciting these histopathologic changes or whether it acts to induce such secondary mediators as platelet activating factor and arachidonate metabolites, which in turn produce the damaging effects that are associated with cachectin administration.

V. THE STRUCTURE OF CACHECTIN/TNF AND LYMPHOTOXIN

Cachectin/TNF is synthesized as a prohormone.[40-42,44,47,49] containing a large and highly conserved amino-terminal domain that is removed in processing to yield the mature polypeptide hormone. In the mouse, the polypeptide sequence is 79 amino acids in length while in the case of human cachectin/TNF, 76 amino acids are appended. Processing involves successive steps of proteolytic cleavage, yielding a number of intermediate molecular forms that are apparent on western blot analysis of medium derived from certain macrophages and macrophage cell lines.[78] Since the propeptide is conserved to the extent of 86% on comparison of the primary structure of mouse and human forms, while the mature polypeptide hormone is conserved to the extent of 79%, it has been widely assumed that the propeptide possesses certain hormonal activities that are yet to be identified. Unlike IL-1 and certain other cytokines, the cachectin propeptide contains a well-defined hydrophobic leader sequence and the protein, once synthesized, is rapidly and efficiently exported from the cell.

In all species thus far examined, cachectin/TNF displays two cysteine residues which are known to be involved in the formation of a single disulfide bond.[25] Two regions of strict conservation have been noted in the cachectin/TNF sequence. The longest of these encompasses amino acids 115 through 130.[78] This region is highly conserved in the lymphotoxin molecule.[39] Lymphotoxin possesses but a single cysteine residue, and therefore contains no disulfide bridge; however, since it competes with cachectin/TNF for binding sites on plasma membrane surfaces,[50] it would seem certain that critical regions of the lymphotoxin molecule closely resemble homologous segments of the TNF molecule. The design of mutant cachectin/TNF molecules, devoid of toxicity to the host, yet in full possession of their ability to induce hemorrhagic necrosis of tumors, has often been discussed. To date, however, such molecules remain purely hypothetical.

VI. CONTROL OF CACHECTIN/TNF BIOSYNTHESIS

Since cachectin/TNF serves an important mediator of endotoxicity and possibly other inflammatory states as well, a detailed understanding of the molecular mechanisms responsible for its biosynthesis assumes considerable importance. Cachectin/TNF is not synthesized by quiescent macrophages and the hormone is undetectable in serum samples obtained from healthy animals; however, as noted above, cachectin/TNF is one of the major secretory products of endotoxin-activated peritoneal macrophages.[22] It may be said that cachectin/TNF secretion rises by a factor of at least 10,000 following induction of LPS.

Measurements of cachectin/TNF gene transcription[79] suggests that the cachectin/TNF mRNA is synthesized in resting macrophages, and only a threefold enhancement of transcriptional activity occurs in response to LPS. This 3-fold enhancement of transcription is associated with a roughly 100-fold increase in the cellular content of cachectin/TNF mRNA. Thus, it may be said that cachectin/TNF expression is chiefly controlled at a posttranscriptional level. In certain instances, cachectin/TNF mRNA may be expressed in considerable abundance, while the protein is not expressed or is expressed at a very low level.[79] This would suggest that certain mechanisms govern the efficiency of cachectin/TNF translation. For example, in macrophages obtained from the endotoxin-resistant C3H/HeJ mouse, exceedingly high concentrations of LPS are required to induce cachectin/TNF mRNA accumulation; however, even when large amounts of the message are expressed, very little cachectin/TNF is actually synthesized, since translation appears to be inefficient. Macrophages obtained from endotoxin-sensitive strains fail to produce cachectin/TNF in response to LPS if pretreated with dexamethasone. In this instance, the biosynthetic blockade also involves both transcriptional and translational components.

The 3'-untranslated segment of the cachectin cDNA was noted to contain a highly conserved sequence element consisting of repeating and overlapping octameric units bearing the sequence TTATTTAT.[49] This AT-exclusive sequence extends for over 30 residues, and is present in murine, rabbit, and human TNF, cDNAs, as well as in the cDNA encoding lymphotoxin, interleukin-1 (IL-1), interferon of all subclasses, GM-CSF, and certain protooncogenes of diverse species origin. Shaw and Kamen[80] showed that the GM-CSF TTATTTAT sequence confers instability upon mRNAs transcribed from globin genes into which the sequence was artificially inserted.[80] This would suggest that the TTATTTAT sequence represents a site that is recognized by a specific ribonuclease, or a site that is inherently unstable in such mRNAs. It is likely that the TTATTTAT sequence plays an important role in the control of cachectin/TNF mRNA levels, and perhaps in the control of cachectin/TNF mRNA translation.

It is also known that certain other cytokines are capable of influencing cachectin/TNF biosynthesis. For example, human peripheral blood monocytes fail to express large quantities of cachectin mRNA or protein unless they are treated with γ-interferon in addition to LPS.[81] Similarly, γ-interferon appears to augment cachectin mRNA and protein biosynthesis by macrophages obtained from C3H/HeJ mice.[82] The role played by γ-interferon *in vivo* remains to be determined, although it is widely suspected that this, or a related cytokine, may be involved in the so called "priming" phenomenon.

VII. THE EFFECT OF CACHECTIN/TNF ON SPECIFIC TISSUES AND CELL TYPES

Cachectin/TNF has now been critically assessed as a mediator of numerous inflammatory processes. In many of these studies, recombinant material was employed, eliminating the possibility that other macromolecular mediators were responsible for the effects observed. Among the tissues responsive to cachectin/TNF, one might make the following, somewhat arbitrary categorizations.

A. OTHER LEUKOCYTES
Cachectin/TNF exerts a profound effect on neutrophils, stimulating their adherence to

endothelial cell surfaces,[83,84] their degranulation,[84] and their production of H_2O_2[84] and superoxide anion.[85] Neutrophils also exhibit enhanced phagocytic activity when exposed to cachectin/TNF[84] and cachectin/TNF has been shown to exert a chemotactic effect on the cells and to augment their ability to kill certain organisms.[86]

Eosinophils are also influenced by cachectin, which enhances their ability to kill schistosomula *in vitro*.[87] Cachectin/TNF also has effects on mononuclear phagocytes, stimulating their production of IL-1[88] and enhancing their ability to kill tumor cells.[89]

B. EFFECTS ON ENDOTHELIAL CELLS

As mentioned earlier, cachectin/TNF appears to allow the egress of fluid from the intravascular compartment. Presumably this is accomplished by the alteration of capillary endothelial permeability. Cachectin/TNF has been reported to be directly cytotoxic to endothelial cells[90] and to cause endothelial cell rearrangement.[91] In addition, it has been noted to alter the normal pattern of antigenic expression by these cells;[92-94] in particular, it augments the expression MHC class I antigens, the H4/18 antigen, and possibly the ICAM-1 (intercellular adhesion molecule) antigen as well. These effects might contribute to a change in cell-cell adhesion and may be related to an increase in permeability.

Cachectin also appears to down-regulate the expression of thrombomodulin by endothelial cells[95] and to prompt the production of a procoagulant activity[95,96] by endothelial cells. Both of these latter effects would be expected to favor hemostasis and may account in some measure for the coagulopathy that frequently accompanies Gram negative sepsis. Moreover, cachectin/TNF induces endothelial cell production of Il-1, which may also elicit many of these effects.[97,98]

Independent of a direct effect on neutrophils, cachectin/TNF has been shown to modify endothelium so as to promote neutrophil adhesion.[83,99] This effect appears to be dependent upon protein synthesis, whereas the aforementioned action of TNF on neutrophils is not.

C. EFFECTS ON FIBROBLASTS, BONE, AND CARTILAGE

Cachectin/TNF appears to have growth-stimulatory effects on certain fibroblastoid lines, while it is overtly cytotoxic to others. Cachectin/TNF influences the expression of certain antigens by fibroblast, including MHC class I antigens.[93] In addition, it seems to prompt the biosynthesis of other proteins, the function of which remains to be identified.[100] Cachectin/TNF also prompts the production of collagenase and prostaglandin E_2 (PGE_2) by primary cultures of human fibroblasts,[101] suggesting that it may play a role in local inflammatory processes or in tissue remolding. Synovial cells similarly respond to cachectin by producing increased quantities of collagenase and PGE_2. This effect of cachectin/TNF, formerly attributed exclusively to IL-1 may also reflect an important role of the hormone in chronic inflammatory disease states.

Cachectin/TNF exhibits osteoclast activating factor (OAF) activity, prompting the release of calcium from bone *in vitro*.[102] It also appears to play a role in the degradation of proteoglycan.[103] These effects, like those on synovial cells, may implicate this hormone as a mediator of destructive processes involving bone and cartilage.

D. EFFECT ON HEMATOPOIETIC PROGENITOR CELLS

Cachectin/TNF is known to induce the production of granulocyte/macrophage colony stimulating factor (GM-CSF) by a number of target cell types.[104] However, in *in vitro* assays, cachectin/TNF appears to suppress the development of myeloid colonies.[105,106] It also seems to suppress erythroid progenitor cells,[106-108] although in both instances, it remains to be seen whether the hormone acts directly or through elicitation of a secondary mediator produced by stromal elements of the marrow. The net effect of cachectin/TNF on hematopoiesis *in vivo* also remains unclear; however, preliminary evidence suggests that the hormone leads to an anemic state in which reticulocytosis is suppressed.[119]

E. EFFECTS ON ADIPOSE TISSUE

Cachectin's marked suppressive effect on adipocyte expression of LPL has already been discussed. The hormone also appears to stimulate glycerol release from adipocytes in culture,[20,109] suggesting that it activates the hormone-sensitive lipase. Cachectin/TNF acts to suppress a whole class of mRNA molecules that are specifically expressed by mature adipocytes, but not by their indifferent precursors.[110] Among these mRNA molecules, those encoding glycerolphosphate dehydrogenase and the fatty acid binding protein and adipsin,[111] a proteolytic enzyme produced by mature adipocytes, have been identified, while other mRNA species encode unknown proteins. Suppression of mRNA expression appears to reflect suppression of transcription;[110] however, as with all of the other bioactivities exhibited by cachectin, the mechanism of signal transduction is entirely unclear.

VIII. THE EFFECT OF CACHECTIN/TNF ON TUMORS *IN VIVO* AND ON TUMOR CELL LINES *IN VITRO*

Cachectin/TNF acts to cause hemorrhagic necrosis of certain transplantable tumors in animal models. This effect is chiefly restricted to tumors that are implanted within the dermis or subcutaneous tissue. Visceral implants or metastatic lesions are less susceptible to destruction by TNF. As noted by Algire et al.,[112] hemorrhagic necrosis occurs through a vascular mechanism. It is likely that both neutrophil adhesion and a coagulative process lead to the selective occlusion of tumor vessels. The basis of this selectivity remains obscure; however, it is quite clear that cachectin/TNF is capable, at high doses, of injuring normal tissues in a manner that closely resembles the injury inflicted upon the tumor mass. Moreover, many tumors that are highly susceptible to hemorrhagic necrosis *in vivo* seem to display little sensitivity to the effects of cachectin/TNF when grown *in vitro*. Thus, the mechanism of cytolysis *in vitro* is likely to be entirely different than the mechanism of hemorrhagic necrosis.

Approximately 30% of transformed cell lines studied appear sensitive to the cytotoxic effect of cachectin/TNF *in vitro*.[133] The mechanism of action of cachectin/TNF has not been established. Interestingly, the cytotoxic effect of cachectin/TNF is greatly potentiated in cells treated with inhibitors of protein or mRNA synthesis.[114] Even nontumorigenic cell lines, which are normally insensitive to the action of cachectin/TNF, can be lysed by the hormone if incubated in the presence of actinomycin D or cycloheximide. This has been taken to suggest that normal cells are endowed with a protective mechanism requiring protein synthesis that allows them to escape lysis.[100,114] Certain tumor cells, on the other hand, may have lost this adaptive mechanism.

IX. THE CACHECTIN/TNF RECEPTOR AND POSTRECEPTOR RESPONSE

Little is known at present concerning the structure of the cachectin/TNF receptor. As indicated above, the receptor has an affinity constant for cachectin/TNF of approximately $3 \times 10^9 \ M^{-1}$. The number of receptors varies considerably depending upon the cell line studied; however, the receptor seems to be present on cells derived from most tissues. Cross-linking studies suggest that the binding subunit of the receptor has a size of approximately 75 kDa.[115-117] Since cachectin/TNF molecules derived from diverse species may compete equally well for binding sites derived from a single species, yet exhibit different specific activity in terms of cytolytic potential,[118] it would appear that receptor occupancy is not the sole determinant of biological effect; e.g., bioactivity may depend upon structural aspects of the cachectin/TNF molecule that are distinct from that portion of the molecule involved in interaction with the receptor. The signal transduced following binding remains entirely unclear.

X. THE BIOLOGICAL ROLE OF CACHECTIN/TNF AND LYMPHOTOXIN

During the past 2 years, a consensus has emerged that cachectin/TNF evolved neither as a "cachectin" per se, nor as an immunosurveillance mechanism designed to eliminate incipient neoplastic disease, but as a general mediator of inflammatory processes. Since cachectin/TNF represents an important component of the inflammatory response, it is likely that its beneficial effects are a subset of those of the inflammatory response as a whole.

Lymphotoxin, which was originally identified as a possible participant in delayed-type hypersensitivity, is particularly interesting in this regard. Since lymphotoxin is elicited in response to specific antigenic stimuli and is not produced by T cells derived from antigen-naive individuals, it may be imagined that this cytokine plays an important role under pathologic circumstances in which chronic or cyclical exposure to an invasive agent is manifested. By contrast, cachectin/TNF production does not seem to require prior exposure to a specific antigen. On the contrary, biosynthesis and release of this cytokine are augmented by exposure to nonspecific "priming" agents, including a variety of facultative intracellular bacteria. The usual circumstances under which cachectin/TNF is produced *in vivo*, and those circumstances in which it plays a beneficial role, are therefore more difficult to imagine. It is possible that this cytokine is called forth to deal with acute, serious infections, whose rapid course does not allow the development of a conventional immune response.

In the years to come, the biochemical mechanisms by which the cytokines exert their varied and important effects will doubtless be explored in great detail. It is to be anticipated that the knowledge gained from these studies may prove useful in our efforts to exploit the inflammatory response for its benefits and to interrupt the inflammatory response for fear of its attendant injuries.

REFERENCES

1. **Filkins, J. P.**, Monokines and the metabolic pathophysiology of septic shock, *Fed. Proc.*, 44, 300, 1985.
2. **Beisel, W. R.**, Metabolic response to infection, *Annu. Rev. Med.*, 26, 9, 1975.
3. **Feldmann, M.**, Lymphokines and interleukins emerge from the primeval soup, *Nature*, 313, 351, 1985.
4. **Franke, F. E.**, Action of toxic doses of the polysaccharide from *Serratia marcescens (Bacillus prodigiosus)* on the dog and guinea pig, *JNCI*, 5, 185, 1944.
5. **Morgan, H. R.**, Pathologic changes produced in rabbits by a toxic somatic antigen derived from *Eberthella typhosa*, *Am. J. Pathol.*, 19, 135, 1942.
6. **Brunson, J. G., Gamble, C. N., and Thomas, L.**, Morphologic changes in rabbits following the intravenous administration of meningicoccal toxin. I. The effects produced in young and in mature animals by a single injection, *Am. J. Pathol.*, 31, 489, 1955.
7. **Berry, L. J., Smythe, D. S., and Young, L. G.**, Effects of bacterial endotoxin on metabolism. I. Carbohydrate depletion and the protective role of cortisone, *J. Exp. Med.*, 110, 389, 1959.
8. **Gilbert, R. P.**, Mechanisms of the hemodynamic effects of endotoxin, *Physiol. Rev.*, 40, 245, 1960.
9. **Maclean, L. D., Mulligan, W. G., McLean, A. P. H., and Duff, J. H.**, Patterns of septic shock in man—a detailed study of 56 patients, *Ann. Surg.*, 166, 543, 1967.
10. **Shwartzman, G.**, Reactivity of malignant neoplasms to bacterial filtrates. I. The effect of spontaneous and induced infections on the growth of mouse sarcoma 180, *Arch. Pathol.*, 21, 284, 1936.
11. **Nishijima, H., Weil, M. H., Shubin, H., and Cavanilles, J.**, Hemodynamic and metabolic studies on shock associated with Gram negative bacteremia, *Medicine*, 52, 287, 1973.
12. **Elin, R. J. and Wolff, S. M.**, Biology of endotoxin, *Annu. Rev. Med.*, 27, 127, 1976.
13. **Fry, D. E., Pearlstein, L., Fulton, R. L., and Polk, H. C., Jr.**, Multiple system organ failure, *Arch. Surg.*, 115, 136, 1980.
14. **Sugarman, H. J., Peyton, J. W. R., and Greenfield, L. J.**, Gram-negative sepsis, *Current Problems in Surgery*, Ravitch, M. M., Year Book Medical Publishers, Chicago, 1981, 408.

15. **Michalek, S. M., Moore, R. N., McGhee, J. R., Rosenstreich, D. L., and Mergenhagen, S. E.,** The primary role of lymphoreticular cells in the mediation of host responses to bacterial endotoxin, *J. Infect. Dis.,* 141, 55, 1980.

16. **Rouzer, C. A. and Cerami, A.,** Hypertriglyceridemia associated with *Trypanosoma brucei brucei* infection in rabbits: role of defective triglyceride removal, *Mol. Biochem. Parasitol.,* 2, 31, 1980.

17. **Guy, M. W.,** Serum and tissue fluid lipids in rabbits experimentally infected with *Trypanosoma brucei, Trans. R. Soc. Trop. Med. Hyg.,* 69, 429, 1975.

18. **Kawakami, M. and Cerami, A.,** Studies of endotoxin-induced decrease in lipoprotein lipase activity, *J. Exp. Med.,* 154, 631, 1981.

19. **Kawakami, M., Pekala, P. H., Lane, M. D., and Cerami, A.,** Lipoprotein lipase suppression in 3T3-L1 cells by an endotoxin-induced mediator from exudate cells, *Proc. Natl. Acad. Sci. U.S.A.,* 79, 912, 1982.

20. **Pekala, P. H., Price, S. R., Horn, C. A., Hom, B. E., Moss, J., and Cerami, A.,** Model for cachexia in chronic disease: secretory products of endotoxin-stimulated macrophages induce a catabolic state in 3T3-L1 adipocytes, *Trans. Assoc. Am. Phys.,* 97, 251, 1984.

21. **Pekala, P. H., Kawakami, M., Angus, C. W., Lane, M. D, and Cerami, A.,** Selective inhibition of synthesis of enzymes for *de novo* fatty acid biosynthesis by an endotoxin-induced mediator from exudate cells, *Proc. Natl. Acad. Sci. U.S.A.,* 80, 2743, 1983.

22. **Beutler, B., Mahoney, J., Le Trang, N., Pekala, P., and Cerami, A.,** Purification of cachectin, a lipoprotein lipase-suppressing hormone secreted by endotoxin-induced RAW 264.7 cells, *J. Exp. Med.,* 161, 984, 1985.

23. **Beutler, B., Milsark, I. W., and Cerami, A.,** Cachectin/tumor necrosis factor: production, distribution, and metabolic fate *in vivo, J. Immunol.,* 135, 3972, 1985.

24. **Beutler, B., Greenwald, D., Hulmes, J. D., Chang, M., Pan, Y.-C.E., Mathison, J., Ulevitch, R., and Cerami, A.,** Identity of tumour necrosis factor and the macrophage-secreted factor cachectin, *Nature,* 316, 552, 1985.

25. **Aggarwal, B. B., Kohr, W. J., Hass, P. E., Moffat, B., Spencer, S. A., Henzel, W. J., Bringman, T. S., Nedwin, G. E., Goeddel, D. V., and Harkins, R. N.,** Human tumor necrosis factor. Production, purification, and characterization, *J. Biol. Chem.,* 260, 2345, 1985.

26. **Coley, W. B.,** The treatment of malignant tumors by repeated inoculations of erysipelas; with a report of ten original cases, *Am. J. Med., Sci.,* 105, 487, 1893.

27. **Coley, W. B.,** Treatment of inoperable malignant tumors with toxins of erysipelas and the *Bacillus prodigiosus, Trans. Am. Surg. Assoc.,* 12, 183, 1894.

28. **Coley, W. B.,** The therapeutic value of the mixed toxins of the streptococcus of erysipelas in the treatment of inoperable malignant tumors, with a report of 100 cases, *Am. J. Med. Sci.,* 112, 251, 1896.

29. **Coley, W. B.,** Further observations upon the treatment of malignant tumors with the mixed toxins of erysipelas and *Bacillus prodigiosus* with a report of 160 cases, *Bull. Johns Hopkins Hosp.,* 65, 157, 1896.

30. **Coley, W. B.,** Late results of the treatment of inoperable sarcoma by the mixed toxins of erysipelas and *Bacillus prodigiosus, Am. J. Med. Sci.,* 131, 375, 1906.

31. **Shear, M. J. and Andervont, H. B.,** Chemical treatment of tumors. III. Separation of hemorrhage-producing fraction of *E. coli* filtrate, *Proc. Soc. Exp. Biol. Med.,* 34, 323, 1936.

32. **Shear, M. J., Perrault, A., and Adams, J. R., Jr.,** Chemical treatment of tumors. VI. Method employed in determining the potency of hemorrhage-producing bacterial preparations, *JNCI,* 4, 99, 1943.

33. **Shear, M. J., Turner, F. C., Perrault, A., and Shovelton, J.,** Chemical treatment of tumors. V. Isolation of the hemorrhage-producing fraction from *Serratia marcescens (Bacillus prodigiosus)* culture filtrate, *JNCI,* 4, 81, 1943.

34. **Kahler, H., Shear, M. J., and Hartwell, J. L.,** Chemical treatment of tumors. VIII. Ultracentrifugal and electrophoretic analysis of the hemorrhage-producing fraction from *Serratia marcescens (Bacillus prodigiosus)* culture filtrate, *JNCI,* 4, 123, 1943.

35. **Hartwell, J. L., Shear, M. J., and Adams, J. R., Jr.,** Chemical treatment of tumors. VII. Nature of the hemorrhage-producing fraction from *Serratia marcescens (Bacillus prodigiosus)* culture filtrate, *JNCI,* 4, 107, 1943.

36. **Shear, M. J.,** Chemical treatment of tumors. IX. Reactions of mice with primary subcutaneous tumors to injection of hemorrhage-producing bacterial polysaccharide, *JNCI,* 4, 461, 1944.

37. **O'Malley, W. E., Achinstein, B., and Shear, M. J.,** Action of bacterial polysaccharide on tumors. II. Damage of sarcoma 37 by serum of mice treated with *Serratia marcescens* polysaccharide, and induced tolerance, *JNCI,* 29, 1169, 1962.

38. **Carswell, E. A., Old, L. J., Kassel, R. L., Green, S., Fiore, N., and Williamson, B.,** An endotoxin-induced serum factor that causes necrosis of tumors, *Proc. Natl. Acad. Sci. U.S.A.,* 72, 3666, 1975.

39. **Aggarwal, B. B., Henzel, W. J., Moffat, B., Kohr, W. J., and Harkins, R. N.,** Primary structure of human lymphotoxin derived from 1788 lymphoblastoid cell line, *J. Biol. Chem.,* 260, 2334, 1985.

40. **Pennica, D., Nedwin, G. E., Hayflick, J. S., Seeburg, P. H., Derynck, R., Palladino, M. A., Kohr, W. J., Aggarwal, B. B., and Goeddel, D. V.**, Human tumor necrosis factor: precursor structure, expression and homology to lymphotoxin, *Nature*, 312, 724, 1984.

41. **Wang, A. M., Creasy, A. A., Ladner, M. B., Lin, L. S., Strickler, J., Van Arsdell, J. N., Yamamoto, R., and Mark, D. F.**, Molecular cloning of the complementary DNA for human tumor necrosis factor, *Science*, 228, 149, 1985.

42. **Shirai, T., Yamaguchi, H., Ito, H., Todd, C. W., and Wallace, R. B.**, Cloning and expression in *Escherichia coli* of the gene for human tumour necrosis factor, *Nature*, 313, 803, 1985.

43. **Pennica, D., Hayflick, J. S., Bringman, T. S., Palladino, M. A., and Goeddel, D. V.**, Cloning and expression in *Escherichia coli* of the cDNA for murine tumor necrosis factor, *Proc. Natl. Acad. Sci. U.S.A.*, 82, 6060, 1985.

44. **Fransen, L., Muller, R., Marmenout, A., Tavernier, J., Van der Heyden, J., Kawashima, E., Chollet, A., Tizard, R., Van Heuverswyn, H., Van Vliet, A., Ruysschaert, M.-R., and Fiers, W.**, Molecular cloning of mouse tumour necrosis factor cDNA and its eukaryotic expression, *Nucl. Acids Res.*, 13, 4417, 1985.

45. **Zilberstein, A., Ruggieri, T., Korn, J. H., and Revel, M.**, Structure and expression of cDNA and genes for human interferon-beta-2, a distinct species inducible by growth-stimulatory cytokines, *EMBO J.*, 5, 2529, 1986.

46. **Nedospasov, S. A., Hirt, B., Shakhov, A. N., Dobrynin, V. N., Kawashima, E., Accolla, R. S., and Jongeneel, C. V.**, The genes for tumor necrosis factor (TNF-alpha) and lymphotoxin (TNF-beta) are tandemly arranged on chromosome 17 of the mouse, *Nucl. Acids Res.*, 14, 7713, 1986.

47. **Ito, H., Yamamoto, S., Kuroda, S., Sakamoto, H., Kajihara, J., Kiyota, T., Hayashi, H., Kato, M., and Seko, M.**, Molecular cloning and expression in *Escherichia coli* of the cDNA coding for rabbit tumor necrosis factor, *DNA*, 5, 149, 1986.

48. **Ito, H., Shirai, T., Yamamoto, S., Akira, M., Kawahara, S., Todd, C. W., and Wallace, R. B.**, Molecular cloning of the gene encoding rabbit tumor necrosis factor, *DNA*, 5, 157, 1986.

49. **Caput, D., Beutler, B., Hartog, K., Brown-Shimer, S., and Cerami, A.**, Indentification of a common nucleotide sequence in the 3′-untranslated region of mRNA molecules specifying inflammatory mediators, *Proc. Natl. Acad. Sci. U.S.A.*, 83, 1670, 1986.

50. **Aggarwal, B. B., Eessalu, T. E., and Hass, P. E.**, Characterization of receptors for human tumour necrosis factor and their regulation by gamma-interferon, *Nature*, 318, 665, 1985.

51. **Ruddle, N. H., Powell, M. B., and Conta, B. S.**, Lymphotoxin, a biologically relevant model lymphokine, *Lymphokine Res.*, 2, 23, 1983.

52. **Conta, B. S., Powell, M. B., and Ruddle, N. H.**, Production of lymphotoxin, IFN-gamma, and IFN-alpha, beta by murine T cell lines and clones, *J. Immunol.*, 130, 2231, 1983.

53. **Mannel, D. N., Moore, R. N., and Mergenhagen, S. E.**, Macrophages as a source of tumoricidal activity (tumor-necrotizing factor), *Infect. Immunol.*, 30, 523, 1980.

54. **Satomi, N., Haranaka, K., and Kunii, O.**, Research on the production site of tumor necrosis factor (TNF), *Jpn. J. Exp. Med.*, 51, 317, 1981.

55. **Matthews, N.**, Tumour-necrosis factor from the rabbit. V. Synthesis *in vitro* by mononuclear phagocytes from various tissues of normal and BCG-injected rabbits, *Br. J. Cancer*, 44, 418, 1981.

56. **Fisch, H. and Gifford, G. E.**, *In vitro* production of rabbit macrophage tumor cell cytoxin, *Int. J. Cancer*, 32, 105, 1983.

57. **Watanabe, N., Sone, H., Neda, H., Niitsu, Y., and Urushizaki, I.**, Mechanisms of production of tumor necrosis factor (TNF): reconstitution experiment with nude mice, *Gan To Kagaku Ryoho*, 11, 1284, 1984.

58. **Takeda, Y., Higuchi, M., Sugimoto, M., Shimoda, O., Jong Woo, H., Shimada, S., and Osawa, T.**, The production of a cytotoxic factor by mouse peritoneal macrophages and macrophage hybridomas treated with various stimulating agents, *Microbiol. Immunol.*, 30, 143, 1986.

59. **Kawakami, M., Ikeda, Y., Le Trang, N., Vine, W., and Cerami, A.**, Studies of conditions and agents that stimulate and inhibit the production of cachectin by macrophages, in *Proceedings of the IUPHAR*, Patton, W., Ed., Macmillan, New York, 1984, 377.

60. **Ruddle, N. H. and Waksman, B. H.**, Cytotoxic effect of lymphocyte-antigen interaction in delayed hypersensitivity, *Science*, 157, 1060, 1967.

61. **Ruddle, N. H. and Waksman, B. H.**, Cytotoxicity mediated by soluble antigen and lymphocytes in delayed hypersensitivity. I. Characterization of the phenomenon, *J. Exp. Med.*, 128, 1237, 1968.

62. **Ruddle, N. H. and Waksman, B. H.**, Cytotoxicity mediated by soluble antigen and lymphocytes in delayed hypersensitivity. II. Correlation of the *in vitro* response with skin reactivity, *J. Exp. Med.*, 128, 1255, 1968.

63. **Ruddle, N. H. and Waksman, B. H.**, Cytotoxicity mediated of soluble antigen and lymphocytes in delayed hypersensitivity. III. Analysis of mechanism, *J. Exp. Med.*, 128, 1267, 1968.

64. **Granger, G. A. and Williams, T. W.**, Lymphocyte cytotoxicity *in vitro*: activation and release of a cytotoxic factor, *Nature*, 218, 1253, 1968.

65. **Ruddle, N. H.,** Delayed hypersensitivity to soluble antigens in mice. II. Analysis *in vitro, Int. Arch. Allerg. Appl. Immunol.,* 58, 44, 1979.

66. **Ruddle, N. H.,** Delayed hypersensitivity to soluble antigens in mice, *Int. Arch. Allergy Appl. Immunol.,* 58, 44, 1979.

67. **Beutler, B., Krochin, N., Milsark, I. W., Goldberg, A., and Cerami, A.,** Induction of cachetin (tumor necrosis factor) synthesis by influenza virus: deficient production by endotoxin-resistant (C3H/HeJ) macrophages, *Clin. Res.,* 34, 491a, 1986.

68. **Aderka, D., Holtmann, H., Toker, L., Hahn, T., and Wallach, D.,** Tumor necrosis factor induction by Sendai virus, *J. Immunol.,* 136, 2938, 1986.

69. **Berent, S. L., Torczynski, R. M., and Bollon, A. P.,** Sendai virus induces high levels of tumor necrosis factor mRNA in human peripheral blood leukocytes, *Nucl. Acids Res.,* 14, 8997, 1986.

70. **Green S., Dobrjansky, A., Chiasson, M. A., Carswell, E., Schwartz, M. K., and Old, L. J.,** Corynebacterium parvum as the priming agent in the production of tumor necrosis factor in the mouse, *JNCI,* 59, 1519, 1977.

71. **Ha, D. K., Gardner, I. D., and Lawton, J. W.,** Characterization of macrophage function in *Mycobacterium lepraemurium*-infected mice: sensitivity of mice to endotoxin and release of mediators and lysosomal enzymes after endotoxin treatment, *Parasite Immunol.,* 5, 513, 1983.

72. **Wood, P. R. and Clark, I. A.,** Macrophages from *Babesia* and malaria infected mice are primed for monokine release, *Parasite Immunol.,* 6, 309, 1984.

73. **Urushizaki, I., Niitsu, Y., and Watanabe, N.,** Definition of tumor-necrosis factor and its production mechanism, *Gan To Kagaku Ryoho,* 11, 1356, 1984.

74. **Haranaka, K., Satomi, N., Sakurai, A., and Haranaka, R.,** Role of first stimulating agents in the production of tumor necrosis factor, *Cancer Immunol. Immunother.,* 18, 87, 1984.

75. **Abe, S., Gatanaga, T., Yamazaki, M., Soma, G., and Mizuno, D.,** Purification of rabbit tumor necrosis factor, *FEBS Lett.,* 180, 203, 1985.

76. **Beutler, B., Milsark, I. W., and Cerami, A.,** Passive immunization against cachectin/tumor necrosis factor (TNF) protects mice from the lethal effect of endotoxin, *Science,* 229, 869, 1985.

77. **Tracey, K. J., Beutler, B., Lowry, S. F., Merryweather, J., Wolpe, S., Milsark, I. W., Hariri, R. J., Fahey, T. J., III., Zentella, A., Albert, J. D., Shires, G. T., and Cerami, A.,** Shock and tissue injury induced by recombinant human cachectin, *Science,* 234, 470, 1986.

78. **Beutler, B. and Cerami, A.,** Cachectin and tumor necrosis factor as two sides of the same biological coin, *Nature,* 320, 584, 1986.

79. **Beutler, B., Krochin, N., Milsark, I. W., Luedke, C., and Cerami, A.,** Control of cachectin (tumor necrosis factor) synthesis: mechanisms of endotoxin resistance, *Science,* 232, 977, 1986.

80. **Shaw, G. and Kamen, R.,** A conserved AU sequence from the 3' untranslated region of GM-CSF mRNA mediates selective mRNA degradation, *Cell,* 46, 659, 1986.

81. **Nedwin, G. E., Svedersky, L. P., Bringman, T. S., Palladino, M. A., and Goeddel, D. V.,** Effect of interleukin 2, interferon-gamma, and mitogens on the production of tumor necrosis factors alpha and beta, *J. Immunol.,* 135, 2492, 1985.

82. **Beutler, B., Tkacenko, V., Milsark, I. W., Krochin, N., and Cerami, A.,** The effect of interferon-gamma on cachectin expression by mononuclear phagocytes: reversal of the lps-d (endotoxin resistance) phenotype, *J. Exp. Med.,* 164, 1791, 1986.

83. **Gamble, J. R., Harlan, J. M., Klebanoff, S. J., Lopez, A. F., and Vadas, M. A.,** Stimulation of the adherence of neutrophils to umbilical vein endothelium by human recombinant tumor necrosis factor, *Proc. Natl. Acad. Sci. U.S.A.,* 82, 8667, 1985.

84. **Klebanoff, S. J., Vadas, M. A., Harlan, J. M., Sparks, L. H., Gamble, J. R., Agosti, J. M., and Waltersdorph, A. M.,** Stimulation of neutrophils by tumor necrosis factor, *J. Immunol.,* 136, 4220, 1986.

85. **Tsujimoto, M., Yokota, S., Vilcek, J., and Weissman, G.,** Tumor necrosis factor provokes superoxide anion generation from neutrophils, *Biochem. Biophys. Res. Commun.,* 137, 1094, 1986.

86. **Djeu, J. Y., Blanchard, D. K., Halkias, D., and Friedman, H.,** Growth inhibition of *Candida albicans* by human polymorphonuclear neutrophils: activation by interferon-gamma and tumor necrosis factor, *J. Immunol.,* 137, 2980, 1986.

87. **Silberstein, D. S. and David, J. R.,** Tumor necrosis factor enhances eosinophil toxicity to *Schistosoma mansoni* larvae, *Proc. Natl. Acad. Sci. U.S.A.,* 83, 1055, 1986.

88. **Bachwich, P. R., Chensue, S. W., Larrick, J. W., and Kunkel, S. L.,** Tumor necrosis factor stimulates interleukin-1 and prostaglandin E2 production in resting macrophages, *Biochem. Biophys. Res. Commun.,* 136, 94, 1986.

89. **Philip, R. and Epstein, L. B.,** Tumour necrosis factor as immunomodulator and mediator of monocyte cytotoxicity induced by itself, gamma-interferon and interleukin-1, *Nature,* 323, 86, 1986.

90. **Sato, N., Goto, T., Haranaka, K., Satomi, N., Nariuchi, H., and Mano Hirano, Y.,** Actions of tumor necrosis factor on cultured vascular endothelial cells: morphologic modulation, growth inhibition, and cytotoxicity, *JNCI,* 76, 1113, 1986.

91. **Stolpen, A. H., Guinan, E. C., Fiers, W., and Pober, J. S.,** Recombinant tumor necrosis factor and immune interferon acts singly and in combination to reorganize human vascular endothelial cell monolayers, *Am. J. Pathol.,* 123, 16, 1986.

92. **Pober, J. S., Bevilacqua, M. P., Mendrick, D. L., Lapierre, L. A., Fiers, W., and Gimbrone, M. A., Jr.,** Two distinct monokines, interleukin 1 and tumor necrosis factor, each independently induce biosynthesis and transient expression of the same antigen on the surface of cultured human vascular endothelial cells, *J. Immunol.,* 136, 1680, 1986.

93. **Collins, T., Lapierre, L. A., Fiers, W., Strominger, J. L., and Pober, J. S.,** Recombinant human tumor necrosis factor increases mRNA levels and surface expression of HLA-A,B antigens in vascular endothelial cells and dermal fibroblasts *in vitro, Proc. Natl. Acad. Sci. U.S.A.,* 83, 446, 1986.

94. **Pober, J. S., Gimbrone, M. A., Jr., Lapierre, L. A., Mendrick, D. L., Fiers, W., Rothlein, R., and Springer, T. A.,** Overlapping patterns of activation of human endothelial cells by interleukin 1, tumor necrosis factor, and immune interferon, *J. Immunol.,* 137, 1893, 1986.

95. **Stern, D. M. and Nawroth, P. P.,** Modulation of endothelial hemostatic properties by tumor necrosis factor, *J. Exp. Med.,* 163, 740, 1986.

96. **Bevilacqua, M. P., Pober, J. S., Majeau, G. R., Fiers, W., Cotran, R. S., and Gimbrone, M. A., Jr.,** Recombinant tumor necrosis factor induces procoagulant activity in cultured human vascular endothelium: characterization and comparison with the actions of interleukin 1, *Proc. Natl. Acad. Sci. U.S.A.,* 83, 4533, 1986.

97. **Nawroth, P., Bank, I., Handley, D., Cassimeris, J., Chess, L., and Stern, D.,** Tumor necrosis factor/cachectin interacts with endothelial cell receptors to induce release of interleukin 1, *J. Exp. Med.,* 163, 1363, 1986.

98. **Libby, P., Ordovas, J. M., Auger, K. R., Robbins, A. H., Birinyi, L. K., and Dinarello, C. A.,** Endotoxin and tumor necrosis factor induce interleukin-1 gene expression in adult human vascular endothelial cells, *Am. J. Pathol.,* 124, 179, 1986.

99. **Pohlman, T. H., Stanness, K. A., Beatty, P. G., Ochs, H. D., and Harlan, J. M.,** An endothelial cell surface factor(s) induced *in vitro* by lipopolysaccharide, interleukin 1, and tumor necrosis factor-alpha increases neutrophil adherence by a CDw18-dependent mechanism, *J. Immunol.,* 136, 4548, 1986.

100. **Kirstein, M. and Baglioni, C.,** Tumor necrosis factor induces synthesis of two proteins in human fibroblasts, *J. Biol. Chem.,* 261, 9565, 1986.

101. **Dayer, J.-M, Beutler, B., and Cerami, A.,** Cachectin/tumor necrosis factor (TNF) stimulates collagenase and PGE2 production by human synovial cells and dermal fibroblasts, *J. Exp. Med.,* 162, 2163, 1985.

102. **Bertolini, D. R., Nedwin, G., Bringman, T., Smith, D., and Mundy, G. R.,** Stimulation of bone resorption and inhibition of bone formation *in vitro* by human tumour necrosis factor, *Nature,* 319, 516, 1986.

103. **Saklatvala, J.,** Tumour necrosis factor alpha stimulates resorption and inhibits synthesis of proteoglycan in cartilage, *Nature,* 322, 547, 1986.

104. **Munker, R., Gasson, J., Ogawa, M., and Koeffler, H. P.,** Recombinant human TNF induces production of granulocyte-monocyte colony-stimulating factor, *Nature,* 323, 79, 1986.

105. **Murphy, M., Loudon, R., Kobayashi, M., and Trinchieri, G.,** Gamma interferon and lymphotoxin, released by activated T cells, synergize to inhibit granulocyte/monocyte colony formation, *J. Exp. Med.,* 164, 263, 1986.

106. **Broxmeyer, H. E., Williams, D. E., Lu, L., Cooper, S., Anderson, S. L., Beyer, G. S., Hoffman, R., and Rubin, B. Y.,** The suppressive influences of human tumor necrosis factors on bone marrow hematopoietic progenitor cells from normal donors and patients with leukemia: synergism of tumor necrosis factor and interferon-gamma, *J. Immunol.,* 136, 4487, 1986.

107. **Lu, L., Welte, K., Gabrilove, J. L., Hangoc, G., Bruno, E., and Hoffman, R.,** Effects of recombinant human tumor necrosis factor alpha, recombinant human gamma-interferon and prostaglandin E on colony formation of human hematopoietic progenitor cells stimulated by natural human pluripotent colony-stimulating factor, pluripoietin alpha, and recombinant erythropoietin in serum-free cultures, *Cancer Res.,* 46, 4357, 1986.

108. **Degliantoni, G., Murphy, M., Kobayashi, M., Francis, M. K., Perussia, B., and Trinchieri, G.,** Natural killer (NK) cell-derived hematopoietic colony-inhibiting activity and NK cytotoxic factor. Relationship with tumor necrosis factor and synergism with immune interferon, *J. Exp. Med.,* 162, 1512, 1985.

109. **Patton, J. S., Shepard, H. M., Wilking, H., Lewis, G., Aggarwal, B. B., Eessalu, T. E., Gavin, L. A., and Grunfeld, C.,** Interferons and tumor necrosis factors have similar catabolic effects on 3T3 L1 cells, *Proc. Natl. Acad. Sci. U.S.A.,* 83, 8313, 1986.

110. **Torti, F. M., Dieckmann, B., Beutler, B., Cerami, A., and Ringold, G. M.,** A macrophage factor inhibits adipocyte gene expression: an *in vitro* model of cachexia, *Science,* 229, 867, 1985.

111. **Min, H. Y. and Spiegelman, B. M.,** Adipsin, the adipocyte serine protease: gene structure and control of expression by tumor necrosis factor, *Nucl. Acids Res.,* 14, 8879, 1986.

112. **Algire, G. H., Legallais, F. Y., and Anderson, B. F.,** Vascular reactions of normal and malignant tissues *in vivo.* V. The role of hypotension on the action of a bacterial polysaccaride on tumors, *JNCI,* 12, 1279, 1952.

113. **Sugarman, B. J., Aggarwal, B. B., Hass, P. E., Figari, I. S., Palladino, M. A., Jr., and Shepard, H. M.,** Recombinant human tumor necrosis factor-alpha: effects on proliferation of normal and transformed cells, *in vitro, Science,* 230, 943, 1985.

114. **Kirstein, M., Fiers, W., and Baglioni, C.,** Growth inhibition and cytotoxicity of tumor necrosis factor in L929 cells is enhanced by high cell density and inhibition of mRNA synthesis, *J. Immunol.,* 137, 2277, 1986.

115. **Scheurich, P., Ucer, U., Kronke, M., and Pfizenmaier, K.,** Quantification and characterization of high-affinity membrane receptors for tumor necrosis factor on human leukemic cell lines, *Int. J. Cancer,* 38, 127, 1986.

116. **Israel, S., Hahn, T., Holtmann, H., and Wallach, D.,** Binding of human TNF-alpha to high-affinity cell surface receptors: effect of IFN, *Immunol. Lett.,* 12, 217, 1986.

117. **Kull, F. C., Jr., Jacobs, S., and Cuatrecasas, P.,** Cellular receptor for ^{125}I-labeled tumor necrosis factor: specific binding, affinity labeling, and relationship to sensitivity, *Proc. Natl. Acad. Sci. U.S.A.,* 82, 5756, 1985.

118. **Smith, R. A., Kirstein, M., Fiers, W., and Baglioni, C.,** Species specificity of human and murine tumor necrosis factor, *J. Biol. Chem.,* 261, 14871, 1986.

119. **Tracey, K., et al.,** unpublished data.

Chapter 11

PRODUCTION OF HEMOPOIETIC COLONY STIMULATING FACTORS BY MURINE T LYMPHOCYTES

Anne Kelso, Nicholas M. Gough, and Donald Metcalf

TABLE OF CONTENTS

I. INTRODUCTION

Multipotential stem cells in fetal liver and adult bone marrow can give rise to all the mature cells of the blood, including erythrocytes, neutrophilic granulocytes, monocytes, eosinophils, megakaryocytes, mast cells, and lymphocytes. The ability of the hemopoietic system both to maintain the supply of mature cells throughout life and to respond to stress by amplifying numbers of a given cell type, suggests that mechanisms must exist to regulate the proliferation and differentiation of cells in each lineage. *In vivo,* hemopoiesis is thought to be controlled by interactions with cells and short-range mediators in the microenvironment and by circulating long-range mediators. *In vitro,* the production and activity of all the nonlymphoid hemopoietic cells can be stimulated by a group of glycoprotein hormones, or colony stimulating factors (CSFs), with distinct as well as overlapping specificities for different lineages.[1]

Table 1 lists the nine murine hemopoietic growth factors which have been shown to be molecularly distinct by biochemical purification and molecular cloning, and shows their major cellular targets and normal cellular sources. These factors are synthesized by several cell types, some of which are widespread throughout the hemopoietic and nonhemopoietic tissues. Identification of producing cells has therefore depended largely on the use of monoclonal cell lines. Evidence that T lymphocytes can synthesize some of these factors came first from *in vitro* studies with immunologically activated lymphoid cells[30-34] and later from various T cell lymphomas,[35,36] hybridomas,[17,37-39] and interleukin-2 (IL-2)-dependent lines and clones,[34,40-49] which could be shown to produce CSFs in the absence of other cell types. Studies with some of these monoclonal T cell populations showed that a single clone could produce several different soluble factors in an apparently coordinated fashion, including the CSFs, IL-2, B cell stimulating factors, and interferon-γ. In most cases, production was not constitutive but depended on activation of the cells with their specific antigen or certain other agents, such as lectins. Because of their inducibility and their high levels of factor synthesis, some of these lines have proved to be potent sources of protein and mRNA for biochemical purification and cDNA cloning of CSFs and other factors.[6,10,17,18,21,24,25]

In this chapter we summarize our work on the production of hemopoietic CSFs by murine T lymphocytes. Two general areas have been studied: clonal heterogeneity in the production of CSFs, and the cellular and molecular control of CSF synthesis. The work has relied largely on the use of polyclonally activated T cell blasts and monoclonal IL-2-dependent T cell lines as model T cell populations. Recently, however, assays have been developed that allow some of these issues to be addressed at the level of the single CSF-secreting cell. The relevance of these studies to hemopoiesis are discussed in the light of recent results on the *in vivo* effects of CSFs.

II. CLONAL ANALYSIS OF CSF PRODUCTION BY T CELLS

Unfractionated spleen or lymph node populations can be stimulated to produce CSFs and other soluble factors by specific antigens, such as allogeneic cells, or some lectins, such as concanavalin A (Con A) and pokeweed mitogen (PWM) (Figure 1).[30-34] CSF production in such primary bulk cultures roughly parallels IL-2 production and T cell proliferation, and can be shown to be largely T cell-derived.[32-34] Conditioned medium (CM) from 7-d cultures of PWM-stimulated spleen cells has been shown by biochemical fractionation to contain at least 3 CSFs: GM-CSF,[56] multi-CSF,[4] and the human-active Eo-CSF[16] which is now known to be equivalent to eosinophil differentiation factor and IL-5.[17,57]

In order to analyze CSF-producing cells at the clonal level, blast cells from mixed leukocyte cultures were cloned by single-cell micromanipulation and assayed for CSF production following Con A stimulation. In one series of experiments with a group of 45 clones

TABLE 1
Murine Hemopoietic Growth Factors

Factor	Sources[a]	Target lineages
Multipotential CSF[2-7] (multi-CSF, IL-3)	T lymphocytes[b]	Multipotential cells Granulocytes Macrophages Eosinophils Megakaryocytes Erythrocytes Mast cells
Granulocyte-macrophage CSF[8-11] (GM-CSF)	T lymphocytes Macrophages Endothelial cells Fibroblasts	Granulocytes Macrophages Eosinophils
Granulocyte CSF[12,13] (G-CSF)	Macrophages	Granulocytes Macrophages
Macrophage CSF[14,15] (M-CSF, CSF-1)	Fibroblasts	Macrophages Granulocytes
Eosinophil CSF[16-18] (Eo-CSF, EDF, BCGF II, IL-5)	T lymphocytes	Eosinophils B lymphocytes
IL-1[19,20]	Macrophages	T lymphocytes B lymphocytes Endothelial cells Fibroblasts
IL-2[21,22]	T lymphocytes	T lymphocytes B lymphocytes
IL-4[23-25]	T lymphocytes	Hemopoietic progenitor cells T lymphocytes B lymphocytes Mast cells
Erythropoietin[26-28]	Kidney[c]	Erythrocytes

[a] The list of sources and target cells is not exhaustive but includes the major, well-documented populations identified in the mouse.

[b] The production of multi-CSF by the myelomonocytic cell line WEHI-3B, which has been used as a source of multi-CSF mRNA and protein in many studies, is aberrant due to insertion of a retroviral element close to the promoter region of this gene.[29]

[c] The identity of erythropoietin-synthesizing cells in the kidney is controversial.

(Table 3),[58] most produced CSF as detected by granulocyte-macrophage colony formation by fetal liver cells (Table 2), with titers varying over a 10^5-fold range. Since no evidence has been found from colony morphology, G-CSF-dependent differentiation assays, or biochemical fractionation[58] for either G-CSF or M-CSF production by T cell clones, the fetal liver GM-stimulating activity was attributed to GM-CSF and/or multi-CSF. The presence of multi-CSF could be assayed independently using the multi-CSF-dependent cell line 32D cl 3. No such assay exists for GM-CSF since all available GM-CSF-responsive populations and lines (such as FDC-P1) also respond to multi-CSF. However, biochemical fractionation[58] and Northern blot hybridization to CSF transcripts[122] have indicated that most, if not all, multi-CSF-producing clones also produce GM-CSF. A third CSF specific for the eosinophil lineage could also be assayed independently by its ability to stimulate pure eosinophil colony formation from human bone marrow cells. Interestingly, these three CSF assays revealed only four combinations of activities among the 45 clones tested (Table 3). There appears to be a hierarchy of CSF synthesis in which positive clones produce GM-CSF only, GM-CSF and multi-CSF only, or GM-CSF, multi-CSF, and Eo-CSF. The finding that clones in all three groups could be positive or negative for IL-2 production is difficult to interpret since

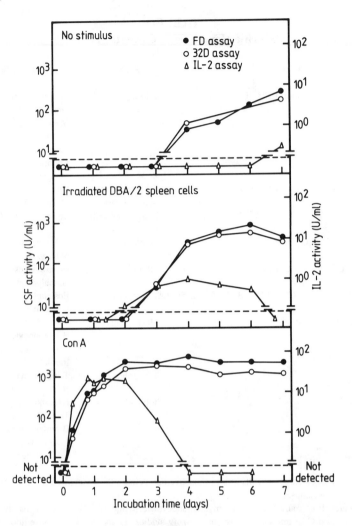

FIGURE 1.   CSF and IL-2 production in lymphoid cell cultures. Spleen cells from C57BL/6 (H-2^b) mice were cultured at 2×10^6 cells/ml in medium alone (top panel), with 1500 rad-irradiated DBA/2 (H-2^d) spleen cells at 2×10^6 cells/ml (middle panel), or 5 µg/ml Con A (bottom panel). At the indicated times, conditioned medium (CM) was harvested and assayed for CSFs in agar cultures of FD or 32D cells, and for IL-2 in a proliferation assay with CTLL (see Table 2 for details). Cultures of irradiated DBA/2 cells alone did not produce detectable CSF or IL-2.

the ability of such IL-2-dependent clones to consume IL-2 interferes with its detection.[48] It should also be noted that the proportion of clones in each group depends on the assay sensitivity. In particular, the Eo-CSF assay used here is thought to be less sensitive than liquid culture assays for eosinophil formation, so that the size of the third group is probably underestimated. Thus, Sanderson et al.[47] found that most IL-3-secreting alloreactive clones produced eosinophil differentiation activity (mainly attributable to Eo-CSF) as detected in the liquid culture assay.

All of the clones tested expressed surface antigens typical of peripheral T cells, being either Thy-1$^+$ Lyt-2$^+$ L3T4$^-$ (and hence H-2 class I-restricted)[60] or Thy-1$^+$ Lyt-2$^-$ L3T4$^+$ (H-2 class II-restricted).[61] No qualitative differences in patterns of CSF or IL-2 production were detected between Lyt-2$^+$ clones (many of which were conventional H-2 class I-reactive

TABLE 2
Assays for CSFs and IL-2

Target cell	Assay method[a]	Activities detected
CBA fetal liver cells[50]	Colony formation	Multi-CSF
		GM-CSF
		G-CSF
		M-CSF
Human bone marrow cells[16]	Colony formation	Eo-CSF
FDC-P1 hemopoietic cell line[51,52]	Colony formation	Multi-CSF
	Proliferation	GM-CSF
32D hemopoietic cell line[52,53]	Colony formation	Multi-CSF
	Proliferation	
CTLL T cell line[54]	Proliferation	IL-2

[a]   Colony assays in agar were performed as described.[1] Proliferation was measured in liquid cultures by [^{3}H]thymidine incorporation in 100 μl microtiter wells or by direct cell counting in 10 μl Terasaki microwells.[55] Titers were determined from dose-response curves and expressed as units (U) per milliliter. In colony assays, 50 U was the CSF concentration stimulating half-maximal colony numbers to develop. In FD and 32D proliferation assays, 50 U was the CSF concentration stimulating half-maximal [^{3}H]thymidine incorporation in 100 μl cultures, or 1 U was the concentration stimulating 50 cells to survive or proliferate in 10 μl cultures, standardized to a reference recombinant IL-3 preparation (Biogen). Calculated in this way, FD and 32D assay titers were roughly equivalent to C57BL/6 bone marrow colony assay units. In the CTLL assay, 1 U was the IL-2 concentration stimulating half-maximal [^{3}H]thymidine incorporation.

TABLE 3
Clonal Analysis of CSF and IL-2 Production by T Cells[a]

GM-CSF and/or multi-CSF	Multi-CSF	Eo-CSF	IL-2	Percent of clones
−	−	−	−	18
+	−	−	−	33
+	−	−	+	13
+	+	−	−	4
+	+	−	+	18
+	+	+	−	2
+	+	+	+	11

[a]   BALB/c or C57BL/6 spleen cells were stimulated with irradiated DBA/2 spleen cells in mixed leukocyte culture for 5 d. Individual blast cells were cloned by micromanipulation into wells containing irradiated DBA/2 spleen cells and EL-4 thymoma CM[59] as a source of IL-2 (average cloning efficiency 23%), and then maintained by passage with the same stimuli. CM from 45 randomly derived clones were prepared by culturing washed cells at 2×10^5 cells/ml with 5 μg/ml Con A for 18 to 24 h. CSF was measured by colony assay with fetal liver cells, 32D cells, and human bone marrow cells.

cytolytic cells) and L3T4$^+$ clones. However, a marked quantitative difference was observed in that L3T4$^+$ clones on average produced CSFs and IL-2 in titers 10- to 100-fold higher than Lyt-2$^+$ clones. Accordingly, a higher proportion of L3T4$^+$ clones produced several or all of the activities measured.[46,58] This finding is consistent with an earlier observation that the precursors of alloreactive cells producing GM-colony stimulating activity were 3- to 4-fold more frequent among Lyt-2$^-$ than among Lyt-2$^+$ normal T cells.[62]

A later series of experiments was performed to take advantage of improved GM-CSF and multi-CSF detection by ^{3}H-thymidine incorporation assays using the hemopoietic cell lines FDC-P1 and 32D cl 3 (Figure 2). In this case, CSF production was detected by all clones and, as before, clones were very heterogeneous with CSF titers varying over a 10^7-

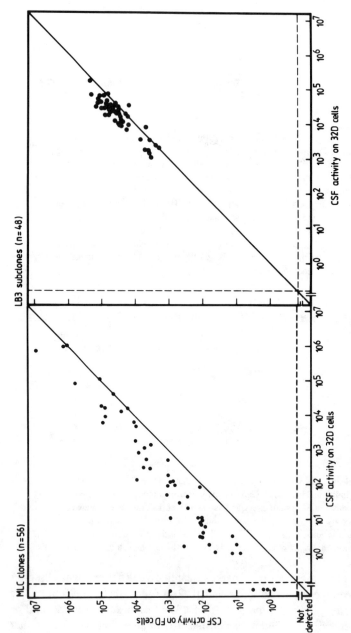

FIGURE 2.   Clonal analysis of CSF production by alloreactive T cells. Single blast cells from 5-d C57BL/6 anti-DBA/2 mixed leukocyte cultures (left panel) (set up as described in Figure 1) or single cells of the clone LB3 (right panel) were cloned by micromanipulation as described in Table 3. After 7 to 10 d incubation, clones were restimulated once for 5 to 7 d, then washed and cultured at 10^6 cells/ml with 5 μg/ml Con A and 100 U/ml highly purified recombinant human IL-2 from *E. coli* (Cetus Corp.).[63] Conditioned medium (CM) was harvested after 48 h incubation and assayed for CSF in proliferation assays with FD or 32D cells.

fold range. Most synthesized multi-CSF, accompanied in at least some cases by GM-CSF (where the FD titer was considerably higher than the 32D titer), while the remainder (11%) produced GM-CSF in the absence of detectable multi-CSF. By comparison, random sub-clones of an established T cell clone, LB3, varied over only a 100-fold range in total CSF titer and all were positive in both assays. Similarly, repeated testing of clones and subclones suggested that these were stable, heritable properties of each clone.

Taken together, these two studies indicate that individual clones can vary widely in their level of CSF production and in the ratios of GM-CSF to multi-CSF and Eo-CSF they produce. No evidence was obtained for distinct subsets of clones producing different factors. Rather, the data suggest that clones comprise a spectrum, from low producers (which produce only GM-CSF) to intermediate producers (which synthesize GM-CSF and multi-CSF in variable ratio) to high producers (which synthesize GM-CSF, multi-CSF, and Eo-CSF). The differences between clones therefore appear to be quantitative rather than qualitative, raising the possibility that improved methods for stimulation and assay of factor production may reveal that all clones can synthesize all factors. Several other studies have also detected production of GM-CSF and/or multi-CSF by a high proportion of Lyt-2[+] and L3T4[+] clones of various antigenic specificities.[42,45-47,49,62,64-66]

A different conclusion was suggested by Mosmann et al.[49] who have identified two distinct groups of lymphokine-producing L3T4[+] clones which differ in their ability to produce IL-2, interferon-γ, and IL-4. Since both groups produce GM-CSF and multi-CSF, and since our results cannot distinguish failure to synthesize IL-2 from IL-2 consumption, the relationship between our clones and those of Mosmann is not clear. An interesting feature of Mosmann's study is the suggestion that different types of antigens may preferentially activate one or other group of L3T4[+] cells and thereby indirectly alter the response of other cells (such as IL-4-induced immunoglobulin isotype switching by B cells). Similarly, Sanderson et al.[66] speculated that the T cell-dependent eosinophilia associated with certain helminth infections in mice may be due to eosinophil differentiation factor (Eo-CSF) production by parasite-reactive T cells, since the frequency of EDF-secreting clones was higher among parasite-reactive clones from infected animals than among alloreactive clones from normal or infected animals.

III. INDUCTION OF CSF SYNTHESIS IN ACTIVATED T CELLS

Several well-characterized T cell clones have been used to analyze CSF production by activated T cells in detail. These include LB3,[58] an alloreactive clone derived from a BALB/c anti DBA/2 mixed leukocyte culture, and E9.D4,[67] an azobenzenearsonate (ABA)-reactive I-A^k-restricted clone derived from lymph node cells of an ABA-immunized CBA mouse, both of which are Thy-1[+] Lyt-2[−] L3T4[+] IL-2-dependent clones. Most of the observations made with these lines have also been made with polyclonally activated T cell blast populations.

Activated T cells, including most T cell clones[41-49] and some lymphomas[35,36] and hybridomas,[38,39] require exogenous stimulation to transcribe and translate detectable amounts of CSFs and other lymphokines. Two pathways for stimulation of CSF synthesis have been identified (Table 4).[55] The first is induced by incubation with Concanavalin A (Con A) and some other lectins (such as wheat germ agglutinin), appropriately presented antigen, or in some cases the antibody F23.1, which binds to a determinant on a subset of variable regions of the β chain of the T cell antigen receptor.[68,69] This group of stimuli induces production of high titers of CSF by LB3 and E9.D4 cells, as detected by FD and 32D proliferation assays. Titers on FD cells are consistently higher than on 32D cells, indicating the presence of both GM-CSF and multi-CSF. Similarly, Northern blot hybridization consistently detects the presence of abundant GM-CSF and multi-CSF transcripts in the same clones activated

TABLE 4
Induction of CSF Synthesis in Activated T Cells[a]

Cells	Stimulus	CSF activity (U/ml)			
		FD assay		32D assay	
		− CsA	+ CsA	− CsA	+ CsA
Clone LB3	Medium	8.8	3.9	<0.8	<0.8
	Con A	144,164	1,780	21,701	8.2
	WGA	44,232	906	4,782	4.4
	IL-2	2,545	2,840	1.6	<0.8
	PMA	557	579	1.3	<0.8
Clone E9.D4	Medium	61	55	<1.1	<1.1
	Con A	628,966	24,055	181,581	1,191
	F23.1	1,324,138	17,986	327,441	491
	IL-2	2,979	3,310	46	42
Con A blasts	Medium	<0.1	<0.1	<0.4	<0.4
	Con A	8,369	3.9	2,055	<0.4
	WGA	3,397	41	379	<0.4
	F23.1	17,723	6.3	8,514	1.4
	IL-2	4.6	1.9	<0.4	<0.4

[a]   Clone cells, or C57BL/6 spleen cells incubated for 3 d with Con A, then for 2 d
with EL-4 CM (Con A blasts), were cultured at 10^6 cells/ml with Con A (10 µg/
ml), wheat germ agglutinin (WGA, 10 µg/ml), F23.1 (plastic-adsorbed, 10 µg/
ml), IL-2 (200 U/ml), or phorbol 12-myristate 13-acetate (PMA, 100 ng/ml) in
the presence or absence of cyclosporin A (CsA, 1 µg/ml). CSF production was
measured after 48 h in proliferation assays with FD or 32D cells.

in these ways, although these and other clones differ in their relative levels of the two
CSFs.[55,70] Most other studies have used stimuli of this type to induce synthesis of CSFs,
IL-2, interferon-γ, B-cell stimulating factors, and other activities by T cells.

The second pathway leading to CSF production is activated by incubation with IL-2. In
most clones, IL-2 preferentially stimulates GM-CSF production, as evidenced by a high
ratio of the FD titer to the 32D titer (Table 4)[55] and by the presence of higher GM-CSF than
multi-CSF mRNA levels. The ratio of GM-CSF to multi-CSF produced in response to IL-
2 varies markedly between clones, but in most cases is higher for IL-2 than for Con A
stimulation of the same clone. The clones shown in Table 4, which were selected for high
CSF production, produce more CSF in response to Con A than to IL-2, but clones can also
be found whose Con A response is similar to or less than the response to IL-2. IL-2-induced
production of B-cell stimulating factors[71,72] and interferon-γ[73] by T cells in the absence of
antigen has also been described.

Both activation pathways can proceed in the absence of DNA synthesis (Figure 3).[55] In
fact, optimal concentrations of Con A and F23.1 for induction of CSF synthesis profoundly
inhibit proliferation by clones and blast populations.[48,123] For the IL-2-dependent pathway,
on the other hand, dose-response curves for the stimulation of proliferation and CSF production are similar (Figure 3) and, in low-density cultures where proliferation is possible,
the kinetics of CSF production parallel population growth. Activation of CSF synthesis by
IL-2, therefore, appears to be mediated, at least in part, through the same pathways as
activation of proliferation. Synergism between IL-2 and Con A or antigen can be observed,
particularly for low-producing clones.[55] An earlier study suggested that IL-2 prolonged the
duration of lymphokine synthesis by T cell clones, perhaps by prolonging cell survival.[74]

Stimuli of the first group (Con A, antigen, antireceptor antibodies) have been reported
to induce in T cells the hydrolysis of phosphatidylinositol (PI) bisphosphate to 1,2-diacyl-

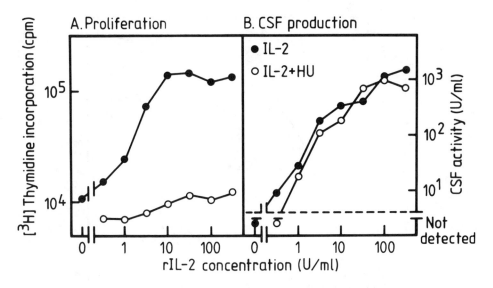

FIGURE 3. CSF production by a T cell clone in response to IL-2. LB3 cells were cultured at 4×10^5 cells/ml with the indicated concentrations of recombinant IL-2 in the presence or absence of 300 μg/ml hydroxyurea (HU). Proliferation was assessed by [³H]thymidine incorporation during the final 6 h of a 24-h incubation (left panel). CM were harvested from parallel cultures after 48 h incubation, passed over Sephadex G25M columns to remove HU, and titrated in an FD proliferation assay (right panel). CSF production in response to 5 μg/ml Con A was 12,220 U/ml in the absence and 10,790 U/ml in the presence of HU.

glycerol and inositol triphosphate, a rise in the concentration of cytoplasmic free calcium, and, by inference, activation of protein kinase C.[75-80] Binding of IL-2 to its receptor apparently activates protein kinase C but does not cause a calcium flux or activate PI breakdown.[77,78,80-82] The finding that the immunosuppressant cyclosporin A, which interferes with calcium-dependent activation pathways in T cells,[83,84] inhibits CSF synthesis induced by Con A or F23.1 but not by IL-2 (Table 4), supports the view that these stimuli activate CSF synthesis via at least two distinct pathways.[125] Phorbol 12-myristate 13-acetate (PMA), an analog of diacylglycerol which directly activates protein kinase C, induces a similar response to IL-2 that is also not inhibited by cyclosporin A. As reported for other lymphokines,[84-86] the effect of cyclosporin A is pretranslational, since it profoundly inhibits the accumulation of GM-CSF and multi-CSF mRNA in cells stimulated with Con A or F23.1.

Experiments with the anti-L3T4 antibody GK1.5, which can inhibit interaction of antigen with its receptor on class II-restricted T cells,[61] are also consistent with two activation pathways. GK1.5 can inhibit CSF synthesis by E9.D4 cells in response to antigen or suboptimal concentrations of Con A or F23.1, but not to IL-2 or PMA.[87,123] The two pathways, therefore, differ in the ratio of GM-CSF to multi-CSF produced and in their inhibition by cyclosporin A and GK1.5. Direct evidence that Con A activates CSF synthesis wholly or partly through the antigen receptor has not been obtained; however, the ability of GK1.5 to inhibit the response to Con A and the finding by others that antigen and Con A induce phosphorylation of a polypeptide associated with the T cell antigen receptor[88,89] support this possibility.

IV. KINETIC ANALYSES OF CSF PRODUCTION BY T CELL CLONES

As for Con A-stimulated normal spleen cells (Figure 1), the production of CSFs by T cell clones is rapid and short-lived (Figure 4).[41,46,48,90,91] Parallel analyses of cytoplasmic CSF mRNA levels reveal the transient accumulation of GM-CSF and multi-CSF transcripts

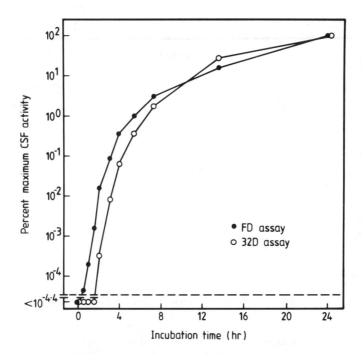

FIGURE 4. Kinetics of CSF production by Con A-stimulated LB3 cells. LB3 cells were cultured at 10^6 cells/ml with 10 μg/ml Con A. At the indicated times, CM were harvested and assayed for CSF in proliferation assays with FD or 32D cells. Maximum titers were 1,079,900 U/ml in the FD assay and 256,470 U/ml in the 32D assay.

over the same period (Figure 5). Clones vary in the rates and duration of synthesis of all the lymphokines, with high-producing clones secreting for longer than low-producing clones. As noted above, IL-2 can prolong the duration of lymphokine synthesis by Con A or antigen-stimulated clones.[74]

Kinetic studies by several groups have suggested that all the lymphokines produced by a clone are produced at similar rates following antigen or lectin stimulation;[46,84,90,91] however, in our own studies, we have noted a consistent difference in the first few hours after Con A or F23.1 stimulation, with expression of the GM-CSF gene being detected up to 3 h earlier than expression of the multi-CSF gene by both mRNA (Figure 5) and CSF (Figure 4) assays.[126] It is not known whether this observation reflects differences in the initiation or rate of transcription itself or in the rate of RNA processing or degradation.

The reason for the cessation of lymphokine synthesis after less than 20 h is not clear. Where a high concentration of Con A or F23.1 is the stimulus, this may be due to clone death. CSF production was also short-lived when a cytolytic anti-H-2^d clone K32[55] was stimulated with H-2^d-expressing P815 tumor cells and IL-2, conditions under which the clone proliferated. In this case, CSF synthesis may have ceased because the clone lysed the stimulating cells within 4 h of their addition. Indeed, as shown in Table 5, readdition of P815 cells 4 or 7 h after a first stimulation under optimal conditions induced a second burst of production equal to the first, regardless of whether the culture medium was changed at the time of restimulation. In a similar system, Harris et al.[78] found that at least 8 h interaction of a cytolytic clone with antigen was required for optimal stimulation of lymphokine synthesis, but even using a persisting stimulus (glutaraldehyde-fixed P815 cells), production ceased within 20 h. The experiment in Table 5 suggests that CSF synthesis can be repeatedly stimulated at the population level, although it does not indicate that each cell can respond

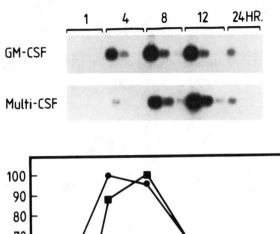

FIGURE 5. Kinetics of accumulation of GM-CSF and multi-CSF mRNA in
Con A-stimulated LB3 cells. LB3 cells were cultured at 10^6 cells/ml with 5
μg/ml Con A. Cytoplasmic polyadenylated RNA, prepared from cells harvested at the indicated times, was fractionated on duplicate 1% agarose gels
as described.[92] For each time point, 1.5, 0.3, and 0.6 μg of RNA were used
(upper panel). GM-CSF and multi-CSF hybridization riboprobes were derived
by *in vitro* transcription[93] of the SP6 GM-CSF and multi-CSF subclones detailed in Barlow et al.[94] The specific activities of the two probes were identical
(about 1×10^9 cpm/μg) and they were used at 5×10^6 cpm/ml of hybridization
solution. Filters were hybridized and washed essentially as described previously.[55] The GM-CSF filter was autoradiographed for 16 h and the multi-CSF
was autoradiographed for 5 d. The intensity of hybridization to each mRNA
species was quantitated by densitometry and expressed as a percent of the
maximum (lower panel).

more than once. There is, therefore, no evidence for a feedback mechanism to limit the
response. The possibility of inhibition by secreted CSFs is rendered unlikely by our failure
to detect GM-CSF or multi-CSF receptors on LB3, and the failure of exogenous CSFs to
affect *de novo* CSF production.[124]

V. CSF PRODUCTION BY SINGLE ACTIVATED T LYMPHOCYTES

To date, it has not been possible to analyze many aspects of T cell function at the clonal
level other than by *in vitro* expansion of cell lines, which may not be representative of
normal activated T cells. An assay for lymphokine production by single T cells would be
useful for analyses of functional heterogeneity among T cells activated by various antigens

TABLE 5

Restimulation of CSF Production by a Cytolytic T cell Clone[a]

Stimulus			CSF production at
at 0 h	at 4 h	at 7 h	25 h (U/ml)
Medium			1.4
IL-2			9.2
P815 + IL-2			80
P815 + IL-2	P815		192
P815 + IL-2		P815	139
P815 + IL-2	P815	P815	216
P815 + IL-2	wash/P815 + IL-2		88
P815 + IL-2	wash/IL-2		14
P815 + IL-2		wash/P815 + IL-2	30
P815 + IL-2		wash/IL-2	8.2

[a]   The clone K32 was cultured at 10^6 cells/ml with or without 50 U/ml recombinant IL-2 and 5×10^5 P815 tumor cells/ml. Cultures were restimulated as indicated with the same concentrations of stimuli with or without washing the K32 cells once. CSF production was measured after a total of 25 h incubation in a proliferation assay with FD cells. Supernatants from cultures of P815 cells or IL-2 alone did not contain detectable CSF.

and of the interaction between T cells and various stimuli in the absence of other cell interactions. The techniques of *in situ* RNA hybridization and immunohistochemistry[95] allow factor-synthesizing cells to be identified in mixed populations and tissue sections, but they have the disadvantages that they measure intracellular levels at a fixed time and cannot easily measure more than one product in each cell. The approach described below is based on the assay of total cumulative production of CSFs by each cell.

The two major limitations in developing a single-cell assay for lymphokine-producing cells are the sensitivity of assays required to detect the product of a single cell and the difficulty of activating T cells in isolation. The first problem necessitated the use of micro-culture proliferation assays using FD and 32D cells, performed in 10 μl volumes and scored microscopically to allow detection of the small cell numbers present at limiting CSF concentrations. These microassays can detect as little as 0.2 U/ml or approximately 10^{-13} *M* CSF (or a total of 10^{-18} mol in 10 μl).[96] The second problem has been overcome in part by using preactivated T cell populations whose requirements for induction of lymphokine synthesis appear less complex than those of resting T cells, and stimuli which do not require presentation on a cell surface.

In a first attempt to establish a single-cell assay, cells of the clone LB3 were activated with Con A. These experiments revealed that Con A was only a weak stimulus for isolated cells because of a requirement for aggregation of the T cells for optimal activation, resulting in a markedly nonlinear relationship between cell density and the apparent frequency and activity of CSF-producing cells.[97] In contrast, the antireceptor antibody F23.1 was found to be an efficient stimulus for isolated cells of the F23.1$^+$ clone E9.D4. Optimal E9.D4 activation depended on immobilization of the antibody by adsorption to the culture wells,[87] perhaps by facilitating multimeric binding and cross-linking of the antigen receptor.[99] The relationships between cell density and both the frequency of CSF-producing cells and total CSF production were linear in this case.

Single-cell assays of F23.1-activated E9.D4 cells have been used in two ways: to determine the relationship between the concentration of stimulating ligand and the frequency and activity of CSF-producing cells (Figure 6), and to compare the production of GM-CSF and multi-CSF by individual cells (Figure 7).[98] As shown in Figure 6, increasing concentrations of immobilized F23.1 stimulated an increasing proportion of single E9.D4 cells to

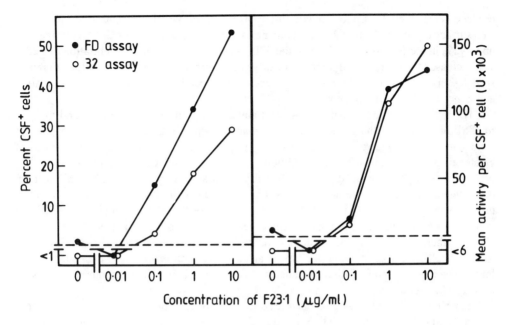

FIGURE 6. Frequency and activity of CSF-producing cells of a T cell clone. Single E9.D4 cells were transferred by micromanipulation into 15 μl volumes in Terasaki microwells previously coated with the indicated concentrations of protein A-purified F23.1 antibody (100 cells/group). After 24 h incubation, 5 μl aliquots of CM were removed and individually titrated in microwell proliferation assays with FD and 32D cells, standardized with purified recombinant IL-3. Wells which contained more than one E9.D4 cell at the time of conditioned medium (CM) harvest were excluded from the analysis. The left panel shows the frequency of cells that produced detectable CSF. The right panel shows the arithmetic mean of the CSF titers produced by positive cells (U/cell).

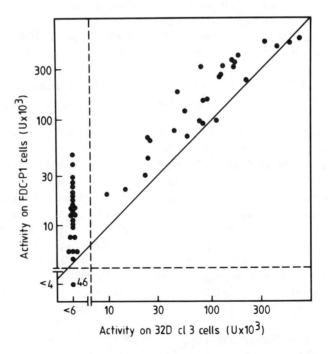

FIGURE 7. CSF production by single F23.1-activated E9.D4 cells. Each dot represents the CSF titer (U/cell) produced by a single E9.D4 cell activated with 10 μg/ml plastic-adsorbed F23.1 from the experiment shown in Figure 6.

produce detectable CSF up to a maximum at 10 μg/ml (at which concentration the culture well surface is saturated with F23.1). In other experiments, frequencies of CSF[+] cells reached up to 92% in the FD assay and 58% in the 32D assay. Increasing the concentration of F23.1 also increased the average CSF titer per positive cell, demonstrating that in contrast to recent speculation,[100] the size of the response of each cell depends on the strength of stimulation and is not an all-or-none phenomenon.

The activities of individual E9.D4 cells stimulated with 10 μg/ml F23.1 and assayed for CSF production in the FD and 32D assays are shown in Figure 7. The two CSF assays were standardized to have the same sensitivity to pure multi-CSF, so that FD:32D ratios of greater than one should reflect the additional presence of GM-CSF. In this and other experiments, many of the positive cells (usually at least half) produced GM-CSF without detectable multi-CSF. The remaining cells produced multi-CSF, but since the FD:32D ratios usually averaged at least 2, it is likely that most or all of these also produced GM-CSF. It is notable that the multi-CSF-negative cells were low to medium producers (0.004 to 0.5 U/cell), whereas the multi-CSF-positive cells were medium to high producers of CSF (0.02 to 0.6 U/cell). As argued above for clones at the population level, these data suggest that low-producing cells preferentially synthesize GM-CSF, whereas high-producing cells synthesize both factors.

The single-cell assay has also been used to measure CSF production by normal T cells preactivated in bulk culture with F23.1 and IL-2. These activated T cell populations comprise essentially 100% Thy-1[+] Lyt-2[+] L3T4[−] F23.1[+] cells, although normal T cells of both the Lyt-2[+] and L3T4[+] phenotypes express the F23.1 determinant.[101] As shown in Figure 8 for multi-CSF production, both micromanipulation and limiting dilution analyses indicate that a substantial proportion of such polyclonally activated Lyt-2[+] cells can synthesize detectable multi-CSF. In other experiments, up to 36% of cells were positive in the FD assay and up to 30% were also positive in the 32D assay. As in the clonal studies described earlier (Figure 2), individual cells differed in their production of GM-CSF and multi-CSF, and multi-CSF was generally a product of high-producing cells. If long-term clones are representative of their normal counterparts, L3T4[+] cells can be expected to express higher frequencies and levels of CSF production than the Lyt-2[+] cells assayed here.[46,58]

VI. MOLECULAR REGULATION OF CSF PRODUCTION IN T CELL CLONES

Although several of the hemopoietic growth factors listed in Table 1 are glycoproteins of similar molecular weight (about 25,000 Da) and many are produced coordinately by a single cell type, they do not display significant nucleotide or amino acid homology and so do not belong to a multigene family.[70,102] Moreover, in most known cases they are encoded on different chromosomes. One notable exception has been identified: by pulsed field gel electrophoresis, the genes encoding GM-CSF and multi-CSF have been mapped within a 230 kb segment of mouse chromosome 11.[94] The relevance of their proximity to the co-ordinate expression of these genes by T cells is unclear, particularly since expression of several unlinked genes (such as IL-2 on human chromosome 4[103] and interferon-γ on human chromosome 12[104]) is similarly controlled. In man, the GM-CSF gene has been localized to chromosome 5, close to the genes encoding M-CSF and the receptors for M-CSF and platelet-derived growth factor, in the 5q 21-33 region whose deletion is associated with certain leukemias.[105,106]

Most of the data available suggest that CSF synthesis by T cells is controlled mainly at the pretranslational level. Thus, in our studies, cumulative levels of cytoplasmic CSF transcripts correlate well with cumulative production of biologically active protein in the 24 h after induction (Figure 5).[126] Others have also described the marked increases in total mRNA

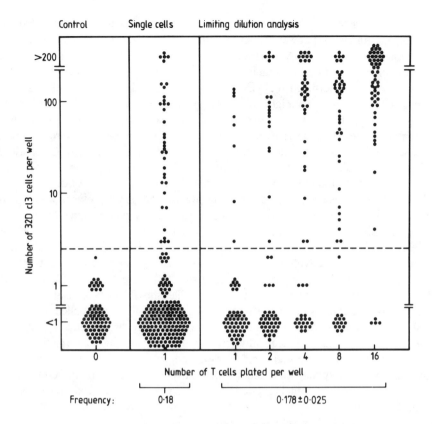

FIGURE 8. Frequency analysis of CSF-producing cells among F23.1-activated lymph node cells. C57BL/6 lymph node cells were cultured at 2×10^6 cells/ml with 10 μg/ml plastic-adsorbed F23.1 and EL-4 CM for 3 d and then in EL-4 CM for a further 2 d. Cells were plated either individually by micromanipulation (middle panel; 200 wells) or at the indicated average numbers by dilution (right panel; 54 wells/group) in 10 μl volumes in Terasaki microwells previously coated with 10 μg/ml F23.1. After 24 h incubation, 5 μl aliquots of CM were removed and added to microwells with 200 32D cells. Each dot represents the number of 32D cells counted after 2 d incubation with each conditioned medium (CM). A minimal estimate of the frequency of multi-CSF-producing E9.D4 cells was obtained from the limiting dilution data by the maximum likelihood method from the Poisson distribution relationship between the number of E9.D4 cells and the logarithm of the fraction of negative cultures (defined by control cultures; left panel).

levels for CSFs and other lymphokines which accompany the production of these factors by polyclonal and monoclonal T cell populations.[84,86,91,107] The relative contributions of transcription, processing and transport from the nucleus, and degradation of mRNA are not known, although evidence for regulation at each of these levels has been reported.[108,109]

The coordinate, inducible expression of several lymphokine genes in cloned T cells has stimulated a search for regulatory sequences common to each of these genes.[11,22,70,102,110-112] For example, Stanley et al.[11,70] and Miyatake et al.[111] have identified several oligonucleotide sequences in common in the immediate 5′-flanking regions of the murine GM-CSF, multi-CSF and IL-2, and the human IL-2 and interferon-γ genes. Although the function of these sequences remains to be established, Gasson et al.[110,112] have shown that the region of 150 bp upstream of the promoter of the human GM-CSF gene, which includes these sequence motifs, is in fact involved in its tissue-specific, lectin-inducible expression in T cells. In the case of the human IL-2 gene, although no data are available about the region actually spanning the corresponding sequence motifs (at around 170 bp 5′ of the promoter), sequences adjacent and either side of this element (between -127 and -145, and -319 and -264)

have been shown to be required for inducible expression.[113] Another level of control is indicated by the finding of Shaw and Kamen[109] that the 3'-untranslated region of the human GM-CSF mRNA contains an AU-rich sequence which, at least in fibroblasts, increases mRNA instability when fused to a rabbit β-globin transcript. Similar sequences have been identified in the 3'-untranslated regions of many other lymphokines, growth factors, and oncogenes, suggesting that this might be a common feature of transiently expressed mRNAs.

Many studies of lymphokine synthesis by T cells have emphasized the similarities in production of different lymphokines; however, our own experiments summarized here have revealed several differences in the production of GM-CSF and multi-CSF by single cells and clones which indicate that they can be differentially regulated.[126] Thus, low-producing cells and clones can be found which synthesize GM-CSF in the absence of detectable multi-CSF (Figure 2), whereas the converse has not been observed. Among clones which produce both factors, preferential production of GM-CSF can be observed in three circumstances: early in the response to Con A or F23.1 (Figures 4 and 5), in a proportion of low-producing cells (Figure 7), and in response to stimulation with IL-2 (Table 2). GM-CSF is not always the major product quantitatively but it is the "preferred" product in each of these cases. Although these observations are likely to reflect several different levels of control, which may be pre- or posttranscriptional, two general mechanisms might be considered.

The first is that expression of the multi-CSF gene is obligatorily linked to that of the GM-CSF gene. Given the close proximity of the two genes on chromosome 11, this linkage could reflect a requirement for sequential changes in chromosome conformation for transcriptional activation, although such a model would not accommodate the coordinate expression of other unlinked lymphokine genes. Alternatively, activation of the GM-CSF gene might result in delivery of a signal required for multi-CSF production. That signal apparently is not the GM-CSF protein itself since inhibition of protein synthesis does not reduce the accumulation of multi-CSF mRNA in Con A-stimulated LB3 cells.[70]

The second proposed mechanism is that the requirements for activation of synthesis of the two CSFs are qualitatively or quantitatively different. A quantitative model in which a stronger signal is required to activate multi-CSF compared with GM-CSF synthesis would accommodate most of the observations described here; however, it would also predict that suboptimal concentrations of Con A or F23.1 would preferentially stimulate GM-CSF production. In fact, dose-response experiments measuring cumulative GM-CSF and multi-CSF production suggest that the thresholds for stimulation are the same.[55]

VII. THE ROLE OF CSF PRODUCTION BY T LYMPHOCYTES *IN VIVO*

The cloning of cDNAs encoding murine GM-CSF and multi-CSF and their expression in mammalian, yeast, and bacterial cells has permitted the large-scale production and purification of recombinant CSFs of both types. Bacterially synthesized, nonglycosylated GM-CSF and multi-CSF exhibit the same specific activity and range of target cell actions *in vitro*[5,6,96,114] and similar *in vivo* half-lives in mice as the corresponding native molecules. For these reasons, it has become feasible to examine the *in vivo* effects of injected recombinant GM-CSF and multi-CSF in normal adult mice.

Following the intraperitoneal injection of recombinant GM-CSF or multi-CSF, 3 times daily for 6 d, of doses varying from 6 to 200 ng, obvious dose-related changes were observed in hemopoietic populations in injected mice. For mice injected with rGM-CSF,[115] only a minor elevation was observed in circulating neutrophil levels but these mice exhibited major rises in the number of peritoneal macrophages, eosinophils, and neutrophils. The largest rice occurred in peritoneal macrophages whose numbers increased from a normal level of 2 to 4 $\times$ 10^6 to up to 100 $\times$ 10^6 per mouse. These cells also exhibited functional activation as assessed by increased phagocytic activity. In addition, mice injected with rGM-CSF showed rises in spleen weight, in the percentages of neutrophils and monocytes in both spleen and bone marrow, and in the content of these cells in the liver and lung.

In mice injected with multi-CSF,[116] similar rises were observed in the levels of peritoneal macrophages, eosinophils, and neutrophils, although macrophage numbers were somewhat lower than those elicited by rGM-CSF. Mice injected with rmulti-CSF exhibited a 2- to 3-fold increase in spleen weight and a dramatic 100-fold rise in spleen mast cell numbers. Rises of lesser magnitude were observed in spleen megakaryocytes and in mast cell numbers in the skin, gut, and lymph nodes. These mice also showed rises in spleen and marrow progenitor cell numbers and rises in the liver content of macrophages and neutrophils.

These various *in vivo* effects were achieved with CSF doses comparable with those used *in vitro* to stimulate the proliferation of hemopoietic cells. Moreover, the cell populations responding *in vivo* were the same as those stimulated *in vitro* by the direct action of the two CSFs. These data therefore strongly support the large body of indirect evidence that the CSFs function *in vivo* as genuine regulators of the production and functional activity of granulocytes, macrophages, and related cell populations.[1]

However, several important questions remain. In particular, it is not yet clear whether GM-CSF and multi-CSF are produced *in vivo* and whether synthesis of these factors by T lymphocytes is physiologically important. Cells bearing specific receptors for GM-CSF or multi-CSF have been identified in normal hemopoietic tissues and receptor expression mirrors the responsiveness of those cells to CSFs *in vitro*.[117,118] GM-CSF can be extracted from normal lymphoid tissues and appears to be a minor component of the GM-colony stimulating activity (together with G-CSF and M-CSF) detected in serum, which fluctuates during infections and hematopoietic stress;[1,119] however, because of the multiplicity of cellular sources of GM-CSF (Table 1), including macrophages and endothelial cells which are also present in lymphoid organs, this CSF may not be of T cell origin. Multi-CSF presents a particular problem because this molecule has not been detected in serum or tissue extracts, except after injection of multi-CSF-secreting leukemic cells, despite the availability of extremely sensitive and specific assays.[1,120] Thus, the sources and distribution of multi-CSF in a normal animal are unknown. It is hoped that histochemistry with monoclonal antibodies or *in situ* mRNA hybridization with nucleic acid probes will resolve these issues.

The low or undetectable circulating levels of CSFs, and indeed of the other T cell-derived lymphokines, can be reconciled with the high concentrations found in T cell culture supernatants, if it is proposed that these molecules remain at the site of production. In this case, T cell production of CSFs is unlikely to be important in the development and maintenance of steady-state hemopoiesis, as the hemopoietic normality of the athymic mouse attests. Instead, antigenic stimulation of T cells in the lymphoid organs would result in local production of CSFs whose effects would be limited to neighboring target cells. Since target cells in the periphery mainly comprise mature cells, the major effects of T cell-derived CSFs may be the enhancement of functional activity (such as macrophage phagocytosis and neutrophil and eosinophil cytotoxicity)[115,116,121] rather than the stimulation of progenitor cell differentiation.

VIII. CONCLUDING REMARKS

The ability of cultured T lymphocytes to synthesize several of the CSFs is now well established. Work from a number of laboratories suggests that most, if not all, T cells which can be clonally expanded *in vitro* can produce both GM-CSF and multi-CSF, as well as other lymphokines. The mechanisms controlling synthesis of these molecules are still largely unknown but cellular, biochemical, and genetic approaches are being used to study clonal heterogeneity among T cells in the production of lymphokines and the membrane receptors, intracellular signaling pathways, and genetic elements involved in the expression of lymphokine genes.

In spite of significant advances in the analysis of CSF production and action *in vitro*, the role of CSF synthesis *in vivo* by T lymphocytes is unknown and indeed the evidence that it occurs at all is slim. Since T cell-derived CSFs apparently do not reach the circulation, resolution of this issue will probably depend on the use of specific antibody and nucleic acid probes to detect CSF synthesized at the site of antigenic stimulation.

ACKNOWLEDGMENTS

We thank Annette Futter, Cathy Quilici, and Yvonne Pattison for their excellent technical assistance, and Trevor Owens, Nicos Nicola, and Francesca Walker for their collaboration. Gifts of recombinant growth factors from Cetus Corporation (IL-2) and Biogen (GM-CSF and multi-CSF), and the F23.1 hybridoma from Dr. M. J. Bevan, are gratefully acknowledged. This work was supported by the Carden Fellowship Fund of the Anti-Cancer Council of Victoria, the National Health and Medical Research Council, Canberra, the Queen Elizabeth Fellowship Fund, and The National Cancer Institute, Bethesda, MD, Grants CA-22556 and CA-25972. N. M. Gough was a member of the Ludwig Institute for Cancer Research, Melbourne Tumour Biology Branch, during this study.

REFERENCES

1. **Metcalf, D.,** *The Hemopoietic Colony Stimulating Factors,* Elsevier, Amsterdam, 1984.
2. **Ihle, J. N., Keller, J., Henderson, L., Klein, F., and Palaszynski, E.,** Procedures for the purification of interleukin 3 to homogeneity, *J. Immunol.,* 129, 2431, 1982.
3. **Clark-Lewis, I., Kent, S. B. H., and Schrader, J. W.,** Purification to apparent homogeneity of a factor stimulating the growth of multiple lineages of hemopoietic cells, *J. Biol. Chem.,* 259, 7488, 1984.
4. **Cutler, R. L., Metcalf, D., Nicola, N. A., and Johnson, G. R.,** Purification of a multipotential colony-stimulating factor from pokeweed mitogen-stimulated mouse spleen cell conditioned medium, *J. Biol. Chem.,* 260, 6579, 1985.
5. **Fung, M. C., Hapel, A. J., Ymer, S., Cohen, D. R., Johnson, R. M., Campbell, H. D., and Young, I. G.,** Molecular cloning of cDNA for murine interleukin-3, *Nature,* 307, 233, 1984.
6. **Yokota, L., Lee, F., Rennick, D., Hall, C., Arai, N., Mosmann, T., Nabel, G., Cantor, H., and Arai, K.,** Isolation and characterization of a mouse cDNA clone that expresses mast-cell growth-factor activity in monkey cells, *Proc. Natl. Acad. Sci. U.S.A.,* 81, 1070, 1984.
7. **Miyatake, S., Yokota, T., Lee, F., and Arai, K.,** Structure of the chromosomal gene for murine interleukin 3, *Proc. Natl. Acad. Sci. U.S.A.,* 82, 316, 1985.
8. **Burgess, A. W., Camakaris, J., and Metcalf, D.,** Purification and properties of colony-stimulating factor from mouse lung-conditioned medium, *J. Biol. Chem.,* 252, 1998, 1977.
9. **Sparrow, L. G., Metcalf, D., Hunkapiller, M. W., Hood, L. E., and Burgess, A. E.,** Purification and partial amino acid sequence of asialo murine granulocyte-macrophage colony stimulating factor, *Proc. Natl. Acad. Sci. U.S.A.,* 82, 292, 1985.
10. **Gough, N. M., Gough, J., Metcalf, D., Kelso, A., Grail, D., Nicola, N. A., Burgess, A. W., and Dunn, A. R.,** Molecular cloning of cDNA encoding a murine haematopoietic growth regulator, granulocyte-macrophage colony stimulating factor, *Nature,* 309, 763, 1984.
11. **Stanley, E., Metcalf, D., Sobieszczuk, P., Gough, N. M., and Dunn, A. R.,** The structure and expression of the murine gene encoding granulocyte-macrophage colony stimulating factor: evidence for utilization of alternative promoters, *EMBO J.,* 4, 2569, 1985.
12. **Nicola, N. A., Metcalf, D., Matsumoto, M., and Johnson, G. R.,** Purification of a factor inducing differentiation in murine myelomonocytic leukemia cells. Identification as granulocyte colony-stimulating factor, *J. Biol. Chem.,* 258, 9017, 1983.
13. **Tsuchiya, M., Asano, S., Kaziro, Y., and Nagata, S.,** Isolation and characterization of the cDNA for murine granulocyte colony-stimulating factor, *Proc. Natl. Acad. Sci. U.S.A.,* 83, 7633, 1986.

14. **Stanley, E. R. and Heard, P. M.,** Factors regulating macrophage production and growth. Purification and some properties of the colony stimulating factor from medium conditioned by mouse L cells, *J. Biol. Chem.,* 252, 4305, 1977.

15. **DeLamarter, J. F., Hession, C., Semon, D., Gough, N. M., Rothenbuhler, R., and Mermod, J.-J.,** Nucleotide sequence of a cDNA encoding murine CSF-1 (macrophage-CSF), *Nucl. Acids Res.,* 15, 2389, 1987.

16. **Metcalf, D., Cutler, R. L., and Nicola, N. A.,** Selective stimulation by mouse spleen cell conditioned medium of human eosinophil colony formation, *Blood,* 61, 999, 1983.

17. **Sanderson, C. J., O'Garra, A., Warren, D. J., and Klaus, G. C. B.,** Eosinophil differentiation factor also has B-cell growth factor activity: proposed name interleukin 4, *Proc. Natl. Acad. Sci. U.S.A.,* 83, 437, 1986.

18. **Kinashi, T., Harada, N., Severinson, E., Tanabe, T., Sideras, P., Konishi, M., Azuma, C., Tominaga, A., Bergstedt-Lindqvist, S., Takahashi, M., Matsuda, F., Yaoita, Y., Takatsu, K., and Honjo, T.,** Cloning of complementary DNA encoding T-cell replacing factor and identify with B-cell growth factor II, *Nature,* 324, 70, 1986.

19. **Mizel, S. B. and Mizel, D.,** Purification to apparent homogeneity of murine interleukin 1, *J. Immunol.,* 126, 834, 1981.

20. **Lomedico, P. T., Gubler, U., Hellmann, C. P., Dukovich, M., Giri, J. G., Pan, Y.-C. E., Collier, K., Semionow, R., Chua, A. O., and Mizel, S. B.,** Cloning and expression of murine interleukin-1 cDNA in *Escherichia coli, Nature,* 312, 458, 1984.

21. **Riendeau, D., Harnish, D. G., Bleackley, R. C., and Paetkau, V.,** Purification of mouse interleukin 2 to apparent homogeneity, *J. Biol. Chem.,* 258, 12114, 1983.

22. **Fuse, A., Fujita, T., Yasumitsu, H., Kashima, N., Hasegawa, K., and Taniguchi, T.,** Organization and structure of the mouse interleukin-2 gene, *Nucl. Acids Res.,* 12, 9323, 1984.

23. **Ohara, J. and Paul, W. E.,** Production of a monoclonal antibody to and molecular characterization of B-cell stimulatory factor-1, *Nature,* 315, 333, 1985.

24. **Noma, Y., Sideras, P., Naito, T., Bergstedt-Lindqvist, S., Azuma, C., Severinson, E., Tanabe, T., Kinashi, T., Matsuda, F., Yaoita, Y., and Honjo, T.,** Cloning of cDNA encoding the murine IgG1 induction factor by a novel strategy using SP6 promoter, *Nature,* 319, 640, 1986.

25. **Lee, F., Yokota, T., Otsuka, T., Meyerson, P., Villaret, D., Coffman, R., Mosmann, T., Rennick, D., Roehm, N., Smith, C., Zlotnik, A., and Arai, K.,** Isolation and characterization of a mouse interleukin cDNA clone that expresses B-cell stimulatory factor 1 activities and T-cell- and mast-cell-stimulating activities, *Proc. Natl. Acad. Sci. U.S.A.,* 83, 2061, 1986.

26. **Cutler, R. L., Johnson, G. R., and Nicola, N. A.,** Characterization of murine erythropoietin, *Exp. Hematol.,* 13, 899, 1985.

27. **McDonald, J. D., Lin, F-K., and Goldwasser, E.,** Cloning, sequencing, and evolutionary analysis of the mouse erythropoietin gene, *Mol. Cell. Biol.,* 6, 842, 1986.

28. **Shoemaker, C. B. and Mitsock, L. D.,** Murine erythropoietin gene: cloning, expression, and human gene homology, *Mol. Cell. Biol.,* 6, 849, 1986.

29. **Ymer, S., Tucker, W. Q. J., Sanderson, C. J., Hapel, A. J., Campbell, H. D., and Young, I. G.,** Constitutive synthesis of interleukin-3 by leukaemia cell line WEHI-3B is due to retroviral insertion near the gene, *Nature,* 317, 255, 1985.

30. **McNeil, T. A.,** Release of bone marrow colony stimulating activity during immunological reactions *in vitro, Nature (London) (New Biol.),* 244, 175, 1973.

31. **Parker, J. W. and Metcalf, D.,** Production of colony-stimulating factor in mixed leucocyte cultures, *Immunology,* 26, 1039, 1974.

32. **Parker, J. W. and Metcalf, D.,** Production of colony-stimulating factor in mitogen-stimulated lymphocyte cultures, *J. Immunol.,* 112, 502, 1974.

33. **Metcalf, D. and Johnson, G. R.,** Production by spleen and lymph node cells of conditioned medium with erythroid and other hemopoietic colony-stimulating activity, *J. Cell. Physiol.,* 96, 31, 1978.

34. **Schreier, M. H. and Iscove, N. N.,** Haematopoietic growth factors are released in cultures of H-2-restricted helper T cells, accessory cells and specific antigen, *Nature,* 287, 228, 1980.

35. **Ralph, P., Broxmeyer, H. E., Moore, M. A. S., and Nakoinz, I.,** Induction of myeloid colony-stimulating activity in murine monocyte tumor cell lines by macrophage activators and in a T-cell line by concanavalin A., *Cancer Res.,* 38, 1414, 1978.

36. **Watson, J. D.,** Biology and biochemistry of T cell-derived lymphokines. I. The coordinate synthesis of interleukin 2 and colony-stimulating factors in a murine T cell lymphoma, *J. Immunol.,* 131, 293, 1983.

37. **Howard, M., Burgess, A., McPhee, D., and Metcalf, D.,** T-cell hybridoma secreting hemopoietic regulatory molecules: granulocyte-macrophage and eosinophil colony-stimulating factors, *Cell,* 18, 993, 1979.

38. **Schrader, J. W., Arnold, B., and Clark-Lewis, I.,** A Con A-stimulated T-cell hybridoma releases factors affecting haemopoietic colony-forming cells and B cell antibody responses, *Nature,* 283, 197, 1980.

39. **Burgess, A. W., Bartlett, P. F., Metcalf, D., Nicola, N. A., Clark-Lewis, I., and Schrader, J. W.,** Granulocyte-macrophage colony-stimulating factor produced by an inducible murine T-cell hybridoma: molecular properties and cellular specificity, *Exp. Hematol.,* 9, 893, 1981.

40. **Nabel, G., Greenberger, J. S., Sakakeeny, M. A., and Cantor, H.,** Multiple biological activities of a cloned inducer T-cell population, *Proc. Natl. Acad. Sci. U.S.A.,* 78, 1157, 1981.

41. **Ely, J. M., Prystowsky, M. B., Eisenberg, L., Quintans, J., Goldwasser, E., Glasebrook, A. L., and Fitch, F. W.,** Alloreactive cloned T cell lines. V. Differential kinetics of IL-2, CSF, and BCSF released by a cloned T amplifier cell and its variant, *J. Immunol.,* 127, 2345, 1981.

42. **Staber, F. G., Hultner, L., Marcucci, F., and Krammer, P. H.,** Production of colony-stimulating factors by murine T cells in limiting dilution and long-term cultures, *Nature,* 298, 79, 1982.

43. **Kelso, A., Glasebrook, A. L., Kanagawa, O., and Brunner, K. T.,** Production of macrophage-activating factor by T lymphocyte clones and correlation with other lymphokine activities, *J. Immunol.,* 129, 550, 1982.

44. **Prystowsky, M. B., Ely, J. M., Beller, D. I., Eisenberg, L., Goldman, J., Goldman, M., Goldwasser, E., Ihle, J., Quintans, J., Remold, H., Vogel, S. N., and Fitch, F. W.,** Alloreactive cloned T cell lines. VI. Multiple lymphokine activities secreted by helper and cytolytic cloned T lymphocytes, *J. Immunol.,* 129, 2337, 1982.

45. **Guerne, P.-A., Piguet, P.-F., and Vassalli, P.,** Production of interleukin 2, interleukin 3, and interferon by mouse T lymphocyte clones of Lyt-2$^+$ and -2$^-$ phenotype, *J. Immunol.,* 132, 1869, 1984.

46. **Kelso, A. and Glasebrook, A. L.,** Secretion of interleukin 2, macrophage-activating factor, interferon, and colony-stimulating factor by alloreactive T lymphocyte clones, *J. Immunol.,* 132, 2924, 1984.

47. **Sanderson, C. J., Strath, M., Warren, D. J., O'Garra, A., and Kirkwood, T. B. L.,** The production of lymphokines by primary alloreactive T-cell clones: a co-ordinate analysis of 233 clones in seven lymphokine assays, *Immunology,* 56, 575, 1985.

48. **Kelso, A. and Metcalf, D.,** The characteristics of colony stimulating factor production by murine T-lymphocyte clones, *Exp. Hematol.,* 13, 7, 1985.

49. **Mosmann, T. R., Cherwinski, H., Bond, M. W., Giedlin, M. A., and Coffman, R. L.,** Two types of murine helper T cell clone. I. Definition according to profiles of lymphokine activities and secreted proteins, *J. Immunol.,* 136, 2348, 1986.

50. **Johnson, G. R. and Metcalf, D.,** Pure and mixed erythroid colony formation *in vitro* stimulated by spleen conditioned medium with no detectable erythropoietin, *Proc. Natl. Acad. Sci. U.S.A.,* 74, 3879, 1977.

51. **Dexter, T. M., Garland, J., Scott, D., Scolnick, E., and Metcalf, D.,** Growth of factor-dependent hemopoietic precursor cell lines, *J. Exp. Med.,* 152, 1036, 1980.

52. **Metcalf, D.,** Molecular control of granulocyte and macrophage production, in *Experimental Approaches for the Study of Hemoglobin Switching,* Stamatoyannopoulos, G. and Nienhuis, A., Eds., Alan R. Liss, New York, 1985, 323.

53. **Greenberger, J. S., Sakakeeny, M. A., Humphries, R. K., Eaves, C. J., and Eckner, R. J.,** Demonstration of permanent factor-dependent multipotential (erythroid/neutrophil/basophil) hematopoietic progenitor cell lines, *Proc. Natl. Acad. Sci. U.S.A.,* 80, 2931, 1983.

54. **Gillis, S., Ferm, M. M., Ou, W., and Smith, K. A.,** T cell growth factor: parameters of production and a quantitative microassay for activity, *J. Immunol.,* 120, 2027, 1978.

55. **Kelso, A., Metcalf, D., and Gough, N. M.,** Independent regulation of granulocyte-macrophage colony-stimulating factor and multi-lineage colony-stimulating factor production in T lymphocyte clones, *J. Immunol.,* 136, 1718, 1986.

56. **Burgess, A. W., Metcalf, D., Russell, S. H. M., and Nicola, N. A.,** Granulocyte/macrophage-, megakaryocyte-, eosinophil- and erythroid-colony-stimulating factors produced by mouse spleen cells, *Biochem. J.,* 185, 301, 1980.

57. **Lopez, A. F., Begley, C. G., Williamson, D. J., Warren, D. J., Vadas, M. A., and Sanderson, C. J.,** Murine eosinophil differentiation factor: an eosinophil-specific colony-stimulating factor with activity for human cells, *J. Exp. Med.,* 163, 1085, 1986.

58. **Kelso, A. and Metcalf, D.,** Clonal heterogeneity in colony stimulating factor production by murine T lymphocytes, *J. Cell. Physiol.,* 123, 101, 1985.

59. **Farrar, J. J., Fuller-Farrar, J., Simon, P. L., Hilfiker, M. L., Stadler, B. M., and Farrar, W. L.,** Thymoma production of T cell growth factor, *J. Immunol.,* 125, 2555, 1980.

60. **Swain, S. L.,** Significance of Lyt phenotypes: Lyt 2 antibodies block activities of T cells that recognize class I major histocompatibility complex antigens regardless of their function, *Proc. Natl. Acad. Sci. U.S.A.,* 78, 7101, 1981.

61. **Dialynas, D. P., Wilde, D. B., Marrack, P., Pierres, A., Wall, K. A., Havran, W., Otten, G., Loken, M. R., Pierres, M., Kappler, J., and Fitch, F. W.,** Characterization of the murine antigenic determinant, designated L3T4a, recognized by monoclonal antibody GK1.5: expression of L3T4a by functional T cell clones appears to correlate primarily with class II MHC antigen-reactivity, *Immunol. Rev.,* 74, 30, 1983.

62. **Kelso, A. and MacDonald, H. R.,** Precursor frequency analysis of lymphokine-secreting alloreactive T lymphocytes. Dissociation of subsets producing interleukin 2, macrophage-activating factor, and granulo-cyte-macrophage colony-stimulating factor on the basis of Lyt-2 phenotype, *J. Exp. Med.,* 156, 1366, 1982.

63. **Rosenberg, S. A., Grimm, E. A., McGrogan, M., Doyle, M., Kawasaki, E., Koths, K., and Mark, D. F.,** Biological activity of recombinant human interleukin-2 produced in *Escherichia coli, Science,* 233, 1412, 1984.

64. **Miller, R. A. and Stutman, O.,** Limiting dilution analysis of T helper cell heterogeneity: a single class of T cell makes both IL 2 and IL 3, *J. Immunol.,* 130, 1749, 1983.

65. **Guerne, P.-A., Piguet, P.-F., and Vassalli, P.,** Positively selected Lyt-2$^+$ and Lyt-2$^-$ mouse T lymphocytes are comparable, after Con A stimulation, in release of IL 2 and of lymphokines acting on B cells, macrophages, and mast cells, but differ in interferon production, *J. Immunol.,* 130, 2225, 1983.

66. **Sanderson, C. J., Warren, D. J., and Strath, M.,** Identification of a lymphokine that stimulates eosinophil differentiation *in vitro.* Its relationship to interleukin 3, and functional properties of eosinophils produced in cultures, *J. Exp. Med.,* 162, 60, 1985.

67. **Owens, T. and Miller, J. F. A. P.,** Interaction *in vivo* between hapten-specific suppressor T cells and *in vitro* cultured helper T cell line, *J. Immunol.,* 138, in press, 1987.

68. **Staerz, U. D., Rammensee, H.-G., Benedetto, J. D., and Bevan, M. J.,** Characterization of a murine monoclonal antibody specific for an allotypic determinant on T cell antigen receptor, *J. Immunol.,* 134, 3994, 1985.

69. **Sim, G. K. and Augustin, A. A.,** Vβ gene polymorphism and a major polyclonal T cell receptor idiotype, *Cell,* 42, 89, 1985.

70. **Kelso, A. and Gough, N.,** Expression of hemopoietic growth factor genes in murine T lymphocytes, in *Lymphokines,* Vol. 13, 1987, 209.

71. **Howard, M., Matis, L., Malek, T. R., Shevach, E., Kell, W., Cohen, D., Nakanishi, K., and Paul, W. E.,** Interleukin 2 induces antigen-reactive T cell lines to secrete BCGF-1, *J. Exp. Med.,* 158, 2024, 1983.

72. **Inaba, K., Granelli-Piperno, A., and Steinman, R. M.,** Dendritic cells induce T lymphocytes to release B cell-stimulating factors by an interleukin 2-dependent mechanism, *J. Exp. Med.,* 158, 2040, 1983.

73. **Farrar, W. L., Birchenall-Sparks, M. C., and Young, H. B.,** Interleukin 2 induction of interferon-γ mRNA synthesis, *J. Immunol.,* 137, 3836, 1986.

74. **Kelso, A., MacDonald, H. R., Smith, K. A., Cerottini, J.-C., and Brunner, K. T.,** Interleukin 2 enhancement of lymphokine secretion by T lymphocytes: analysis of established clones and primary limiting dilution microcultures, *J. Immunol.,* 132, 2932, 1984.

75. **Taylor, M. V., Metcalfe, J. C., Hesketh, T. R., Smith, G. A., and Moore, J. P.,** Mitogens increase phosphorylation of phosphoinositides in thymocytes, *Nature,* 312, 462, 1984.

76. **Truneh, A., Albert, F., Golstein, P., and Schmitt-Verhulst, A.,** Early steps of lymphocyte activation bypassed by synergy between calcium ionophores and phorbol ester, *Nature,* 313, 318, 1985.

77. **Imboden, J. B., Weiss, A., and Stobo, J. D.,** Transmembrane signalling by the T3-antigen receptor complex, *Immunol. Today,* 6, 328, 1985.

78. **Harris, D. T., Kozumbo, W. J., Cerutti, P., and Cerottini, J.-C.,** Molecular mechanisms involved in T cell activation. I. Evidence for independent signal-transducing pathways in lymphokine production vs proliferation in cloned cytotoxic T lymphocytes, *J. Immunol.,* 138, 600, 1987.

79. **Kozumbo, W. J., Harris, D. T., Gromkowski, S., Cerottini, J.-C., and Cerutti, P. A.,** Molecular mechanisms involved in T cell activation. II. The phosphatidylinositol signal-transducing mechanism mediates antigen-induced lymphokine production but not interleukin 2-induced proliferation in cloned cytotoxic T lymphocytes, *J. Immunol.,* 138, 606, 1987.

80. **Cantrell, D., Davies, A. A., Londei, M., Feldman, M., and Crumpton, M. J.,** Association of phosphorylation of the T3 antigen with immune activation of T lymphocytes, *Nature,* 325, 540, 1987.

81. **Farrar, W. L. and Anderson, W. B.,** Interleukin-2 stimulates association of protein kinase C with plasma membrane, *Nature,* 315, 233, 1985.

82. **Mills, G. B., Cheung, R. K., Grinstein, S., and Gelfand, E.,** Interleukin 2-induced lymphocyte proliferation is independent of increases in cytosolic-free calcium concentrations, *J. Immunol.,* 134, 2431, 1985.

83. **Metcalfe, S.,** Cyclosporine does not prevent cytoplasmic calcium changes associated with lymphocyte activation, *Transplantation,* 38, 161, 1984.

84. **Wiskocil, R., Weiss, A., Imboden, J., Kamin-Lewis, R., and Stobo, J.,** Activation of a human T cell line: a two-stimulus requirement in the pretranstational events involved in the coordinate expression of interleukin 2 and γ interferon genes, *J. Immunol.,* 134, 1599, 1985.

85. **Elliott, J. F., Lin, Y., Mizel, S. B., Bleackley, R. C., Harnish, D. G., and Paetkau, V.,** Induction of interleukin 2 messenger RNA inhibited by cyclosporin A, *Science,* 226, 1439, 1984.

86. **Granelli-Piperno, A., Inaba, K., and Steinman, R. M.,** Stimulation of lymphokine release from T lymphoblasts. Requirement for mRNA synthesis and inhibition by cyclosporin A, *J. Exp. Med.,* 160, 1792, 1984.

87. **Owens, T. and Fazekas de St. Groth, B.,** Participation of L3T4 in T cell activation in the absence of class II MHC: inhibition by anti-L3T4 antibodies is a function both of epitope density and mode of presentation of anti-receptor antibody, *J. Immunol.,* 138, 2402, 1987.

88. **Samelson, L. E., Harford, J., Schwartz, R. H., and Klausner, R. D.,** A 20-kDa protein associated with the murine T-cell antigen receptor is phosphorylated in response to activation by antigen or concanavalin A, *Proc. Natl. Acad. Sci. U.S.A.,* 82, 1969, 1985.

89. **Oettgen, H. C., Pettey, C. L., Maloy, W. L., and Terhorst, C.,** A T3-like protein complex associated with the antigen receptor on murine T cells, *Nature,* 320, 272, 1986.

90. **Fazekas de St. Groth, B., Thomas, W. R., McKimm-Breschkin, J. L., Clark-Lewis, I., Schrader, J. W., and Miller, J. F. A. P.,** P cell stimulating factor release: a useful assay of T cell activation *in vitro, Int. Arch. Allergy Appl. Immunol.,* 79, 169, 1986.

91. **Herold, K. C., Lancki, D. W., Dunn, D. E., Arai, K., and Fitch, F. W.,** Activation of lymphokine genes during stimulation of cloned T cells, *Eur. J. Immunol.,* 16, 1533, 1986.

92. **Gough, N. M.,** Core and e antigen synthesis in rodent cells transformed with hepatitis B virus DNA is associated with greater than genome length viral messenger RNAs, *J. Mol. Biol.,* 165, 683, 1983.

93. **Melton, D. A., Krieg, P. A., Rebagliati, M. R., Maniatis, T., Zinn, K., and Green, M. R.,** Efficient *in vitro* synthesis of biologically active RNA and RNA hybridization probes from plasmids containing a bacteriophage SP6 promoter, *Nucl. Acids Res.,* 12, 7035, 1984.

94. **Barlow, D. P., Bucan, M., Lehrach, H., Hogan, B. L. M., and Gough, N. M.,** Close genetic and physical linkage between the murine haemopoietic growth factor genes GM-CSF and multi-CSF (IL-3), *EMBO J.,* 6, 617, 1987.

95. **Steinmann, G., Conlon, P., Hefeneider, S., and Gillis, S.,** Serological visualization of interleukin 2, *Science,* 220, 1188, 1983.

96. **Metcalf, D., Burgess, A. W., Johnson, G. R., Nicola, N. A., Nice, E. C., DeLamarter, J., Thatcher, D. R., and Mermod, J.-J.,** *In vitro* actions on hemopoietic cells of recombinant murine GM-CSF purified after production in *Escherichia coli:* comparison with purified native GM-CSF, *J. Cell. Physiol.,* 128, 421, 1986.

97. **Kelso, A.,** An assay for colony-stimulating factor (CSF) production by single T lymphocytes: estimation of the frequency of cells producing granulocyte-macrophage CSF and multi-lineage CSF within a T lymphocyte clone, *J. Immunol.,* 136, 2930, 1986.

98. **Kelso, A. and Owens, T.,** Production of two hemopoietic growth factors is differentially regulated in single T lymphocytes activated with an anti-T cell receptor antibody, *J. Immunol.,* 140, 1159, 1988.

99. **Meuer, S. C., Hodgdon, J. C., Hussey, R. E., Protentis, J. P., Schlossman, S. F., and Reinherz, E. L.,** Antigen-like effects of monoclonal antibodies directed at receptors on human T cell clones, *J. Exp. Med.,* 158, 988, 1983.

100. **Gill, R. G., Babcock, S. K., and Lafferty, K. J.,** A quantitative analysis of antigen-triggered lymphokine production by activated T cells, *J. Immunol.,* 138, 1130, 1987.

101. **Crispe, I. N., Bevan, M. J., and Staerz, U. D.,** Selective activation of Lyt 2$^+$ precursor T cells by ligation of the antigen receptor, *Nature,* 317, 627, 1985.

102. **Arai, K., Yokota, T., Miyajima, A., Arai, N., and Lee, F.,** Molecular biology of T-cell-derived lymphokines: a model system for proliferation and differentiation of hemopoietic cells, *BioEssays,* 5, 166, 1986.

103. **Seigel, L. J., Harper, M. E., Wong-Staal, F., Gallo, R. C., Nash, W. G., and O'Brien, S. J.,** Gene for T-cell growth factor: location on human chromosome 4q and feline chromosome B1, *Science,* 223, 175, 1984.

104. **Naylor, S. L., Sakaguchi, A. Y., Shows, T. B., Law, M. L., Goeddel, D. V., and Gray, P. W.,** Human immune interferon gene is located on chromosome 12, *J. Exp. Med.,* 157, 1020, 1983.

105. **Le Beau, M. M., Westbrook, C. A., Diaz, M. O., Larson, R. A., Rowley, J. D., Gasson, J. C., Golde, D. W., and Sherr, C. J.,** Evidence for the involvement of GM-CSF and FMS in the deletion (5q) in myeloid disorders, *Science,* 231, 984, 1986.

106. **Pettenati, M. J., Le Beau, M. M., Lemons, R. S., Kawasaki, E. S., Larson, R. A., Sherr, C. J., Diaz, M. O., and Rowley, J. D.,** Assignment of *CSF-1* to 5q33.1: evidence for clustering of genes regulating hematopoiesis and for their involvement in the 5q$^-$ anomaly, *Proc. Natl. Acad. Sci. U.S.A.,* in press, 1987.

107. **Efrat, S., Pilo, S., and Kaempfer, R.,** Kinetics of induction and molecular size of mRNAs encoding human interleukin-2 and γ-interferon, *Nature,* 297, 236, 1982.

108. **Efrat, S. and Kaempfer, R.,** Control of biologically active interleukin 2 messenger RNA formation in induced human lymphocytes, *Proc. Natl. Acad. Sci. U.S.A.,* 81, 2601, 1984.

109. **Shaw, G. and Kamen, R.,** A conserved AU sequence from the 3' untranslated region of GM-CSF mRNA mediates selective mRNA degradation, *Cell,* 46, 659, 1986.

110. **Chan, J. Y., Slamon, D. J., Nimer, S. D., Golde, D. W., and Gasson, J. C.,** Regulation of expression of human granulocyte/macrophage colony-stimulating factor, *Proc. Natl. Acad. Sci. U.S.A.,* 83, 8669, 1986.

111. **Miyatake, S., Otsuka, T., Yokoto, T., Lee, F., and Arai, K.**, Structure of the chromosomal gene for granulocyte-macrophage colony stimulating factor: comparison of the mouse and human genes, *EMBO J.*, 4, 2561, 1985.

112. **Nimer, S. D., Chan, J., Golde, D. W., and Gasson, J. C.**, Identification of regulatory sequences in the 5' flanking region of GM-CSF gene (abstract), *J. Cell. Biochem.*, 11A(Suppl.), 219, 1987.

113. **Fujita, T., Shibuya, H., Ohashi, T., Yamanishi, K., and Taniguchi, T.**, Regulation of human interleukin-2 gene: functional DNA sequences in the 5' flanking region for the gene expression in activated T lymphocytes, *Cell*, 46, 401, 1986.

114. **Hapel, A. J., Fung, M. C., Johnson, R. M., Young, I. G., Johnson, G., and Metcalf, D.**, Biologic properties of molecularly cloned and expressed murine interleukin-3, *Blood*, 65, 1453, 1985.

115. **Metcalf, D., Begley, C. G., Williamson, D. J., Nice, E. C., DeLamarter, J., Mermod, J.-J., Thatcher, D., and Schmidt, A.**, Hemopoietic responses in mice injected with purified recombinant murine GM-CSF, *Exp. Hematol.*, 15, 1, 1987.

116. **Metcalf, D., Begley, C. G., Johnson, G. R., Nicola, N. A., Lopez, A. F., and Williamson, D. J.**, Effects of purified bacterially synthesized murine multi-CSF (IL-3) on hematopoiesis in normal adult mice, *Blood*, 68, 46, 1986.

117. **Walker, F. and Burgess, A. W.**, Specific binding of radioiodinated granulocyte-macrophage colony-stimulating factor to hemopoietic cells, *EMBO J.*, 4, 933, 1985.

118. **Nicola, N. A. and Metcalf, D.**, Binding of iodinated multipotential colony-stimulating factor (interleukin-3) to murine bone marrow cells, *J. Cell. Physiol.*, 128, 180, 1986.

119. **Burgess, A. W. and Metcalf, D.**, Characterization of a serum factor stimulating the differentiation of myelomonocytic leukemic cells, *Int. J. Cancer*, 26, 647, 1980.

120. **Garland, J. M., Aldridge, A., Wagstaffe, J., and Dexter, T. M.**, Studies on the *in vivo* production of a lymphokine activity, interleukin 3 (IL-3) elaborated by lymphocytes and a myeloid leukaemic line *in vitro* and the fate of IL-3 dependent cell lines, *Br. J. Cancer*, 48, 247, 1983.

121. **Lopez, A. F., Williamson, D. J., Gamble, J. R., Begley, C. G., Harlan, J. M., Klebanoff, S. J., Waltersdorph, A., Wong, G., Clark, S. C., and Vadas, M. A.**, Recombinant human granulocyte-macrophage colony-stimulating factor stimulates *in vitro* mature human neutrophil and eosinophil function, surface receptor expression, and survival, *J. Clin. Invest.*, 78, 1220, 1986.

122. **Gough, N. M. and Kelso, A.**, unpublished data.

123. **Kelso, A. and Owens, T.**, The role of CD4 in antigen-independent activation of isolated single T lymphocytes, *Cell. Immunol.*, 116, 99, 1988.

124. **Nicola, N. A., Walker, F., and Kelso, A.**, unpublished data.

125. **Kelso, A. and Gough, N. M.**, Differential inhibition by cyclosporin A reveals two pathways for activation of lymphokine synthesis in T cells, *Growth Factors*, 1, in press, 1989.

126. **Gough, N. M. and Kelso, A.**, GM-CSF expression is preferential to multi-CSF (IL-3) expression in murine T lymphocyte clones, *Growth Factors*, in press, 1989.

Chapter 12

LYMPHOKINES AND TUMOR IMMUNITY*

Marion C. Cohen

TABLE OF CONTENTS

I. INTRODUCTION

Lymphokines, as hormone-like products of lymphocytes, are involved in a wide variety of immunologic and inflammatory responses via their effects on cell proliferation, movement, differentiation, and activation. They are protein or glycoprotein in nature, and generally have molecular weights ranging from 10,000 to 70,000 Da. These mediators fall into two discrete categories: afferent lymphokines are involved in the inductive phase of the immune response, while efferent, or effector lymphokines, are involved in various effector manifestations of host defense. Effector lymphokines include those that mediate inflammatory responses and those that are directly cytotoxic to target cells. Afferent lymphokines are considered to be involved mainly in the various processes that lead to functionally active lymphocytes and lymphocyte products.

The role of lymphokines as regulators of these events has been well documented, however, it has also been found that lymphokines can regulate nonimmunologic and non-inflammatory cell types as well.[1] Of particular interest is their role in affecting tumor cells. Most of the work in tumor immunity has focused on the cytotoxic events that lead to the actual destruction of tumor cells by lymphokines. More recently, however, lymphokines have been shown to be capable of modifying the functions of tumor cells that are involved in the expression of their malignant potential. This raises the possibility that there are other ways to control the spread of a tumor that do not involve cell killing. Both of these aspects of tumor immunity are discussed.

II. CELL-MEDIATED IMMUNE RESPONSES

The earliest studies of the role of lymphokines in tumor immunity were performed to assess the immune status of patients with cancer. These involved both analyses of their cell-mediated immune status in general as well as their reactivity against tumor-associated antigens in particular. These studies have been reviewed recently.[2] Generally, these studies involved the production of lymphokines by lymphocytes from tumor-bearing animals or patients with cancer in response to extract prepared from the tumors in question, or the ability of these lymphocytes to respond to mitogen stimulation. Target cells were usually peritoneal exudate cells or leukocytes obtained from normal blood. Some studies also examined the sera of patients with tumors for lymphokines. The results obtained from various laboratories are inconsistent because of the lack of standardization in antigen preparation and differences in techniques, as well as different methods of statistical evaluation. For these reasons these tests cannot be used for immunodiagnosis or monitoring of cell-mediated immune reactions in patients with cancer at the present time.

III. CYTOTOXIC LYMPHOKINES

As stated above, most studies of cell-mediated immunity in neoplastic diseases focus on events which lead to destruction of tumor cells. Lymphokines participate in cytotoxic reactions in three ways: (1) directly (lymphotoxins); (2) indirectly by expanding or inducing effector populations of lymphocytes (γ-interferon, γ-IFN, interleukin-2, IL-2); and (3) indirectly by activating effector inflammatory cells such as macrophages (macrophage activating factor(s)).

A. LYMPHOTOXIN

Lymphotoxin (LT) was first defined as a protein released from T cells after activation with mitogen or specific antigen that killed syngeneic rat or mouse primary fibroblasts as well as a continuous mouse fibroblast line, L929.[3,4] More recently it has been found that other cell types, including tumor cells, are also sensitive to LT.[5-10] LT has been described in a number of species including mouse, rat, guinea pig, Syrian hamster, and human.[3,4,11]

LT is not one molecule but is, in fact, a heterogeneous family of molecules with regard to both size, charge, and antigenicity, and certain forms are unstable.[12] LT forms have been organized into five discrete molecular weight classes with some of them containing multiple subclasses.[6,13-17] Some members of the different molecular weight classes have been found to be interrelated and form a system of subunits which can assemble and disassemble.[13,18,19] It has become clear that individual LT forms may have roles other than direct cell lysis. LT has been implicated in cytolytic T lymphocyte-mediated cytotoxicity,[20,21] antibody-dependent cell-mediated cytotoxicity (ADCC),[22] and natural killer (NK) cell cytotoxicity reactions.[23-25] In addition, it has been found that LT can synergize with other lymphokines such as IFN to increase its growth inhibitory effects[10,26-30] and inhibit hematopoietic colony formation.[31]

Both partially purified preparations of human LT as well as material purified to homogeneity have been reported.[32-34] In addition, it has been possible to purify some of the subunit forms as well.[12] Recently, Gray et al.[35] succeeded in the cloning and expression of DNA sequences encoding human LT. Their data suggest that human LT is encoded by a single gene. In this study it was also found that tumor necrosis followed the injection of recombinant or natural lymphotoxin into Meth A transplants in CB6F1 mice.

LT-containing supernatants appear to exert multiple effects on target cells *in vitro*. These range from reversible growth inhibition at low concentrations to irreversible growth inhibition at intermediate concentrations and cytolysis at high concentrations.[36] There are some reports that LT causes more effective cytostasis and cytolysis of tumor cells than primary cells.[37,38] Attempts have been made to define the mechanism by which LT exerts its effects, however, most of the studies to date have been performed utilizing partially purified preparations so that the results are not conclusive. There is evidence that LT binds to its target cells,[39] that it causes alterations in plasma membrane lipids and protein turnover,[40,41] and that it results in changes in the cell membrane and cytoskeleton.[42] Okamoto and Mayer[43] have described an increase in calcium uptake by target cells, although other studies have shown that LT-induced cytotoxicity is observed in calcium-free medium and over a range of calcium concentrations thus arguing against cell death being due to a massive influx of calcium into the cell.[44] Recently, it was found that LT supernatants cause release of DNA from targets in discretely sized multiples of 200 bp.[45]

It has been almost impossible to recover cell-free lymphotoxins after specific reactions between immune lymphocytes and target cells. Therefore, it must be assumed either that lymphotoxins, if generated by such interactions, are present in smaller quantities than those usually generated by antigen- or mitogen-stimulated lymphocytes or that the production and consumption of lymphotoxins occur in the limited area adjacent to the area of contact.

B. TUMOR NECROSIS FACTOR

Tumor necrosis factor (TNF) is a factor secreted by macrophages, and is therefore a monokine, not a lymphokine. It has been found to cause necrosis of some tumors *in vivo* and is cytotoxic or cytostatic to tumor cells in tissue culture. TNF has been found to share significant homology with LT as well as to be encoded by the same chromosome.[46,47] Nonetheless, it has been shown that the TNF and LT genes, while closely linked, are independently regulated.[48] TNF was originally identified as an activity present in the sera of mice treated sequentially with Bacillus Calmette-Guerin and endotoxin.[49] This activity caused hemorrhagic necrosis of Meth A sarcomas *in vivo* as well as inhibition of the growth of certain murine and human tumor cells *in vitro*.[50-53] TNF has also been identified in supernatants prepared from cells of human origins[54] and when purified has been found to be separable from IFNs α, β, and γ. However, its action is synergistic with IFN[53,55,56] although there is some evidence that under appropriate conditions it can lead to regression of tumors without additional factors.[57] The mode of action of TNF has not been identified, but it has been suggested that its antitumor effect results from an indirect mechanism related to the growth of the implanted tumors rather than to direct cytotoxic effects.[58] In addition, ^{31}P-NMR studies have shown that injection of tumors with TNF results in significant and rapid alterations in the spectral profiles of phosphorylmonoesters and phosphoryldiesters as well as an increase in intratumor pH.[59]

In addition, cachectin, a macrophage product which reduces lipoprotein lipase activity in cultured adipocytes, is thought to contribute to the cachectic state in cancer and chronic infections[60-62] and appears to be involved in the pathogenesis of endotoxic shock.[63] It is also likely to be TNF based on cell source, subunit molecular weight, and N-terminal amino acid sequence.[61] Thus, the evidence is increasing that the cytotoxic and growth inhibitory effects of TNF on tumor cells may be only a small part of the role TNF plays in metabolic and inflammatory processes. Nonetheless, it is clear that a proportion of tumor cells are TNF susceptible and this soluble factor could play a role in cytotoxic events involving neoplastic cells.[64]

C. INTERFERON-γ

IFN-γ was first described by Wheelock[65] as an IFN-like protein produced by human mononuclear cells exposed to phytohemagglutinin (PHA). The aim of the experiments was to study IFN induction by viruses in white blood cells and PHA was used to agglutinate and remove red blood cells from fresh human blood. However, in the absence of virus, cultures of human blood cells exposed to PHA also produced a factor with antiviral activity. Unlike typical IFN, the activity found in these cultures was destroyed by exposure to pH 2. Other investigators confirmed that various mitogens and bacterial products could stimulate IFN production in lymphocytes[66] and that IFN could be induced in sensitized lymphocytes exposed to specific antigens.[67] In 1973, Youngner and Salvin[68] observed that this IFN was antigenically distinct from that produced in response to viruses or double-stranded RNA. In addition it was noted that its production occurs together with other lymphokine activities.[69]

Human IFN-γ has been cloned and sequenced and appears to be encoded by a single gene.[70] The human gene has been localized to chromosome 12.[71] IFN-γ appears to have a number of important biological activities including induction of class II histocompatibility antigens,[72-74] induction of immunoglobulin Fc receptors,[75,76] activation of NK[77,78] and cytotoxic T lymphocytes,[79] inhibition of cell growth,[80] and, most important for this review, activation of macrophages for tumor cell cytotoxicity and antimicrobial activity.[70] Debate continues as to whether IFN-γ is the well-known macrophage activating factor (MAF) defined previously in a variety of *in vitro* and *in vivo* systems,[81] as described in a subsequent section of this chapter, as it has been difficult to separate these factors by physicochemical characterization. For example, using human monocytes as effector cells and K-562 targets, Sadlik et al.[82] found MAF and IFN-γ to be identical by a number of different criteria, including FPLC, monoclonal anti-IFN-γ antibody, and analysis of human T-cell clones. In contrast, however, it has also been found that lymphokines distinct from IFN-γ can induce macrophage tumoricidal activity.[83-86] Thus, it would appear that IFN-γ is MAF, but the converse is not necessarily true. In other words, IFN-γ is one of a class of MAFs. The existence of multiple MAFs is hardly surprising, given the large number of macrophage functions "available" for activation, including production of complement, prostaglandins, IL-1, and matrix components, as well as cytotoxicity, phagocytosis, immunologic presentation, and wound healing.

The association of IFN-γ as a MAF for tumor cytotoxicity began in the early 1970s when it was noticed in several laboratories that macrophages isolated from animals undergoing allograft or tumor rejection, or recovering from facultative intracellular pathogen infection, were capable of killing a variety of neoplastic cells *in vitro* and that a lymphokine was required for induction of this tumoricidal activity.[87] It was not until it was possible to construct T cell hybridomas that the question of whether MAF and IFN-γ were identical could be better resolved. Some studies have reported the production of murine T cell hybridomas which show coordinate production of both MAF and IFN-γ.[88,89] Other groups have reported the presence of MAF activity without antiviral activity in supernatants derived from T cell hybridomas.[83,85,90,91] Nonetheless, it has been shown that IFN-γ is sufficient to activate macrophages for killing.[92,93]

D. MACROPHAGE ACTIVATING FACTOR(S)

Supernatants from cultures of stimulated lymphocytes have been shown to contain factors that are able to induce tumoricidal activity in macrophages *in vitro*.[94-97] As stated above, IFN-γ is an MAF, but investigators have described MAF activity in supernatants found to be free of IFN.[83-86] The *in vitro* assay systems that have been developed vary as to the source of macrophages, the length of the assays, and the use of adherent vs. nonadherent target cells. These factors may account for the observed differences between MAFs.[98] In addition, given the multiplicity of known macrophage functions, it may well turn out that discrete MAFs exist for the activation of one or a limited subset of macrophage properties. The availability of recombinant MAFs from a variety of sources would provide an answer to this question. Recently, it has been found that partially purified MAF derived from a B-lymphoblastoid cell line was capable of reducing the size of some tumors during a phase I clinical trial.[99]

E. INTERLEUKIN 2

IL-2, a lymphokine produced by T lymphoid cells,[100] has a broad range of immuno-regulatory activities *in vitro*, which appear to result from its ability to expand subpopulations of T cells that bear IL-2 receptors.[101] IL-2 can induce the release of other lymphokines such as IFN-γ and B cell growth factors, as well as activate cytotoxic and helper T-cells.[102-106] It has been shown that incubation of either murine splenocytes or human peripheral blood lymphocytes from normal or tumor-bearing hosts in lymphokine preparations containing IL-2 leads to the generation of lymphoid cells capable of lysing fresh autologous or syngeneic tumor cells in chromium-release assays.[107-110] The relationship between these lymphokine-activated killer (LAK) cells, NK cells, and cytotoxic T lymphocytes is still a matter of controversy. Evidence from several different laboratories indicates that many of the characteristics of LAK cell activity can be attributed to stimulation of NK cells by IL-2 and that T cells play only a minor role.[111] It has also been suggested that the cytotoxic effector cell population consists of several different cell types that contribute to the overall cytotoxicity.[112] In any event, the use of IL-2 and IL-2-activated lymphoid cells for the immunotherapy of animal and human tumors has had some success.[113] The major drawback in translating success in treating animal neoplasms to the treatment of human disease has been the toxic side-effects resulting from IL-2 administration in high doses.[114-115] The most important dose-limiting toxic effect is the "vascular leak syndrome", which results in accumulation of extracellular fluid, including ascites, hydrothorax, and pulmonary edema. Recently, there has been a report that IL-2 administration in lower doses on a prolonged schedule may have acceptable toxicity and still induce antitumor responses.[116]

F. INTERLEUKIN 1

IL-1 is a major mediator of the body's responses to microbial invasion, inflammation, immunological reactions, and tissue injury. It was first described as a product of activated phagocytic cells, but is now known to be synthesized by a wide variety of cells including synovial fibroblasts; keratinocytes and Langerhans cells of the skin; mesangial cells of the kidney; B lymphocytes; NK cells; astrocytes and microglial cells of the brain; vascular endothelial and smooth muscle cells; corneal, gingival, and thymic epithelial cells; and some T lymphocyte lines.[117] As such, it is properly described as a cytokine rather than a lymphokine. Moreover, it participates in what has been described as a network of cytokine-induced cytokines which may be important for the augmentation or suppression of various biological properties during host responses to infection or inflammation. For example, IL-1 stimulates the production of IL-2, the IFNs, IL-3, and other colony stimulating factors (CSFs) as well as IL-6.[117]

Two biochemically distinct but structurally related IL-1 molecules have been identified and called IL-1α (pI 5.0) and IL-1β (pI 7.0). Human IL-1α and IL-1β cDNA show 26% homology between their amino acid sequences and 45% homology in their nucleotide sequences.[117] It has been suggested that the major difference between the two species is that the primary translation product of IL-1α is biologically active, while the primary transcript of Il-1β is not biologically active under the same conditions.[118] Another possibility is that the primary transcription product of IL-1α is cleaved to a smaller active form more efficiently than IL-1β and that such cleavage could occur during *in vitro* translation or during the prolonged bioassay of IL-1 activity.[119]

The role of IL-1 in controlling tumor cell growth has not been studied extensively. Macrophages have been reported to exhibit a more prolonged and active tumoricidal state in response to IL-1.[120] Furthermore, it has been shown that purified IL-1 is itself directly cytocidal for some tumor target cells.[121] Thus, it has been suggested that IL-1 could exert antitumor effects by a variety of mechanisms:

1. By augmenting the production of lymphokines such as IL-2, IFN, or TNF which are already known to exert antitumor effects[122-124]
2. By enhancing the activities of cytotoxic T lymphocytes (CTL), NK cells, or monocytes[120,125]
3. By interacting synergistically with IL-2 and IFN to promote CTL and NK activities[126]
4. Perhaps by directly inhibiting the growth of some tumor cells[121,127,128]

IV. NONCYTOTOXIC LYMPHOKINES

A. JOB DESCRIPTION FOR A MALIGNANT CELL

To envision the types of tumor behavior-modifying lymphokine activities that could be protective for the organism, it is necessary to examine the neoplastic process from the point of view of the tumor cell itself. A tumor cell is essentially a parasite, and to live well and prosper it must possess a number of important skills and capabilities. It must:

1. Survive and proliferate locally
2. Invade adjacent tissue
3. Induce supporting stroma and obtain a warm and nourishing blood supply
4. Gain access to the circulation
5. Leave the circulation at a new site
6. Colonize the new location
7. Survive and proliferate at the new site

A lymphokine that can influence one or more of these tumor cell properties could be of potential importance in controlling the growth and spread of malignant cells. We have initially focused on three areas: tumor cell movement, the attachment of tumor cells to endothelium, and regulation of tumor cell proliferation by noncytotoxic means. We have been able to demonstrate the existence of lymphokines that interfere with all of these activities. All are relatively small molecules, with molecular weights of less than 10,000

Da. As such, they appear to represent a previously unrecognized class of lymphokines, since purification procedures until recently usually involved at least one dialysis step in which the pore size of the tubing allowed these factors to be lost in the discarded dialysate.

B. TUMOR MIGRATION INHIBITION FACTOR (TMIF)

We first determined that an ascitic tumor, the P815 mastocytoma, maintained by serial intraperitoneal passage in DBA/2 mice, was capable of migrating from capillary tubes in the presence of RPMI 1640 medium supplemented with serum.[129] The pattern observed was analogous to that seen when inflammatory cells migrate from capillary tubes and was a suitable assay system for the analysis of effects of lymphokines on tumor cell movement. Supernatants with known macrophage migration inhibitory activity (MIF) were prepared from antigen- or mitogen-activated lymphocytes or from long-term lymphoblastoid T- and B-cell lines.[130] Tumor cell migration was inhibited by supernatants of human or murine origin, however, guinea pig MIF-containing supernatants had no effect on the tumor cells.

The observation that migration inhibition of tumor cells was reversible on prolonged incubation (48 to 72 h) provided the first evidence that the effect we were seeing was not due to cytotoxicity. Lack of cytotoxicity in this system was confirmed by trypan blue exclusion studies and radiochromium release experiments.

These studies were extended to other murine ascites tumors including Ehrlich ascites, Hepatoma 129, and Sarcoma 37, as well as the Walker carcinosarcoma which is of rat origin.[131] We also found that dissociated tumor cells from solid neoplasms were inhibited by lymphokine-containing supernatants.[132] More recently, we found that tumor cells from spontaneous human neoplasms are targets for this activity.[133] For these latter experiments we used an agarose microdroplet technique, rather than the capillary tube method, to minimize the number of cells required for assay.[134] This observation suggests that the results obtained in the various model systems may be applicable to humans.

We initially assumed that the inhibition of tumor cell migration that we were observing was due to conventional MIF; however, data obtained from Diaflo ultrafiltration studies indicated that this was not the case. Supernatants prepared from RPMI 8392, one of the long-term lymphoblastoid cell lines, were passed sequentially through PM 30, PM 10, and DM 5 membranes and the retentates concentrated 3-fold. When tested against guinea pig macrophages, the inhibitory activity was found in the PM 10 retentate, indicating a molecular weight greater than 10,000 Da. However, inhibitory activity for mastocytoma cells was found in the DM 5 retentate, indicating a molecular weight of 5000 to 10,000 Da.[131]

This result strongly suggested that the migration inhibitory lymphokine was distinct from MIF and was consistent with our finding that guinea pig lymphocytes could make MIF but could not make the factor affecting tumor cells. In addition, we had previously reported that lymphocytes from C57B1/6 mice cannot generate MIF activity in the absence of serum;[135] however, they can still generate the tumor-affecting factor under these conditions.[131] For these reasons, we believed that this factor represented a new lymphokine, which we named tumor migration inhibition factor, or TMIF.

Our next series of experiments were designed to characterize TMIF and to compare it to other lymphokines known to affect cell migration.[136] The targets of these mediators are inflammatory cells, endothelial cells,[137] and fibroblasts (unpublished observations). Since the efferent lymphokines have not been purified to homogeneity, indirect means must be used to determine whether two factors are the same or different. A single procedure that inhibits one but not the other is not adequate, as the observed results could be due to differences in assay sensitivity. Thus, it is necessary to find reciprocal conditions, such that one experimental procedure destroys one activity without affecting the other, and another experimental procedure does the opposite. As we described eariler, guinea pig-derived lymphokine preparations have MIF but not TMIF activity, and serum-free C57B1/6 mouse-derived lymphokine preparations have TMIF but not MIF activity. In addition, the Amicon ultrafiltration studies resulted in one fraction with MIF and no TMIF, and another with TMIF and no MIF.

We next performed a variety of other characterization procedures. For example, it is known that MIF is inhibited by fucose and rhamnose.[138] Under conditions in which MIF is inhibited by these sugars, TMIF is not. We found that diisopropyl fluorophosphate (DFP) inhibited TMIF but had no effect on MIF, thereby establishing another reciprocal pair for the suppression of MIF and TMIF. DFP can also inhibit leukocyte inhibition factor (LIF), which can inhibit the migration of neutrophils.[139] However, LIF has a molecular weight of approximately 68,000 Da, and it is inhibited by *N*-acetyl-D-galactosamine, whereas TMIF is not. Thus, TMIF is also distinct from LIF.

We have succeeded in producing hybridomas from Concanavalin A (Con A)-stimulated murine spleen cells fused with BW5147, an HAT-sensitive AKR lymphoma that itself does not produce TMIF or MIF.[140] We have obtained several lymphokine-secreting hybridomas, most of which produced both MIF and TMIF. However, one established line makes only TMIF providing further evidence that MIF and TMIF are distinct.

As stated above, TMIF can inhibit the migration of a variety of tumor cells. In addition, we wished to determine whether this factor is unique for neoplastic cells. It is difficult to obtain samples of normal cells that migrate well in the capillary tube or agarose microdroplet assay systems so that a systematic comparison between normal and neoplastic cells that are matched as to cell type (e.g., fibrosarcoma cells and fibroblasts) has not been performed. However, even if the effect by TMIF were not confined to neoplastic cells, it might be expected to exert a differential effect on tumor cells *in vivo* since, under most circumstances, normal cells do not demonstrate local invasiveness or distant dissemination.

Despite these difficulties, to study the effect of TMIF on at least one type of non-neoplastic cell other than an inflammatory cell, we used endothelial cells as migrating target cells. Endothelial cells were obtained from calf pulmonary arteries and cultured according to standard procedures.[141] Their identity as endothelial cells was established by the detection of Factor VIII antigen by indirect immunofluorescence.[142] Migration was studied utilizing the agarose microdroplet technique. Using lymphokine preparations from human lympho-blastoid cell lines, we found that we could inhibit endothelial cell migration reversibly but that this activity tracked with MIF activity through the various characterization procedures.[136] Preparations with TMIF activity, but devoid of other lymphokine activities, were without effect on endothelial cell migration.

We also wished to explore the possible *in vivo* role of TMIF. Mice were immunized with Ehrlich ascites tumor cells and challenged intravenously with a KCl extract of the tumor. Both MIF and TMIF activities were detected in sera collected 6 and 24 h following challenge.[143] We also studied the sera of tumor-bearing mice. Animals were injected with 10^7 tumor cells intraperitoneally, and their sera were tested for MIF and TMIF activities at 3, 5, 7, 9, 11, and 13 d following inoculation. Serum MIF and TMIF activities appeared by day 7 and persisted; however, under these conditions the animals generally die by day 15. Thus, it appears that the presence of endogenous TMIF is not sufficient to protect the host from death. For TMIF to limit tumor spread *in vivo*, it would probably need to be present earlier in the course of tumor growth.

To demonstrate that TMIF could produce a measurable effect *in vivo*, we examined a model analogous to the macrophage disappearance reaction (MDR). In the MDR, the injection of MIF into the peritoneal cavity of animals bearing a macrophage-rich peritoneal exudate leads to a transient reduction in the number of macrophages recoverable from the peritoneal cavity.[144] In the analogous procedure using tumor cells and TMIF,[145] we incubated 10^7 tumor cells for 3 h at 37°C with an unfractionated lymphokine-containing supernatant, the fraction containing MIF activity, the fraction containing TMIF activity, or control medium. The cells were washed and resuspended in 1 ml of the solution in which they had been incubated. They were then injected intraperitoneally into normal mice. Cells were harvested from the peritoneal cavity at various times following injection. Significantly fewer cells were recovered from the animals injected with TMIF-treated tumor cells at 3 h following injection. Although this indicates an *in vivo* effect of TMIF, it is without therapeutic significance, since by 24 h there was no difference between the experimental and control animals. It should be noted that only the partially purified TMIF had this effect. The whole supernatant, although positive in *in vitro* assays did not influence the tumor cells in the peritoneal cavity.

To rule out the possibility that the effect observed was due to an influx of inflammatory cells, supernatants were prepared as described above and injected into the peritoneal cavities of normal mice. The peritoneal cavity was washed at 0, 3, and 24 h following injection, and the total number of cells was determined. Differential cell counts were performed using Giemsa-stained smears. MIF-containing preparations caused an influx of inflammatory cells into the peritoneal cavity, while the fractions with TMIF activity did not. Thus, the effect observed on tumor cells *in vivo* was not due to an inflammatory response to that mediator in the peritoneal cavity. In addition, these results provide yet another distinction between TMIF and MIF.

C. TUMOR BINDING INHIBITION FACTOR (TBIF)

As described above, the ability of TMIF to inhibit tumor cell migration is demonstrable *in vitro*. Furthermore, TMIF can be detected *in vivo* and can exert *in vivo* effects. Thus, it is a good candidate for a factor that has a protective role *in vivo*, as it could inhibit local invasiveness or metastasis. Since the latter involves passage of tumor cells acros endothelium and the first step in such passage must involve attachment, we began a series of studies to determine whether TMIF, or a related lymphokine, could influence the interaction of tumor cells with endothelium *in vitro*.

Endothelial cell monolayers from bovine pulmonary arteries were prepared in 12-well tissue culture plates.[141,142] Tumor cells and endothelium were incubated at 37°C for 30 to 60 min in the presence of either lymphokine-containing or control preparations, followed by 3 washes to remove nonadherent cells. Tumor cell attachment was quantitated either by direct visual count of adherent cells by light microscopy or by the use of tumor cells labeled with radioactive chromium.[146] By either technique we found that when tumor cells were incubated with endothelium in the presence of lymphokine-containing supernatants, binding was markedly suppressed. Decreases of approximately 40 to 70% were found, depending on experimental conditions.[147]

Further analysis of this phenomenon suggested that the effect was due to both diminished attachment and increased dissociation. The responsible agent appears to be of approximately the same molecular weight as TMIF, and it is found in both lymphoblastoid cell lines and mitogen-activated lymphocyte preparations. To exert its inhibitory effect on tumor cell binding to endothelium it must be present during the entire incubation period. It is effective only at 37°C.

As previously described, we have succeeded in producing a hybridoma that secretes TMIF in the absence of MIF.[140] We also found that all hybridomas with TMIF activity had tumor cell-endothelial cell binding inhibitory activity as well. However, BW5147, the fusion partner, was also found to secrete this activity, although it lacked TMIF activity. This latter observation suggests that TMIF and the binding inhibitory factor (which we have called tumor binding inhibition factor, or TBIF) are distinct. Formal proof, other than purification to homogeneity of each, would require the demonstration of a reciprocal effect, i.e., a line producing TMIF in the absence of TBIF, to show that the dissociation in BW5147 is not due merely to a difference in assay sensitivity.

During the course of these experiments, it became apparent that it was impossible to achieve 100% binding of tumor cells to endothelium, even in the absence of lymphokine or with very small numbers of tumor cells. This suggests both functional heterogeneity of tumor cells and the possibility that specific site attachments rather than nonspecific forces are involved in binding. We have begun to identify cell adhesion molecules which appear to be involved in the attachment of tumor cells to endothelium. In any event, although lymphokines that influence cell surface tension have been reported,[148] it is more likely that the lymphokine responsible for the suppression acts at the level of the binding site itself.

We recently extended these studies by investigating the attachment of tumor cells to frozen tissue sections. In agreement with Netland and Zetter,[149] we have found significant binding of tumor cells to these preparations. However, we have not found a correlation between binding to different tissues and the *in vivo* capacity of the tumor to metastasize to the organs from which the tissue was obtained. Our examination of the localization of binding in the lung revealed that tumor cells adhere primarily to lining cells of alveoli, but the preparations did not allow us to distinguish between endothelial and epithelial cell sites. In the liver, tumor cells adhere to both sinusoidal lining cells and parenchymal cells. In other organs, parenchymal cell binding is seen as well. Thus, this assay may reflect both endothelial and parenchymal attachment.

D. CYTOSTATIC ACTIVITY AGAINST TUMOR CELLS

As we have noted, we have been unable to detect lymphokine-mediated cytotoxicity for any of the tumor cells used as targets under our experimental conditions. This is based on trypan blue exclusion, radiochromium release, and, in the case of migration inhibition, reversibility of effect. However, it was still possible that these preparations could be growth inhibitory or cytostatic. We, therefore, undertook studies based on a standard thymidine incorporation assay.[150] In these studies P815 mastocytoma cells were placed in culture in the presence of lymphokine-containing or control preparations for various time periods. Three hours prior to termination of the incubation, ^{3}H-thymidine was added to each culture. At 24 h, thymidine incorporation was 70% less in the presence of lymphokine than in control cultures. At 48 h, there was no difference. Viability was greater than 90% in these studies, with no differences between experimental and control preparations. Initial sizing experiments showed that the responsible factor is of approximately the same molecular weight as TMIF and TBIF. In analogy with the other noncytotoxic factors that we have described, we have called this activity tumor proliferation inhibition factor (TPIF). However, we have not yet demonstrated this activity in mitogen- or antigen-activated lymphocyte cultures, which would be necessary if this effect were to be ascribed to a lymphokine. In any event, the size data strongly suggest that the observed results are not due to an effect of dilute lymphotoxin, since no lymphotoxin activity has been reported in this size range.

Another question was raised by these results. It was possible that the migration inhibition findings that we had observed were actually due to inhibition of proliferation, and that the smaller spreading patterns observed were due to a decrease in the number of cells rather than to diminished motility. This is unlikely since the MIF assay is relatively insensitive to target cell numbers. However, to test the possibility directly, we allowed tumor cells to migrate out of the capillary tubes in the presence or absence of hydroxyurea, an agent known to interfere with cell proliferation. Thymidine uptake was diminished by more than 90% by 1 mM hydroxyurea and abolished by 2 mM hydroxyurea. Nevertheless, no difference in migration area was observed between preparations containing these concentrations of hydroxyurea and control preparations. Thus, migration inhibition assays and thymidine incorporation assays would appear to measure separate phenomena.

V. SUMMARY AND CONCLUSIONS

In this chapter, we have described a number of soluble mediators which affect neoplastic cells. These include several which lead to tumor cell killing as well as a family of low molecular weight lymphokines that we have identified that modify a number of tumor cell functions. We have found that lymphokine preparations of human or murine origin contain a protein, TMIF, that can reversibly inhibit the migration of a variety of tumor cells. Both serially passaged animal tumors and spontaneous human neoplasms respond to TMIF. Determination of physicochemical characteristics, including molecular weight, enzyme inactivation profile, and noncoordinate production by hybridomas, has led to the conclusion that TMIF is distinct from the lymphokines that inhibit the migration of non-neoplastic cells. TMIF can be detected *in vivo* and can modify the behavior of tumor cells *in vivo*.

In addition, TMIF-containing preparations can inhibit the binding of tumor cells to endothelial monolayers. Preliminary evidence suggests that TMIF and TBIF may be separable. Finally, although migration inhibition by TMIF is not associated with cytotoxicity, partially purified TMIF preparations are cytostatic for tumor cells. Cytostasis is not the cause of the observed results in the migration assay, and these properties are therefore functionally distinct.

These three activities, appearing within a narrow range of molecular weights, different from those of other known lymphokines, suggest the existence of a distinct class of mediators with the common function of influencing functional properties of tumor cells. Further characterization of this set of lymphocyte-derived effector molecules will require purification of the various factors to homogeneity. These mediators may have therapeutic potential, since the tumor cell functions that they regulate are those involved in the expression of malignant potential. In addition, studies are underway to determine whether the *in vitro* responsiveness of tumor cells to these factors might correlate with their *in vivo* biologic behavior. Finally, detection of these lymphokines in the serum or urine from patients with neoplasms could be useful in the detection of cancer and/or monitoring of occult tumor metastases or tumor recurrence.

REFERENCES

1. **Cohen, M. C., Gutowski, J. K., and Cohen, S.,** Inflammatory lymphokines in hypersensitivity reactions, in *The Reticuloendothelial System,* Vol. 9, Phillips, S. M. and Escobar, M. R., Eds., Plenum Press, New York, 1986, 209.
2. **Szigeti, R.,** Application of migration inhibition techniques in tumor immunology, *Adv. Cancer Res.,* 43, 241, 1985.
3. **Ruddle, N. H. and Waksman, B. H.,** Cytotoxicity mediated by soluble antigen and lymphocytes in delayed hypersensitivity. III. Analysis of mechanism, *J. Exp. Med.,* 128, 1267, 1968.
4. **Granger, G. A. and Williams, T. W.,** Lymphocyte cytotoxicity *in vitro:* activation and release of a cytotoxic factor, *Nature,* 218, 1253, 1968.
5. **Sawada, J.-I., Shiori-Nakano, K., and Osawa, T.,** Cytotoxic activity of purified guinea pig lymphotoxin against various cell lines, *Jpn. J. Exp. Med.,* 46, 263, 1976.
6. **Granger, G. A., Yamamoto, R. S., Fair, D. S., and Hiserodt, J. C.,** The human LT system. I. Physical-chemical heterogeneity of LT molecules released by mitogen activated human lymphocytes *in vitro, Cell. Immunol.,* 38, 388, 1976.
7. **Smith, M. E., Laudico, R., and Papermaster, B. W.,** A rapid quantitative assay for lymphotoxin, *J. Immunol. Methods,* 14, 243, 1977.
8. **Rundell, J. O. and Evans, C. H.,** Species specificity of guinea pig and human lymphotoxin colony inhibitory activity, *Immunopharmacology,* 3, 9, 1981.
9. **Granger, G. A., Yamamoto, R. S., Devlin, J. J., and Klostergaard, J.,** Lymphotoxins: a multicomponent system of cell-lytic lymphocyte-released effector molecules, *Lymphokine Res.,* 1, 45, 1982.

10. **Powell, M. B., Conta, B. S., Horowitz, M., and Ruddle, N. H.,** The differential inhibitory effect of lymphotoxin and immune interferon on normal and malignant lymphoid cells, *Lymphokine Res.,* 4, 13, 1985.

11. **Evans, C. H.,** Lymphotoxin: an immunological hormone with anticarcinogenic and antitumor activity, *Cancer Immunol. Immunother.,* 12, 181, 1982.

12. **Devlin, J. J., Klostergaard, J., Orr, S. L., Yamamoto, R. S., Masunaka, I. K., Plunkett, J. M., and Granger, G. A.,** Lymphotoxins: after fifteen years of research, in *Lymphokines,* Vol. 9, Pick, E., Ed., Academic Press, Orlando, FL, 1984, 313.

13. **Walker, S. M., Lee, S. C., and Lucas, Z. J.,** Cytotoxic activity of lymphocytes: heterogeneity of cytotoxins in supernatants of mitogen-activated lymphocytes, *J. Immunol.,* 116, 807, 1976.

14. **Hiserodt, J. and Granger, G. A.,** *In vitro* lymphocyte cytotoxicity. II. Unstable lymphotoxins (Beta-LT) secreted and inactivated by mitogen-stimulated human lymphocytes, *Cell. Immunol.,* 26, 211, 1976.

15. **Lee, S. C. and Lucas, Z. J.,** Regulatory factors produced by lymphocytes. I. The occurrence of multiple alpha-lymphotoxins associated with ribonuclease activity, *J. Immunol.,* 117, 283, 1976.

16. **Hiserodt, J. C., Fair, D. S., and Granger, G. A.,** Identification of multiple cytolytic components associated with the beta-LT class of lymphotoxins released by mitogen-activated human lymphocytes *in vitro, J. Immunol.,* 117, 1503, 1976.

17. **Hiserodt, J. C., Prieur, A.-M., and Granger, G. A.,** In vitro lymphocyte cytotoxicity. Evidence of multiple cytotoxic molecules secreted by mitogen activated human lymphoid cells *in vitro, Cell. Immunol.,* 24, 277, 1976.

18. **Yamamoto, R. S., Hiserodt, J. C., Lewis, J. E., Carmack, C. E., and Granger, G. A.,** The human LT system. II. Immunological relationship of LT molecules released by mitogen activated human lymphocytes *in vitro, Cell. Immunol.,* 38, 403, 1978.

19. **Hiserodt, J. C., Yamamoto, R. S., and Granger, G. A.,** The human LT system. III. Characterization of a high molecular weight LT class (complex) composed of the various smaller molecular weight LT classes and subclasses in association with Ig-like molecules, *Cell. Immunol.,* 38, 417, 1978.

20. **Ware, C. F. and Granger, G. A.,** Mechanisms of lymphocyte-mediated cytotoxicity. The effects of anti-human lymphotoxin antisera on the cytolysis of allogenic B cell lines by MLC-sensitized human lymphocytes *in vitro, J. Immunol.,* 126, 1919, 1981.

21. **Sawada, J. and Osawa, T.,** Characterization of lectin-induced cellular cytotoxicity mediated by mouse spleen cells and the role of lymphotoxin, *Immunology,* 41, 325, 1981.

22. **Kondo, L. L., Rosenau, W., and Wara, D. W.,** Role of lymphotoxin in antibody-dependent cell-mediated cytotoxicity (ADCC), *J. Immunol.,* 126, 1131, 1981.

23. **Wright, S. C. and Bonavida, B.,** Selective lysis of NK-sensitive target cells by a soluble mediator released from murine spleen cells and human peripheral blood lymphocytes, *J. Immunol.,* 126, 1516, 1981.

24. **Yamamoto, R. S., Weitzen, M. L., Miner, K. M., Devlin, J. J., and Granger, G. A.,** in *NK Cells and Other Natural Effector Cells,* Herberman, R. B., Ed., Academic Press, New York, 1982, 969.

25. **Farram, E. and Targan, S. R.,** Identification of human natural killer soluble cytotoxic factor(s) (NKCF) derived from NK-enriched lymphocyte populations: specificity of generation and killing, *J. Immunol.,* 130, 1252, 1983.

26. **Williams, T. W. and Bellanti, J. A.,** *In vitro* synergism between interferons and human lymphotoxin: enhancement of lymphotoxin-induced target cell killing, *J. Immunol.,* 130, 518, 1983.

27. **Stone-Wolfe, D. S., Yip, Y. K., Kelker, H. C., Le, J., Henriksen-Sestefano, D., Rubin, B. Y., Rinderknecht, E., Aggarwal, B. B., and Vilcek, J.,** Interrelationships of human interferon-gamma with lymphotoxin and monocyte cytotoxin, *J. Exp. Med.,* 159, 828, 1984.

28. **Lee, S. H., Aggarwal, B. B., Rinderknecht, E., Assisi, F., and Chiu, H.,** The synergistic anti-proliferative effect of interferon and human lymphotoxin, *J. Immunol.,* 133, 1083, 1984.

29. **Conta, B. S., Powell, M. B., and Ruddle, N. H.,** Activation of Lyt-1$^+$ and Lyt-2$^+$ T cell cloned lines: stimulation of proliferation, lymphokine production and self destruction, *J. Immunol.,* 134, 2185, 1985.

30. **Aderka, D., Novick, D., Hahn, T., Fischer, D. G., and Wallach, D.,** Increase of vulnerability to lymphotoxin in cells infected by vesicular stomatitis virus and its further augmentation by interferon, *Cell. Immunol.,* 9, 218, 1985.

31. **Murphy, M., Loudon, R., Kobayashi, M., and Trinchieri, G.,** Interferon and lymphotoxin, released by activated T cells, synergize to inhibit granulocyte/monocyte colony formation, *J. Exp. Med.,* 164, 263, 1986.

32. **Papermaster, B.-W., Gilliland, C. D., McEntire, J. E., Smith, M. E., and Buchok, S. J.,** Lymphokine-mediated immunotherapy studies in mouse tumor systems, *Cancer,* 45, 1248, 1980.

33. **Orr, S., Plunkett, M., Masunaka, I., and Granger, G. A.,** Purification and peptide characterization of human alpha-lymphotoxin obtained from the human lymphoblastoid cell line IR 3.4 *Lymphokine Res.,* 3(Abstr.) 264, 1984.

34. **Aggarwall, B. B., Henzel, W. J., Moffat, B., Kohr, W. J., and Harkinds, R. N.,** Primary structure of human lymphotoxin derived from 1788 lymphoblastoid cell line, *J. Biol. Chem.,* 260, 2334, 1985.

35. **Gray, P. A., Aggarwal, B. B., Benton, C. V., Benton, V., Bringman, T. S., Henzel, W. J., Jarret, J. A., Leung, D. W., Moffat, B., Ng, P., Svedersky, L. P., Palladino, M. A., and Nedwin, G. E.,** Cloning and expression of cDNA for human lymphotoxin, a lymphokine with tumor necrosis activity, *Nature,* 312, 721, 1984.

36. **Jeffes, E. W. B. and Granger, G. A.,** Relationship of cloning inhibition factor, "lymphotoxin" factor, and proliferation inhibition factor release *in vitro* by mitogen-activated human lymphocytes, *J. Immunol.,* 114, 64, 1975.

37. **Evans, C. H., Cooney, A. M., and DiPaola, J. A.,** Colony inhibition mediated by nonimmune leukocytes *in vitro* and skin reactivity *in vivo* as indices of tumorigenicity of guinea pig cultures transformed by chemical carcinogens, *Cancer Res.,* 35, 1045, 1975.

38. **Evans, R., Rabin, E. S., and DiPaolo, J.,** The susceptibility of guinea pig cells to the colony-inhibitory activity of lymphotoxin during carcinogenesis, *Cancer Res.,* 37, 898, 1977.

39. **Tsoukas, C. D., Rosenau, W., and Baxter, J. D.,** Cellular receptors for lymphotoxin: correlation of binding and cytotoxicity in sensitive and resistant target cells, *J. Immunol.,* 116, 184, 1976.

40. **Rosenau, W., Burke, G. C., and Anderson, R.,** Effects of lymphotoxin on target-cell plasma-membrane lipids, *Cell. Immunol.,* 60, 144, 1981.

41. **Rosenau, W. and Burke, G. C.,** Lymphotoxin-induced changes in target-cell plasma-membrane protein: enhancement of synthesis and content, *Cell. Immunol.,* 67, 14, 1982.

42. **Leopardi, E., Friend, D. S., and Rosenau, W.,** Target cell lysis: ultrastructural and cytoskeletal alterations, *J. Immunol.,* 133, 3429, 1984.

43. **Okamoto, M. and Mayer, M. M.,** Studies on the mechanism of action of guinea pig lymphotoxin. II. Increase of calcium uptake rate in LT-damaged target cells, *J. Immunol.,* 120, 279, 1978.

44. **Rosenau, W., Oie, S., and Burke, G. C.,** Calcium in lymphotoxin-mediated cytolysis: cellular pools, fluxes, and role of extracellular concentration, *Cell. Immunol.,* 95, 450, 1985.

45. **Schmid, D. S., Tite, J. P., and Ruddle, N. H.,** DNA fragmentation: manifestation of target cell destruction mediated by cytotoxic T-cell lines, lymphotoxin-secreting helpter T-cell clones, and cell-free lymphotoxin-containing supernatant, *Proc. Natl. Acad. Sci. U.S.A.,* 83, 1881, 1986.

46. **Pennica, D., Nedwin, G. E., Hayflick, J. S., Seeburg, P. H., Derynck, R., Palladino, M. A., Kohr, W. J., Aggarwal, B. B., and Goeddel, D. V.,** Human tumour necrosis factor: precursor structure, expression and homology to lymphotoxin, *Nature,* 316, 552, 1984.

47. **Nedwin, G. E., Naylor, S. L., Sakaguchi, A. Y., Smith, D., Jarrett-Nedwin, J., Pennica, D., Goeddel, D. V., and Gray, P. W.,** Human lymphotoxin and tumor necrosis factor genes: structure, homology and chromosomal localization, *Nucl. Acids Res.,* 13, 6361, 1985.

48. **Cuturi, M. C., Murphy, M., Costa-Giomi, M. P., Weinmann, R., Perussia, B., and Trinchieri, G.,** Independent regulation of tumor necrosis factor and lymphotoxin production by human peripheral blood lymphocytes, *J. Exp. Med.,* 165, 1581, 1987.

49. **Carswell, E. A., Old, L. J., Kassel, R. L., Green, S., Firoe, N., and Williamson, B.,** An endotoxin-induced serum factor that causes necrosis of tumors, *Proc. Natl. Acad. Sci. U.S.A.,* 72, 3666, 1975.

50. **Mannel, D. N., Meltzer, M. S., and Mergenhagen, S. E.,** Generation and characterization of a lipopolysaccharide-induced and serum-derived cytotoxic factor for tumor cells, *Infect. Immunol.,* 28, 204, 1980.

51. **Haranaka, K. and Satomi, N.,** Cytotoxic activity of tumor necrosis factor on human cancer cells *in vitro,* *Jpn. J. Exp. Med.,* 51, 191, 1981.

52. **Kull, F. C., Jr. and Cuatrecacas, P.,** Preliminary characterization of the tumor cell cytotoxin in tumor necrosis serum., *J. Immunol.,* 126, 1279, 1981.

53. **Williamson, B. D., Carswell, E. A., Rubin, B. Y., Prendergast, J. S., and Old, L. J.,** Human tumor necrosis factor produced by human B-cell lines: synergistic cytotoxic interaction with human interferon, *Proc. Natl. Acad. Sci. U.S.A.,* 80, 5397, 1983.

54. **Old, L. J.,** Tumor necrosis factor (TNF), *Science,* 230, 630, 1985.

55. **Sugarman, B. J., Aggarwal, B. B., Hass, P. E., Figari, I. S., Palladino, M. A., Jr., and Shepard, H. M.,** Recombinant human tumor necrosis factor-a: effects on proliferation of normal and transformed cells *in vitro,* *Science,* 230, 943, 1985.

56. **Balkwill, F. R., Lee, A., Aldam, G., Moodie, E., Thomas, J. A., Tavernier, J., and Fiers, W.,** Human tumor xenografts treated with recombinant human tumor necrosis factor alone or in combination with interferons, *Cancer Res.,* 46, 3990, 1986.

57. **Creasey, A. A., Reynolds, M. T., and Laird, W.,** Cures and partial regression of murine and human tumors by recombinant human tumor necrosis factor, *Cancer Res.,* 46, 5687, 1986.

58. **Manda, T., Shimomura, K., Mukumoto, S., Kobayashi, K., Mizota, T., Hirai, O., Matsumoto, S., Oku, T., Nishigaki, F., Mori, J., and Kikuchi, H.,** Recombinant human tumor necrosis factor α: evidence of an indirect mode of antitumor activity, *Cancer Res.,* 47, 3703, 1987.

59. **Poda, F., Carpinelli, G., Di Vito, M., Giannini, M., Proietti, E., Fiers, W., Gresser, I., and Belardelli, F.,** Nuclear magnetic resonance analysis of tumor necrosis factor-induced alterations of phospholipid metabolites and pH in Friend leukemia cell tumors and fibrosarcomas in mice, *Cancer Res.,* 47, 6481, 1987.

60. **Pekala, P. H., Lane, M. D., Cerami, A., and Kawakami, M.,** Lipoprotein lipase suppression in 3T3-L1 cells by an endotoxin-induced mediator from exudate cells, *Proc. Natl. Acad. Sci. U.S.A.,* 79, 912, 1982.

61. **Beutler, B., Mahoney, J., LeTrang, N., Pekala, P., and Cerami, A.,** Purification of cachectin, a lipoprotein lipase suppressing hormone secreted by endotoxin-induced RAW 2;64.7 cells, *J. Exp. Med.,* 161, 984, 1985.

62. **Beutler, B. and Cerami, A.,** Cachectin, a monokine implicated as a mediator of cachexia and shock, in *Lymphokines,* Vol. 14, Pick, E., Ed., Academic Press, San Diego, 1987, 203.

63. **Beutler, B., Milsark, I. W., and Cerami, A.,** Passive immunization against cachectin/tumor necrosis factor protects mice from lethal effect of endotoxin, *Science,* 229, 869, 1985.

64. **Matthews, N. and Neale, M. L.,** Studies on the mode of action of tumor necrosis factor on tumor cells *in vitro,* in *Lymphokines,* Vol. 14, Pick, E., Ed., Academic Press, San Diego, 1987, 223.

65. **Wheelock, E. F.,** Interferon-like virus-inhibitor induced in human leukocytes by phytohemagglutinin, *Science,* 149, 310, 1965.

66. **Friedman, R. and Cooper, H.,** Stimulation of interferon production in human lymphocytes by mitogens, *Proc. Soc. Exp. Biol. Med.,* 125, 901, 1967.

67. **Green, J. A., Cooperband, S. R., and Kibrick, S.,** Immune specific induction of interferon production in cultures of human blood lymphocytes, *Science,* 164, 1415, 1969.

68. **Youngner, J. S. and Salvin, S. B.,** Production and properties of migration inhibitory factor and interferon in the circulation of mice with delayed hypersensitivity, *J. Immunol.,* 111, 1914, 1973.

69. **Salvin, S. B., Youngner, J. S., and Lederer, W. H.,** Migration inhibitory factor and interferon in the circulation of mice with delayed hypersensitivity, *Infect. Immunol.,* 7, 68, 1973.

70. **Vilcek, J., Gray, P. W., Rinderknecht, E., and Sevastopoulos, C. G.,** Interferon γ: a lymphokine for all seasons, in *Lymphokines,* Vol. 11, Pick, E., Ed., Academic Press, Orlando, FL, 1985, 1.

71. **Naylor, S. L., Sakaguchi, A. Y., Shows, T. B., Law, M. L., Goeddel, D. V., and Gray, P. W.,** Human immune interferon gene is located on chromosome 12, *J. Exp. Med.,* 157, 1020, 1983.

72. **Sonnenfeld, G., Meruelo, D., McDevitt, H. O., and Merigan, T. C.,** Effect of type I and type II interferons on murine thymocyte surface antigen expression: induction or selection?, *Cell. Immunol.,* 57, 427, 1981.

73. **Steeg, P. G., Moore, R. N., Johnson, H. M., and Oppenheim, J. J.,** Regulation of murine macrophage Ia antigen expression by a lymphokine with immune interferon activity, *J. Exp. Med.,* 156, 1780, 1982.

74. **King, D. P. and Jones, P. P.,** Induction of Ia and H-2 antigens on a macrophage cell line by immune interferon, *J. Immunol.,* 131, 315, 1983.

75. **Guyre, P. M., Morganelli, P. M., and Miller, R.,** Recombinant immune interferon increases immunoglobulin G Fc receptors on cultured human mononuclear phagocytes, *J. Clin. Invest.,* 72, 393, 1983.

76. **Perussia, B., Dayton, E. T., Lazarus, R., Fanning, V., and Trinchieri, G.,** Immune interferon induces the receptor for monomeric IgG1 on human monocytic and myeloid cells, *J. Exp. Med.,* 158, 1092, 1983.

77. **Weigent, D. A., Langford, M. P., Fleischmann, W. R., Jr., and Stanton, G. J.,** Potentiation of lymphocyte natural killing by mixtures of alpha or beta interferon with recombinant gamma interferon, *Infect. Immunol.,* 40, 35, 1983.

78. **Svedersky, L. P., Shepard, H. M., Spencer, S. A., Shalaby, M. R., and Palladino, M. A.,** Augmentation of human natural cell-mediated cytotoxicity by recombinant human interleukin 2, *J. Immunol.,* 133, 714, 1984.

79. **Farrar, W. L., Johnson, H. M., and Farrar, J. J.,** Regulation of the production of immune interferon and cytotoxic T lymphocytes by interleukin 2, *J. Immunol.,* 126, 1120, 1981.

80. **Le, J., Yip, Y. K., and Vilcek, J.,** Cytolytic activity of interferon-gamma and its synergism with 5-fluorouracil, *Int. J. Cancer,* 34, 495, 1984.

81. **Boraschi, D. and Tagliabue, A.,** Multiple modulation of macrophage functions by lymphokines: different effects of interferon and macrophage activating factor, in *Lymphokines,* Vol. 9, Pick, E., Ed., Academic Press, New York, 1984, 71.

82. **Sadlik, J. R., Hoyer, M., Leyko, M. A., Horvat, R., Parmely, M., Whitacre, C., Zwilling, B., and Rinehart, J. J.,** Lymphocyte supernatant-induced human monocyte tumoricidal activity: dependence on the presence of γ-interferon, *Cancer Res.,* 45, 1940, 1985.

83. **Erickson, K. L., Cicurel, L., Gruys, E., and Fidler, I. J.,** Murine T-cell hybridomas that produce lymphokine with macrophage-activating factor activity as a constitutive product, *Cell. Immunol.,* 72, 195, 1982.

84. **Meltzer, M. S., Benjamin, W. R., and Farrar, J. J.,** Macrophage activation for tumor cytotoxicity: induction of macrophage tumoricidal activity from lymphokines from EL-4, a continuous T cell line, *J. Immunol.,* 129, 2802, 1982.

85. **Ratliff, T. L., Thomasson, D. L., McCool, R. E., and Catalona, W. J.,** T-cell hybridoma production of macrophage activation factor. I. Separation of MAF from interferon gamma, *J. Reticuloendothelial Soc.,* 31, 393, 1982.

86. **Kleinerman, E. A., Schroit, J., Fogler, W. E., and Fidler, I. J.,** Tumoricidal activity of human monocytes activated *in vitro* by free and liposome-encapsulated human lymphokines, *J. Clin. Invest.,* 72, 304, 1983.

87. **Schreiber, R. D. and Celada, A.,** Molecular characterization of interferon γ as a macrophage activating factor, in *Lymphokines,* Vol. 11, Pick, E., Ed., Academic Press, Orlando, FL, 1985, 87.

88. **Schreiber, R. D., Altman, A., and Katz, D. H.,** Indentification of a T cell hybridoma that produces large quantities of macrophage-activating factor, *J. Exp. Med.,* 156, 677, 1982.

89. **Zlotnick, A., Roberts, W. K., Vasil, A., Blumenthal, E., Larosa, F., Leibson, H. J., Endres, R. O., Graham, S. O., White, J., Hill, J., Henson, P., Klein, J. R., Bevan, M. J., Marrack, P., and Kappler, J. W.,** Coordinate production by a T cell hybridoma of gamma interferon and three other lymphokine activities: multiple activities of a single lymphokine?, *J. Immunol.,* 131, 794, 1983.

90. **Ratliff, T. L., Thomasson, D. L., McCool, R. E., and Catalona, W. J.,** Production of macrophage activation factor by a T-cell hybridoma, *Cell. Immunol.,* 68, 311, 1982.

91. **Krammer, P. H., Echtenacher, B., Gemsa, D., Hamann, U., Hultner, L., Kaltmann, B., Kees, U., Kubelka, C., and Marucci, F.,** Immune-interferon (IFN-γ), macrophage-activating factors (MAFs), and colony-stimulating factors (CSFs) secreted by T cell clones in limiting dilution microcultures, long-term cultures, and by T cell hybridomas, *Immunol. Rev.,* 76, 5, 1983.

92. **Pace, J. L., Russell, S. W., Torres, B. A., Johnson, H. M., and Gray, P. W.,** Recombinant mouse γ interferon induces the priming step in macrophage activation for tumor cell killing, *J. Immunol.,* 130, 2011, 1983.

93. **Schultz, R. M. and Kleinschmidt, W. J.,** Functional indentity between murine γ interferon and macrophage activating factor, *Nature,* 305, 239, 1983.

94. **Lohmann-Matthes, M. L., Schipper, H., and Fisher, H.,** Macrophage-mediated cytotoxicity against allogeneic target cells *in vitro, Eur. J. Immunol.,* 2, 45, 1972.

95. **Fidler, I. J.,** Activation *in vitro* of mouse macrophages by syngeneic, allogeneic, or xenogeneic lymphocyte supernatants, *JNCI,* 55, 1159, 1975.

96. **Ruco, L. P. and Meltzer, M. S.,** Macrophage activation for tumor cytotoxicity: induction of tumoricidal macrophages by supernatants of PPD-stimulated Bacillus Calmette-Guerin-immune spleen cell cultures, *J. Immunol.,* 119, 889, 1977.

97. **Sharma, S. D. and Piessens, W. F.,** Tumor cell killing by macrophages activated *in vitro* with lymphocyte mediators, *Cell. Immunol.,* 38, 264, 1978.

98. **Taramelli, D., Varesio, L., Holden, H. T., and Herberman, R. B.,** Studies on the activation of cytotoxicity and/or suppressor activity in murine macrophages by lymphokines, lipopolysaccharide, and polyinosinic-polycytidylic acid, in *Lymphokines,* Vol. 8, Pick, E., Ed., Academic Press, New York, 1983, 175.

99. **Reynolds, R. D., Khojasteh, A., Papermaster, B. W., and McEntire, J. E.,** Phase I clinical trial of MAF containing preparation of RPMI-1788 B-cell human lymphoblastoid lymphokine in advanced cancer patients, *Lymphokine Res.,* 5, S165, 1986.

100. **Morgan, D. A., Ruscetti, F. W., and Gallo, R.,** Selective *in vitro* growth of T lymphocytes from normal human bone marrows, *Science,* 193, 1007, 1976.

101. **Robb, R. J., Munck, A., and Smith, K. A.,** T cell growth factor receptors, *J. Exp. Med.,* 154, 1455, 1981.

102. **Strotter, H., Rude, E., and Wagner, H.,** T-cell factor (interleukin-2) allows *in vivo* induction of T helper cells against heterologous erythrocytes in athymic (nu/nu) mice, *Eur. J. Immunol.,* 10, 719, 1980.

103. **Wagner, H., Hardt, C., Heeg, K., Rollinghoff, M., and Pfizenmaier, K.,** T-cell derived helper factor allows *in vivo* induction of cytotoxic T cells in nu/nu mice, *Nature,* 284, 278, 1980.

104. **Gillis, S. and Smith, K.,** Long-term culture of tumour-specific cytotoxic T-cells, *Nature,* 268, 154, 1977.

105. **Yamamoto, J. K., Farrar, W. L., and Johnson, H. M.,** Interleukin 2 regulation of mitogen induction of immune interferon (IFN γ) in spleen cells and thymocytes, *Cell. Immunol.,* 66, 333, 1982.

106. **Howard, M., Matis, L., Malek, T. R., Shevach, E., Kell, W., Cohen, D., Nakanishi, K., and Paul, W. E.,** Interleukin-2 induces antigen-reactive T cell lines to secrete BCGF-1, *J. Exp. Med.,* 158, 2024, 1983.

107. **Yron, I., Wood, T. A., Spiess, P. J., and Rosenberg, S. A.,** *In vitro* growth of murine T cells. V. The isolation and growth of lymphoid cells infiltrating syngeneic solid tumors, *J. Immunol.,* 125, 238, 1980.

108. **Lotze, M. T., Grimm, E. A., Mazumder, A., Strausser, J. L., and Rosenberg, S. A.,** *In vitro* growth of cytotoxic human lymphocytes. IV. Lysis of fresh and cultured autologous tumor by lymphocytes cultured in T cell growth factor (TCGF), *Cancer Res.,* 41, 4420, 1981.

109. **Grimm, E. A., Mazumder, A., Zhang, H. Z., and Rosenberg, S. A.,** Lymphokine-activated killer cell phenomenon: lysis of natural killer-resistant fresh solid tumor cells by interleukin-2-activated autologous human peripheral blood lymphocytes, *J. Exp. Med.,* 155, 1823, 1982.

110. **Rosenstein, M., Yron, I., Kaufmann, Y., and Rosenberg, S. A.,** Lymphokine activated killer cells: lysis of fresh syngeneic NK-resistant murine tumor cells by lymphocytes cultured in interleukin-2, *Cancer Res.,* 44, 1946, 1984.

111. **Herberman, R. B., et al.,** Lymphokine-activated killer cell activity. Characteristics of effector cells and their progenitors in blood and spleen, *Immunol. Today,* 8, 178, 1987.

112. **Ortaldo, J. R., Mason, J., and Overton, R.,** Lymphokine-activated killer cells. Analysis of progenitors and effectors, *J. Exp. Med.,* 164, 1193, 1986.

113. **Rosenberg, S. A. and Lotze, M. T.,** Cancer immunotherapy using interleukin-2 and interleukin-2-activated lymphocytes, *Annu. Rev. Immunol.,* 4, 681, 1986.

114. **Rosenberg, S. A., Lotze, M. T., Muul, L. M., Leitman, S., Chang, A. E., Ettinghausen, S. E., Matoryl, Y. L., Skibber, J. M., Shiloni, E., Vetto, J. T., Seipp, C. A., Simpson, C., and Reichert, C. M.,** Observation on the systemic administration of autologous lymphokine-activated killer cells and recombinant interleukin-2 to patients with metastatic cancer, *N. Engl. J. Med.,* 313, 1485, 1985.

115. **Rosenberg, S. A., Lotze, M. T., Muul, L. M., Chang, A. E., Avis, F. P., Leitman, S., Linehan, W. N., Robertson, C. N., Lee, R. E., Rubin, J. T., Seipp, C. A., Simpson, C. G., and White, D. E.,** A progress report on the treatment of 157 patients with advanced cancer using lymphokine-activated killer cells and interleukin-2 or high-dose interleukin-2 alone, *N. Engl. J. Med.,* 316, 889, 1987.

116. **Sosman, J. A., Kohler, P. C., Hank, J., Moore, K. H., Bechhofer, R., Storer, B., and Sondel, P. M.,** Repetitive weekly cycles of recombinant human interleukin-2: responses of renal carcinoma with acceptable toxicity, *JNCI,* 80, 60, 1988.

117. **Dinarello, C. A.,** Biology of interleukin 1, *FASEB J.,* 2, 108, 1988.

118. **March, C., Mosley, B., Larsen, A., Cerretti, D. P., Braedt, G., Price, V., Gillis, S., Henney, C. S., Kronheim, S. R., Grabstein, K., Conlon, P. J., Hopp, T. P., and Cosman, D.,** Cloning, sequence and expression of two distinct human interleukin-1 complementary DNAs, *Nature,* 315, 641, 1985.

119. **Oppenheim, J. J., Kovacs, E. J., Matsushima, K., and Durum, S. K.,** There is more than one interleukin 1, *Immunol. Today,* 7, 45, 1986.

120. **Onozaki, K., Matsushima, K., Kleinerman, E. S., Saito, T., and Oppenheim, J. J.,** Role of interleukin 1 in promoting human monocyte-mediated tumor cytotoxicity, *J. Immunol.,* 135, 314, 1985.

121. **Onozaki, K., Matsushima, K., Aggarwal, B. B., and Oppenheim, J. J.,** Human interleukin 1 is a cytocidal factor for several tumor cell lines, *J. Immunol.,* 135, 3962, 1985.

122. **Smith, K. A., Lachman, L. B., Oppenheim, J. J., and Favata, M. F.,** The functional relationship of the interleukins, *J. Exp. Med.,* 151, 1551, 1980.

123. **Kasahara, T., Mukaida, N., Hatake, K., Motoyoshi, K., Kawai, T., and Shiori-Nakano, K.,** Interleukin 1 (IL 1)-dependent lymphokine production of human leukemic T cell line HSB.2 subclones, *J. Immunol.,* 134, 1682, 1985.

124. **Philip, R. and Epstein, L. B.,** Tumour necrosis factor as immunomodulator and mediator of monocyte cytotoxicity induced by itself, gamma-interferon and interleukin-1, *Nature,* 323, 86, 1986.

125. **Farrar, J. J., Benjamin, W. R., Hilfiker, M. L., Howard, M., Farrar, W. L., and Fuller-Farrar, J.,** The biochemistry, biology, and role of interleukin 2 in the induction of cytotoxic T cell and antibody-forming B cell responses, *Immunol. Rev.,* 63, 129, 1982.

126. **Dempsey, R. A., Dinarello, C. A., Mier, J. W., Rosenwasser, L. J., Allegretta, M., Brown, T. E., and Parkinson, D. R.,** The differential effects of human leukocytic pyrogen/lymphocyte activating factor, T cell growth factor, and interferon on human natural killer activity, *J. Immunol.,* 129, 2504, 1982.

127. **Gaffney, E. V. and Tsai, S. C.,** Lymphocyte-activating and growth-inhibitory activities for several sources of native and recombinant interleukin 1, *Cancer Res.,* 46, 3834, 1986.

128. **Lachman, L. B., Dinarello, C. A., Llansa, N. D., and Fidler, I. J.,** Natural and recombinant human interleukin 1β is cytotoxic for human melanoma cells, *J. Immunol.,* 136, 3098, 1986.

129. **Cohen, M. C., Zeschke, R., Bigazzi, P. E., Yoshida, T., and Cohen, S.,** Mastocytoma cell migration *in vitro:* inhibition by MIF-containing supernatants, *J. Immunol.,* 114, 1641, 1975.

130. **Yoshida, T., Kuratsuji, T., Takada, A., Takada, Y., Minowada, J., and Cohen, S.,** Lymphokine-like factors produced by human lymphoid cell lines with B or T cell surface markers, *J. Immunol.,* 117, 548, 1976.

131. **Cohen, M. C., Goss, A., Yoshida, T., and Cohen, S.,** Inhibition of migration of tumor cells *in vitro* by lymphokine-containing supernatants, *J. Immunol.,* 121, 840, 1978.

132. **Donskoy, M., Forouhar, F., and Cohen, M. C.,** Lymphokine-induced migration inhibition of murine tumor cells derived from solid neoplasms, *Cancer Res.,* 44, 3870, 1984.

133. **Cohen, M. C., Forouhar, F., Donskoy, M., and Cohen, S.,** *In vitro* migration of tumor cells from human neoplasms: inhibition by lymphokines, *Clin. Immunol. Immunopathol.,* 34, 94, 1985.

134. **Adelman, N., Hasson, M., Masih, N., and Cohen, M. C.,** Correlation between agarose microdroplet and capillary tube procedures as assays for migration inhibition of target cells, *J. Immunol. Methods,* 34, 235, 1980.

135. **Adelman, N., Cohen, S., and Yoshida, T.,** Strain variations in murine MIF production, *J. Immunol.,* 121, 209, 1978.

136. **Cohen, M. C.,** Characterization of the lymphokine responsible for migration-inhibitory activity against tumor cells, *Cancer Res.,* 42, 2135, 1982.

137. **Cohen, M. C., Picciano, P. T., Douglas, W. J., Yoshida, T., Kreutzer, D. L., and Cohen, S.,** Migration inhibition of endothelial cells by lymphokine-containing supernatants, *Science,* 215, 301, 1982.

138. **Rocklin, R. E.,** Role of monosaccharides in the interaction of two lymphocyte mediators with their target cells, *J. Immunol.,* 116, 816, 1976.

139. **Rocklin, R. E. and Rosenthal, A. S.,** Evidence that human leukocyte inhibitory factor (LIF) is an esterase, *J. Immunol.,* 119, 249, 1977.

140. **Cohen, M. C. and Lazarus, M.,** Production of lymphokines affecting tumor cells by T-T hybridomas, *Cell. Immunol.,* 93, 541, 1985.

141. **Picciano, P. T., Johnson, B., Walenga, R. W., Donovan, M., Bormann, B. J., Douglas, W. H. J., and Kreutzer, D. L.,** Effects of D-valine on pulmonary artery endothelial cell morphology and function in cell culture, *Exp. Cell Res.,* 151, 134, 1984.

142. **Ryan, U. S., Clements, E., Habliston, D., and Ryan, J. W.,** Isolation and culture of pulmonary artery endothelial cells, *Tissue Cell,* 10, 535, 1978.

143. **D'Silva, H., Cohen, M., Yoshida, T., and Cohen, S.,** Serum migration inhibitory activity against macrophages and tumor cells, *Clin. Immunol. Immunopathol.,* 23, 77, 1982.

144. **Sonozaki, H. and Cohen, S.,** The macrophage disappearance reaction. II. Mediation by lymphocytes which lack complement receptors, *Cell. Immunol.,* 3, 644, 1972.

145. **D'Silva, H., Munger, W., Cohen, M. C., and Cohen, S.,** The tumor disappearance reaction: an *in vivo* effect of a noncytotoxic lymphokine active against tumor cells, *Clin. Immunol. Immunopathol.,* 34, 326, 1985.

146. **Kramer, R. H. and Nicolson, G. L.,** Interactions of tumor cells with vascular endothelial cell monolayers: a model for metastatic invasion, *Proc. Natl. Acad. Sci. U.S.A.,* 76, 5704, 1979.

147. **Cohen, M. C., Mecley, M., Antonia, S. J., and Picciano, P. T.,** Adherence of tumor cells to endothelial monolayers: inhibition by lymphokines, *Cell. Immunol.,* 95, 247, 1985.

148. **Thrasher, S. G., Yoshida, T., van Oss, C. J., Cohen, S., and Rose, N. R.,** Alteration of macrophage interfacial tension by supernatants of antigen-activated lymphocyte cultures, *J. Immunol.,* 110, 321, 1973.

149. **Netland, P. A. and Zetter, B. R.,** Organ-specific adhesion of metastatic tumor cells *in vitro, Science,* 224, 1113, 1984.

150. **Antonia, S. J., Cohen, S., and Cohen, M. C.,** The elaboration of a small molecular weight cytostatic factor by lymphoblastoid lines and activated lymphocytes, *Lymphokine Res.,* 301, 1986.

Chapter 13

LYMPHOKINES AND CYTOKINES IN THE REPARATIVE PROCESS

Theresa H. Piela and Joseph H. Korn

TABLE OF CONTENTS

I. INTRODUCTION

The formation of scar tissue, whether in response to mechanical injury, as part of the healing phase of inflammatory reactions, or as a pathologic event in immunological and other disease states, is a complex process involving the interaction of many types of cells and their extracellular products. Any discussion of the reparative phase of most inflammatory reactions must center on the regulation of connective tissue metabolism, as it is through this regulation that orderly repair processes take place.

The reparative functions of connective tissue cells are now known to be governed, in part, by local factors, many of which are produced by immune cells in response to a variety of stimuli. Through the use of modern biochemical and molecular biological techniques, these factors are being identified, molecularly cloned, and made available in pure form in sufficient quantities to explore the mechanisms by which they act on diverse cell types. Our understanding of these local factors and how they may regulate cell functions has revealed the concept of a communications network between connective tissue cells and cells of the immune system which is responsible for both the initiation and resolution of inflammatory reactions. This communication is not necessarily unidirectional, as is discussed in this chapter. This chapter attempts to focus on the regulation of fibroblast (FB) and endothelial cell (EC) responses by the more well-characterized lymphokines and cytokines that are produced in inflammatory lesions.

II. FIBROBLASTS IN THE REPARATIVE PROCESS

A. FIBROBLAST MIGRATION AND ATTACHMENT

The accumulation of fibroblastic cells at sites of tissue injury is an initial step in the reparative process. Accumulation, along with proliferation and accompanying matrix deposition, is a central part of the general healing process. The movement of FB into areas of inflammation is a directed migration and occurs via a chemotactic response. One of the earliest reports describing the release of chemotactic factors for fibroblasts by human lymphocytes demonstrated that activation of the lymphocytes by stimulation with either specific antigen or nonspecific mitogen was required.[1] This chemotaxin, elaborated by activated T lymphocytes and called lymphocyte-derived chemotactic factor for fibroblasts (LDCF-F), is distinct from the monocyte chemotaxin, MDCF-F. Through the generation of chemotactic signals, activated lymphocytes, when found in areas of inflammation, may be a primary means by which fibroblasts are recruited. Specific factors released by cells other than those of T cell lineage also demonstrate chemotactic activity for fibroblasts. Platelet-derived growth factor (PDGF), released by platelets at sites of tissue injury, has been shown to be chemotactic not only for fibroblasts[2,3] but also for leukocyte populations.[4]

Substrate and cell attachment factors such as the interstitial collagens and fibronectins possess potent chemotactic properties for fibroblasts.[5-7] Fibronectins comprise a class of high molecular weight glycoproteins which are present in connective tissue, basement membranes, amniotic fluid, and plasma.[8] Fibronectin has an important role in wound healing[9,10] and there is a correlation between the appearance of fibronectin and subsequent fibrosis.[11]

Intact collagens and collagen fragments are chemotactic for fibroblasts.[12] Human dermal fibroblasts will also bind to chemotactic ^{14}C-labeled collagen-derived peptides,[13] implying a receptor-mediated chemotactic response. It can logically be inferred that the degradation and release of breakdown products of collagens and fibronectins that occurs at inflammatory sites are additional recruitment signals for fibroblasts.

Fibroblasts will adhere to such extracellular matrices as fibronectin and collagen, conferring a degree of mechanical stability. Recently, much attention has focused on these cell-substrate interactions. The tripeptide Arg-Gly-Asp is common to fibronectin, vitronectin,

TABLE 1
Cytokines Influencing Fibroblast Accumulation

Factor(s)	Fibroblast response	Ref.
PDGF (platelets, monocytes)		2, 3, 7
Collagen (fibroblasts)		5, 12
Fibronectin (fibroblasts, monocytes)		5, 6, 7
TGFβ (lymphocytes, monocytes, platelets)	Chemotaxis	49
Complement components		163
Lymphocyte-derived chemotactic factor (lymphocytes)		1
Monocyte-derived chemotactic factor (monocytes)		1, 23
FGF (bovine pituitary, hypothalamus, cartilage, bone, monocytes)		36, 39
PDGF		50, 51
IL-1 (monocytes, endothelial cells)	Growth (+)	
TNFα (monocytes)		32, 33
TGFβ		50, 51
Monocyte-derived growth factor (monocytes)		3
IFN-α, -β, -γ (lymphocytes, monocytes, fibroblasts)		54—56
IL-1	Growth (−)	59—62
PGE$_2$ (monocytes, platelets, fibroblasts)		59, 60

fibrinogen, and collagen, all of which function as cellular adhesion substrates, and appears to be an essential sequence necessary for cell attachment. Cellular surface receptors for each of these substrates are, however, distinct both in structure and specificity, and it appears that variations to the Arg-Gly-Asp sequences may account for this specificity. The tetra-peptide Arg-Gly-Asp-Ser is reported to be the minimal sequence present in fibronectin responsible for cell attachment, whereas Arg-Gly-Asp-Val is required for binding specifically to vitronectin. Substrates that have been derivatized with synthetic peptides containing such sequences will bind certain types of fibroblastic cells[14] with subsequent focal contact formation. These types of experiments are being used to isolate and characterize the cell surface receptors responsible for substrate adhesion.[15] Factors contributing to fibroblast migration and affecting other fibroblast functions are summarized in Table 1.

B. FIBROBLAST PROLIFERATION

The proliferation of fibroblastic cells has also been shown to be regulated by soluble immune cell-derived mediators. Early studies showed that monocytes were required *in vivo* for normal wound healing[16] and that monocytes *in vitro* released factors that stimulated fibroblast proliferation.[17] Products released by activated mononuclear cells are known to increase several fibroblast metabolic activities such as glucose uptake and lactate production[18] and collagen synthesis.[19,20] More recent studies have shown that components of mononuclear cell supernatants can both stimulate and suppress fibroblast proliferation.

1. Growth Factors

Monocyte-macrophages *in vitro* release factors which are mitogenic for fibroblasts.[21] Alveolar macrophages, when stimulated with immune complexes, produce a PDGF-like molecule,[22] macrophage-derived growth factor for fibroblasts, which is both mitogenic and chemotactic for fibroblasts.[3,23] PDGF is considered to be the principal mitogen found in mammalian serum for cells of mesenchymal origin.[24]

Another monocyte/macrophage product, IL-1 is a 17,000 Da factor which is essential for T cell activation,[25] and has been cloned and expressed in bacteria.[26] Two IL-1 species, IL-1α and IL-1β, are distinct molecules derived from separate genes but sharing similar, if not identical, activities.[27] Both bind to the same high affinity fibroblast receptor.[28] Both native and recombinant IL-1 have been reported to be directly mitogenic for fibroblasts.[29]

Tumor necrosis factor-alpha, TNFα, also derived from macrophages/monocytes, was originally described as a mediator of lipopolysaccharide (LPS)-induced hemorrhagic necrosis of tumors in animals. The cDNA for TNF has been cloned[30,31] and the recombinant protein has been shown to be a mitogenic signal for fibroblasts.[32,33]

Fibroblast growth factors (FGFs) have been isolated from several sources and have recently been purified. Two major forms of FGF have been identified, a cationic form and an anionic form,[34] which apparently bind to the same cell surface receptor.[35] The cationic form, called basic FGF, was initially isolated from bovine pituitary,[36] and both basic and acidic (anionic form) FGF are readily isolated from brain.[34,37,38] Acidic FGF is sometimes referred to as endothelial cell growth factor and possesses angiogenic properties as well.[39]

The family of transforming-growth factors (TGFs) are polypeptides that are known to cause certain cell types to express a transformed phenotype.[40,41] Two forms of TGF (α and β) have been identified which are structurally and antigenically distinct and which recognize different cell surface receptors.[41,42] TGFβ, which has been purified and partially sequenced and cloned[43-45] is found in several tissue and cell types, including T cells, monocytes, platelets, and some tumors.[44,46] TGFβ, which has no known homology to other factors yet described[47] is secreted by both activated T[43] and B cells.[48] TGFβ is chemotactic for fibroblasts[49] and, in conjunction with epidermal growth factor (EGF), has been shown to enhance fibroblast proliferation.[50] TGFβ is reported to be even more effective than EGF in stimulating epidermal regeneration.[51] In *in vivo* studies, TGFβ potentiates wound healing; the accumulation of cells, collagen, and total protein in experimental wounds is augmented by systemic administration of TGFβ.[52]

2. Growth Suppressive Factors

Mononuclear cells also elaborate cytokines which suppress fibroblast proliferation. The family of molecules known as interferons (IFNs) include γ or immune IFN (derived from activated T cells), IFN-β (a product of monocytes, fibroblasts, and other cells), and α or nonimmune IFN (produced by both monocyte and lymphocyte populations). IFN-α and -β, although distinct molecular species, bind to a common cell surface receptor. IFN-γ binds to a different fibroblast cell surface receptor; the receptor-ligand complex is rapidly internalized and cell surface IFN-γ receptors are rapidly replenished.[53] Originally defined by virtue of their antiviral properties, the effects of IFN on immune responses and on connective tissue cell metabolism may be of greater import. Recombinant IFNs of each type have been shown to suppress the proliferation of fibroblasts and other cells.[54-56] Whether previously identified lymphocyte products which suppress fibroblast proliferation[57,58] are distinct molecules or are, in fact, one of the IFN species is unknown.

Interleukin-1 (IL-1), which is directly mitogenic for fibroblasts, can also suppress fibroblast proliferation.[59-62] This suppression can be reversed by indomethacin or other cyclooxygenase inhibitors and is mediated by its stimulatory effect of fibroblast prostaglandin E_2 (PGE_2) synthesis. PGE, in turn, suppresses fibroblast proliferation by augmenting intracellular cAMP. Exogenous PGE has a similar effect[59] which suggests that at sites of inflammation, monocyte, or platelet-derived PGE may also limit fibroblast proliferation.

3. Regulatory Networks for Control of Proliferation

Regulatory networks exist for the regulation of fibroblast growth. The antagonistic direct and indirect effects of IL-1 have already been noted. It has been suggested that different lymphokines, released at different stages of inflammation may favor proliferation during the early stages of tissue repair, followed by a shift toward growth inhibition as healing nears completion.[58] In one study, IFN-γ suppressed fibroblast proliferation initially, but then stimulated fibroblast replication; the mechanisms responsible for this bimodal effect are unclear.[63]

The interactions of cytokines with immune cells may promote or suppress the production of specific factors regulating fibroblast proliferation. IFN-γ, while directly suppressing fibroblast proliferation, stimulates the release of the fibroblast mitogen, IL-1, from monocytes.[64,65] The production of IFN-γ in turn, may be regulated by peptide growth factors.[66] IL-1, by its actions on lymphocytes, may lead to further release of lymphokines affecting fibroblast growth. Overall, it appears that activated immune cells can produce both positive and negative regulatory signals for fibroblast proliferation. The balance of signals may depend on the state of immune cell activation, the nature of infiltrating immune cells and the responding fibroblast population, and the extent to which local nonimmune factors govern the relative importance of direct and indirect cytokine effects. The complex interaction of these signals may ultimately determine whether proliferation or suppression of growth is observed.

C. SYNTHESIS OF MATRIX

Following the arrival of fibroblasts at sites of inflammation, they progressively lay down new matrix components such as collagens, fibronectin, and proteoglycans. Here again, fibroblast biosynthesis is subject to regulatory influences from immune cells.

1. Collagen

Collagen is the most prevalent of all connective tissue proteins and is the primary structural component of organs and tissues. The collagen fibrils are formed extracellularly by the association of several collagen molecules, each of which consists of three polypeptide chains intertwined to form a helical structure. The fibril is composed of collagen molecules arranged in an overlapping configuration and fibril strength is augmented through the formation of intermolecular cross-links.

The regulation of fibroblast collagen synthesis is crucial for orderly repair processes to take place. Inappropriate activation of fibroblasts leading to excessive collagen deposition is associated with such pathological conditions as scleroderma and pulmonary fibrosis. T cell regulation of fibroblast collagen synthesis, as has been seen for fibroblast growth regulation, is dependent upon both positive and negative signals, and may, in fact, be growth-state dependent.[67]

Lymphocyte products have generally been reported to stimulate fibroblast collagen synthesis. Johnson and Ziff[20] were the first to demonstrate that PHA-activated T lymphocytes produced a factor that induced fibroblast collagen synthesis. Antigen-specific T cells, when appropriately stimulated, also caused both fibroblast proliferation and increased collagen production, thereby suggesting that both fibroblast proliferation and increased collagen deposition may be a result of a specific antigenic challenge.[68,69]

Mononuclear cell supernatants and alveolar macrophages have been reported to depress collagen synthesis,[70] an effect which appears to be mediated in part via stimulation of prostaglandin E_2 (PGE_2) production.[60,71] This suggests that the net effect of mononuclear cell supernatants on collagen production may depend inversely on the extent to which PGE_2 synthesis is stimulated. IL-1, a major component of mononuclear cell supernatants, has been shown to directly increase collagen synthesis by dermal and synovial fibroblasts.[71] A specific lymphokine, 55 kDa in size, which directly suppresses collagen synthesis has been identified and is termed "collagen synthesis inhibitory factor" (CSIF).[72,73]

The IFNs are probably the most significant group of molecules involved in the suppression of collagen synthesis. Recently, both IFN-α and -γ have been reported as specific cytokines that suppress fibroblast collagen synthesis[56,74] and do so by regulation at the transcriptional level.[75] Several *in vitro* studies have shown that IFN-γ-mediated suppression of collagen synthesis is correlated with a decrease in collagen mRNA.[75,76] *In vivo* evidence of IFN-γ-mediated down-regulation of collagen has been reported in the mouse. Subcutaneously implanted osmotic pumps induced the formation of large fibrous capsules around the pump. In mice implanted with pumps delivering recombinant murine IFN-γ (2 $\times$ 10^3 U/h for 14 d), capsule formation and its collagen content was markedly decreased.[77]

TGFβ has been shown to stimulate fibroblast collagen synthesis as well as proliferation.[50] The regulation of fibroblast collagen synthesis by TGFβ also takes place at the transcriptional level.[78,79] The *in vitro* effects of TGFβ on collagen synthesis have been replicated *in vivo*. When injected subcutaneously into newborn mice, TGFβ induces a rapid increase in connective tissue formation.[80]

2. Glycosaminoglycans

Fibroblasts are major producers of glycosaminoglycans (GAG), an important part of the extracellular matrix. Enhanced GAG deposition occurs as an early step in the processes of connective tissue repair and may be important in the regulation of cellular proliferation and differentiation.[81] The synthesis of GAG matrix by fibroblasts can be influenced by immune mediators. Supernatants of Concanavalin A (Con A) activated MNC cultures have been shown to stimulate both fibroblast GAG synthesis and murine thymocyte proliferation,[82] suggesting an active role for IL-1 in fibroblast GAG regulation. More recently, using human recombinant IL-1β Yaron et al.[83] have shown that human synovial fibroblast cultures are highly sensitive to IL-1 induction of increased GAG synthesis (up to 500%).

3. Matrix Degradation (Table 2)

In addition to the building up of connective tissue matrices such as collagen and proteoglycans, fibroblasts have a role in their degradation as well. Fibroblasts have been shown to secrete both collagenase and other proteases, largely under the control of immune cell-derived cytokines. The monocyte product, IL-1, appears to be the major effector molecule for stimulating fibroblasts to increase synthesis and secretion of collagenase.[84-86] Fibroblasts also make a collagenase inhibitor, tissue inhibitor of metalloproteinases (TIMP), and the production of both inhibitor and collagenase are coordinately regulated by IL-1.[87] TNF, like IL-1, also stimulates fibroblast collagenase.[88] Lymphokine-activated human monocytes/macrophages themselves secrete substantial amounts of collagenase,[89] as well as other lysosomal enzymes, elastase, and prostaglandins,[90,91] all of which are involved in tissue destruction.

D. FIBROBLAST HETEROGENEITY AND SELECTION

Mediators released by mononuclear cells may not only directly affect fibroblast metabolism but may lead to a subsequent, apparently permanent alteration of existing fibroblast subpopulations. Korn[92] has demonstrated that even a short-term exposure of human fibroblasts *in vitro* to supernatants of mitogen-activated mononuclear cells can lead to persistent enhancement of PGE$_2$ metabolism. The enhanced PGE$_2$ synthetic response to IL-1-containing mononuclear cell culture supernates persisted for as long as 19 cell generations after the original exposure to the mononuclear cell products.

Similar observations of persistently altered cell phenotypes following cytokine exposure have recently been reported by Worrall et al.[93] and Duncan and Berman.[94] Worrall et al. showed that short-term exposure of fibroblasts to mononuclear cell products led to persistent and propagable increases in glycosaminoglycan synthesis.[93] In studies of IFN effects on collagen synthesis, Duncan and Berman[94] demonstrated that transient exposure of high collagen producing scleroderma cell lines to IFNs resulted in persistently reduced collagen synthesis. Similar exposure of normal fibroblasts to IFNs led to only transient suppression of collagen synthesis; collagen synthesis returned to pretreatment levels during subsequent culture. Effects of cytokines on fibroblast metabolism may, therefore, depend on the makeup of the responding fibroblast population.

It has been suggested that a permanent alteration of connective tissue metabolism could

TABLE 2
Cytokines Influencing Fibroblast Matrix Synthesis and Degradation

Factor(s)	Fibroblast response	Ref.
IL-1	Prostaglandin E$_2$	57, 60, 61
TNFα		88
IL-1		71
TGFβ	Collagen (+)	50, 80
Partially characterized cytokines		20, 68, 69
IFN-γ		56, 74, 77
IFN-α	Collagen (−)	74
Collagen synthesis inhibitory factor (lymphocytes)		72, 73
IL-1	Collagenase	84—86
TNFα		88
IL-1	Proteoglycans	82, 83

TABLE 3
Cytokines Influencing Interactions of Fibroblasts with Immune Cells

Factor(s)	Fibroblast response	Ref.
IFN-γ	Ia expression	100, 101
IL-1	Release of other cytokines	111, 112
TNFα	Release of other cytokines	113
IFN-γ	Adhesiveness for lymphocytes	120
IL-1	Adhesiveness for lymphocytes	121

arise via a clonal selection.[59,92] Cloned fibroblast populations derived from a single parent line have demonstrated metabolic heterogeneity. Biosynthesis of PGE$_2$, collagenase, and tissue factor by fibroblast substrains derived by limiting dilution cloning varied five- to tenfold and each metabolic phenotype was stable over multiple weeks in culture.[95,96] High producer phenotypes for each of the cell products examined appeared to segregate independently. Finally, different fibroblast substrains were differentially sensitive to growth modulatory effects of immune derived cytokines.[96] These studies demonstrate that the potential exists for an immunologic "selection" of sorts, which may lead to expansion or suppression of certain cell subpopulations when fibroblasts are exposed, even transiently, to inflammatory mediators.

E. EFFECTS OF FIBROBLASTS ON IMMUNE CELLS (TABLE 3)

Many earlier studies of the effects of mononuclear cell supernatants on fibroblast metabolism took a one-way approach, that is, the role of the fibroblast was viewed as a passive target cell for lymphocyte-derived mediators, essentially ignoring cell-cell interactions. Lymphocyte-fibroblast coculture experiments sought to more closely reflect *in vivo* conditions. Using such a coculture system, Hibbs et al.[97] were able to demonstrate that fibroblast-derived collagen accumulation both quantitatively and qualitatively reflected the changes observed during wound healing and in stages of early inflammation. A similar coculture system was used to show that communication between the two cell types was bi-directional, in that lymphocytes cocultured with fibroblasts displayed a short-term suppression of PHA-induced mitogenesis; the fibroblast-mediated suppression was a result of immune cell directed increases in fibroblast PGE synthesis.[98]

Antigen presentation to T lymphocytes depends upon the recognition of class II major histocompatibility complex (MHC) antigens collectively referred to as Ia antigens. Cell surface Ia antigen expression is an essential requirement for accessory cells such as macrophages, B cells, and dendritic cells for effective antigen presentation. Ia synthesis and expression on such accessory cells is not constitutive, but can be up-regulated by a soluble product of activated T cells, now known to be IFN-γ.[99]

IFN-γ has been shown to induce surface Ia expression on fibroblastic cells leading to the prediction that they may also possess accessory cell function.[100,101] Recently, Geppert and Lipsky[102] have shown that IFN-γ treated dermal fibroblasts can function only as an incomplete antigen-presenting-cell (APC). Although they are able to take up and process antigen effectively, they lack an additional signal necessary for antigen-induced T cell proliferation and IL-2 production. This additional signal can be supplied by coculture with ECs, IL-1, or IL-2,[102,103] thus demonstrating that expression of surface Ia and the capacity to process antigen effectively are necessary but not in themselves sufficient for a cell to function as an APC.

Fibroblasts have been found to express Ia antigens at sites of inflammation[104,105] possibly due to the local release of IFN-γ. Local production of IL-1 by ECs or other cells may allow fibroblasts to serve as antigen presenting cells. The further activation of immune processes may lead, in turn, to greater Ia expression by connective tissue cells. Evidence suggests a correlation between the quantity of Ia antigens expressed in lesions and the extent and velocity of the immune response.[106]

F. FIBROBLAST-DERIVED CYTOKINES

Not only do fibroblastic cells respond to the regulatory signals derived from other cells, but they are also capable of releasing their own modulatory factors. Monocytes/macrophages not only produce colony stimulating activity (CSA)[107,108] and burst promoting activity (BPA),[109] but monocyte conditioned medium has been found to contain a nondialyzable factor which is able to induce neonatal foreskin fibroblasts to release their own CSA and BPA,[110] whereas such release by unstimulated fibroblasts is negligible. The responsible monocyte factor has recently been identified as IL-1.[111,112] IL-1 and TNF have been shown to induce normal human lung fibroblasts to synthesize granulocyte macrophage-colony stimulating factor (GM/CSF) mRNA and protein in a dose-dependent manner.[113] It can be inferred that, at sites of inflammation, GM/CSF may be synthesized locally in response to TNF and IL-1 released by macrophages. It has been proposed that the major role of monocyte/macrophages in granulopoiesis is not through their own production of CSA, but in their recruitment of other cells, such as fibroblasts, to do so.[110] Similarly, the growth stimulatory effect of macrophages on fibroblasts may be mediated, in large part, via induction of fibroblast growth stimulatory autokines.

IFN-β2 (IL-6) is another cytokine that can be released by fibroblastic cells. It is distinct from the other IFNs in that its expression by fibroblasts can be increased by other cytokines such as TNF and IL-1[114,115] It is now known that IFN-β2 and the immunoglobulin-inducing cytokine BSF-2 are identical;[116] therefore, its synthesis by connective tissue cells during inflammation may lead to enhanced local antibody synthesis.

G. ADHESION OF LYMPHOCYTES TO FIBROBLASTS

Another aspect of fibroblast participation in local immune reactions may be that of maintaining lymphocyte localization in inflamed connective tissues. The adhesion of lymphocytes to endothelium has been regarded as an initial step in the process of lymphocyte migration from the blood to lymphoid and inflammatory tissues, and adhesion-related molecules on the surface of endothelial cells can be regulated by lymphokines such as IL-1, TNF, and IFN-γ[117-119] (Section III.D). We have demonstrated the existence of similar adhesive interactions between human dermal fibroblasts and human peripheral blood T cells, which can be upregulated by exposure of the fibroblasts to IFN-γ.[120] This up-regulation proceeds in a dose-dependent fashion and appears to be independent of Ia induction. Non-adherent T cells which are collected at the end of adhesion assays demonstrate a reduced capacity to adhere to a second monolayer of IFN-γ-treated fibroblasts, suggesting the depletion of a distinct T cell subpopulation. This adhesiveness may be relevant *in vivo* in areas of tissue inflammation and in the localization of lymphocytes subsequent to their emigration through the vascular endothelium.

A cell adhesion molecule designated ICAM-1 has been described and is found on the surface of many hematopoietic and nonhematopoietic cells, including fibroblasts.[121] Monoclonal antibody to ICAM-1 can inhibit PHA-stimulated T cell blasts and a T lymphoma cell line from binding to human dermal fibroblasts. A complementary adhesion molecule on activated lymphocytes, LFA-1, is involved in binding to ICAM.[121]

III. ENDOTHELIAL CELLS

The repair of damaged vasculature and the provision of a new vascular supply to proliferating connective tissue structures is a critical event in reparative processes. The role of endothelium is, therefore, intimately associated with all aspects of tissue development, repair, and inflammation. The directed movement and proliferation of ECs is central to the process of angiogenesis and EC have been shown to possess numerous other specialized functions as well. The availability of the technical means by which EC can be propagated *in vitro* has led to a greater understanding of the factors which control both their migration and proliferation.

A. ENDOTHELIAL CELL PROLIFERATION

A family of endothelial cell growth factors (ECGFs) have been described that are mitogenic for EC *in vitro*. They have been isolated from such diverse origins as brain,[112] retina, eye, and other tissues.[123] Many of these growth factors show a strong affinity for heparin and the use of heparin-affinity chromatography has facilitated their isolation and purification. Collectively, these are known as the heparin-binding growth factors. Heparin and heparin-like molecules appear to potentiate the proliferative effects of ECGFs and have been shown to increase the binding of ECGF to EC receptors. Many of the characteristics and functional mechanisms of ECGFs and their interactions with heparin and the EC are not well understood at the present time. Chemotactic and proliferation factors for EC have been found in tumor cell conditioned medium,[124] fibroblast cell cultures,[125] and wound fluids[126] and remain to be characterized.

Additionally, products of lymphocytes and macrophages affect EC functions such as migration[127] and proliferation.[128,129] IL-1 enhances the proliferation of EC[128] and may be a major pathway by which macrophages induced EC growth and vascular proliferation. IFN-γ has been reported to inhibit the mitogenic effects of ECGF on EC in a dose-dependent manner.[130] This inhibition was associated with a decrease in the number of ECGF binding sites on the surface of the EC, therefore, the action of IFN-γ may be mediated via receptor modulation.

B. ENDOTHELIAL CELL-DERIVED CYTOKINES

Human umbilical vein EC have been shown to express mRNA for the β-chain of PDGF and to constitutively produce molecules with PDGF-like activity.[131,132] This EC-derived factor is antigenically related to PDGF and is able to compete with ^{125}I PDGF for binding to the PDGF receptor.[133] Harlan et al.[134] have shown that physiologic concentrations of α-thrombin, which is generated at sites of vascular injury and has numerous effects on EC metabolism, induced a time and dose-dependent increase in the release of PDGF-like activity from cultured EC. These authors suggested that PDGF activity released from EC would be a longer-lasting supplement to the PDGF released from platelets during the initial phase of vascular injury.

ECs, like monocytes, are able to synthesize and secrete IL-1-like molecules after an exposure to endotoxin.[135] EC cultured with either endotoxin or TNF express mRNA and protein synthesis of both IL-1α and IL-1β.[136] Miossec and Ziff[137] have reported that although IFN-γ had no effect on EC IL-1 production, it enhanced EC IL-1 synthesis after endotoxin challenge, an effect analogous to IFN-γ enhancement of IL-1 release by endotoxin-stimulated monocytes. Therefore, EC may serve as both a source and a target for IL-1.

ECs have been known to release hematopoietic factors with burst promoting activity (BPA)[138] and colony stimulating activity (CSA)[139,140] and the production of these factors can be increased by incubation of the EC in monocyte-conditioned medium.[141] This monocyte-derived factor was operationally designated MRA (monocyte recruiting activity). Bagby et al.[142] have shown that MRA and IL-1 are biologically, biophysically, and immunologically identical, thereby implicating IL-1 as a mediator by which granulopoiesis may be regulated *in vivo*. The CSA released by IL-1-stimulated EC has recently been identified by Sieff et al.[143] as GM-CSF. GM-CSF is a multilineage hematopoietin which induces the proliferation of myeloid and erythroid progenitors.[144] TNFα has also been shown to stimulate human EC to produce GM-CSF,[143,145] and Munker et al.[113] demonstrated GM-CSF mRNA and protein in EC stimulated with TNF.

C. ENDOTHELIAL CELLS AND COAGULATION

ECs possess both procoagulant and anticoagulant properties. Under normal physiologic conditions, procoagulant activity is suppressed, however, disturbances to the EC can lead to a shift in this homeostatic balance toward active procoagulant activity. *In vitro* evidence supports the hypothesis that changes in the EC may account for thrombogenesis at sites of immune vascular injury. The initiation of thrombogenesis and the laying down of fibrin provides a stroma for fibroblast migration and proliferation.

Tissue factor is an initiator of blood coagulation which catalyzes the cleavage of factor X and factor IX by factor VIIa. Tissue factor expression by ECs can be increased by a number of stimuli. Treatment of EC with IL-1 results in rapidly enhanced tissue factor expression. This effect of IL-1 on EC can be dissociated from effects of IL-1 on PGE and prostacyclin (PGI$_2$) metabolism as tissue factor production is insensitive to such agents as hydrocortisone, indomethacin, and exogenous arachidonic acid.[146] Endotoxin is another agent by which EC are induced to increase tissue factor expression. Moore et al.[147] have shown that the increase in tissue factor is accompanied by a sustained and dose-dependent suppression of thrombomodulin activity (which is anticoagulant); both effects would favor intravascular coagulation. As endotoxin also leads to IL-1 release by monocytes, inflammation resulting from bacterial infection provides a potent stimulus for thrombogenesis.

D. IMMUNE PROPERTIES OF ENDOTHELIAL CELLS

Exposure of ECs to IFN-γ induces the expression of Ia antigens on the EC surface,[101,148] a critical event in rendering them competent as antigen presenting cells. Ia expression is not strictly an *in vitro* phenomenon, as EC express Ia antigens at sites of inflammatory lesions.[104,105] Cultured human EC can effectively replace macrophages as accessory cells and have been shown to be able to present soluble antigen to T cells in an HLA-DR-restricted manner.[149] Human EC have been shown to function as accessory cells in T cell proliferative responses of mitogen-stimulated T lymphocytes.[150] Shore et al.[151] have shown that EC can substitute for monocytes in T cell-dependent B cell differentiation and also demonstrated that the addition of small numbers of EC to cultures of peripheral blood mononuclear cells enhanced IL-2 production. It appears that not only are EC capable of accessory cell functions, but they may possess other immune modulatory functions as well.

Both structural and functional changes of EC, leading to an increased adhesiveness for lymphocytes and certain lymphoid-derived cell lines, have been reported after exposure to different immune cell-derived soluble mediators. As has been mentioned, adhesion related molecules on the surface of ECs which have been collectively called ELAMs (endothelial-leukocyte adhesion molecules) can be up-regulated by IL-1, TNF, and IFN-γ.[117-119,152,153] EC-leukocyte adhesion is thought to be of importance in regulating the passage of lymphocytes from the circulation into the areas of inflammation.

Recirculating lymphocytes enter lymph nodes and Peyer's patches from the blood by adhering to and migrating through specialized endothelial walls of postcapillary high endothelial venules (HEV).[154] HEV recognition by lymphocytes appears to be a specific receptor-mediated phenomenon and "homing receptors" on lymphocyte subpopulations have been identified. Distinct homing receptors responsible for lymphocyte adhesion to either Peyer's patches or lymph node HEV have been identified in the mouse and specific monoclonal antibodies have been produced. One such antibody, MEL-14, blocks lymphocyte adhesion to lymph node HEV, while others specifically block adhesion to Peyer's patch HEV.[155] In the mouse, certain lymphomas adhere selectively to only one kind (lymph node or Peyer's patch) of HEV[155] supporting a concept of lymphocyte populations precommitted to certain target areas. The adhesion related molecules present on lymphocytes and ECs thus contribute to controlled migration and distribution of immune cells.

IV. WOUND REPAIR

The interaction of fibroblasts, endothelium, and mononuclear cells in reparative processes occurs in both immunologically based inflammatory reactions and in simple wound healing. Over 1 decade ago, Leibovich and Ross[16] demonstrated that guinea pigs made monocytopenic by treatment with antimacrophage serum failed to heal skin wounds normally. Simple surgical skin wounds result in vascular injury, activation of blood coagulation, and release of platelet-derived growth factors including PDGF, thus providing a stimulus for fibroblast replication. The deposition of fibrin forms a substrate for further fibroblast and epidermal cell migration. Remodeling of the connective tissue matrix leads to release of chemotactic peptides from collagen and fibronectin with recruitment of fibroblasts and mononuclear cells. Monocyte-derived cytokines such as IL-1 stimulate fibroblast proliferation, matrix synthesis, and synthesis of degradative enzymes which allow the progression of remodeling and repair of tissue.

Abnormal repair may be associated with either defective or excessive connective tissue function. An example of the former would be scurvy, a deficiency of ascorbic acid, where both vascular repair and collagen synthesis are defective;[156] ascorbic acid is a cofactor for lysyl and prolyl hydroxylase activity and stimulates collagen production.[157,158] Hydrocortisone stimulates fibroblast proliferation but suppresses collagen synthesis;[159] treatment with glucocorticoids *in vivo* leads to impaired wound healing. In certain individuals, wound healing is characterized by excessive collagen accumulation and formation of keloids. The factors responsible for this abnormality are unclear but may relate to abnormal responses of fibroblasts to hormones or cytokines.[160]

V. PATHOLOGIC FIBROSIS

Excessive accumulation of fibroblasts and/or matrix characterizes certain inflammatory disorders. These entities include such states as idiopathic pulmonary fibrosis, scleroderma, and rheumatoid arthritis. The pathogenesis of these disorders has been recently reviewed.[161,162] The pathologic accumulation of fibroblasts and collagen in these disorders results from the interplay of multiple processes. In immune complex-mediated inflammation, complement components may be chemotactic for fibroblasts.[163] Release of degradative enzymes by neutrophils and monocytes leads to generation of chemotactic fragments of collagen and fibronectin. Activation of monocytes by complexes leads to tissue factor generation, activation of the coagulation system, and fibrin deposition. To the extent that such processes are sustained, e.g., the continuing localized immune complex disease of rhematoid synovitis, fibroblast activation continues. Sustained inflammation and release of cytokines by mononuclear cells at inflammatory sites also promotes continued fibroproliferation and matrix synthesis.

The continuation of fibrotic processes even after inflammation and immune events have subsided, as with keloid formation, represents a failure to terminate normal reparative processes. The persistence, during *in vitro* culture, of metabolic abnormalities in fibroblasts isolated from lesional tissue in some of these disorders (scleroderma, rheumatoid arthritis)[161] may represent acquired defects in regulatory responses to normal growth factors or overgrowth or selection of normally occurring subpopulations as discussed earlier. While a great deal has been learned about the cytokines that stimulate connective tissue repair, our understanding of the factors responsible for termination of the healing process is less substantial.

VI. CONCLUSION

Immune-cell derived cytokines play a critical role in reparative processes. They function in the accumulation of fibroblastic cells and in the stimulation of these cells for synthesis of matrix components. Immune cytokines also play an important role in modulating EC function and in the regulation of blood coagulation; the latter, in turn, further influences connective tissue function. In addition, by modulation of lymphocyte and monocyte homing and function, fibroblasts and ECs serve as effector cells in influencing the course of immune and inflammatory reactions.

ACKNOWLEDGMENTS

Supported by USPHS grants AR 32343 and AR 20621, the Medical Research Service of the Veterans Administration, and the Arthritis Foundation. Dr. Piela is supported by a postdoctoral training grant (USPHS-AR 07475).

REFERENCES

1. **Postlethwaite, A. E., Snyderman, R., and Kang, A. H.,** The chemotactic attraction of human fibroblasts to a lymphocyte-derived factor, *J. Exp. Med.,* 144, 1188, 1976.
2. **Seppa, H. E. J., Grotendorst, G. R., Seppa, S. I., Schiffmann, E., and Martin, G. R.,** The platelet-derived growth factor is a chemoattractant for fibroblasts, *J. Cell. Biol.,* 92, 584, 1982.
3. **Kohler, N. and Lipton, A.,** Platelets as a source of fibroblast growth promoting activity, *Exp. Cell. Res.,* 87, 297, 1974.
4. **Deul, T. F., Senior, R. M., Huang, J. S., and Griffin, G. L.,** Chemotaxis of monocytes and neutrophils to platelet-derived growth factor, *J. Clin. Invest.,* 69, 1046, 1982.
5. **Gauss-Muller, V., Kleinman, H. K., Martin, G. R., and Schiffman, E.,** Role of attachment factors and attractants in fibroblast chemotaxis, *J. Lab. Clin. Med.,* 96, 1071, 1980.
6. **Postlethwaite, A. E., Keski-Oja, J., Balian, G., and Kang, A. H.,** Induction of fibroblast chemotaxis by fibronectin, *J. Exp. Med.,* 153, 494, 1981.
7. **Seppa, H., Seppa, S., and Yamada, K. M.,** The cell binding fragment of fibronectin and platelet-derived growth factor are chemoattractants for fibroblasts, *J. Cell. Biol.,* 87, 323a, 1980.
8. **Yamada, K. M. and Olden, K.,** Fibronectins-adhesive glycoproteins of cell surface and blood, *Nature,* 275, 179, 1978.

9. **Clark, R., Lanigan, J., Dellapelle, P., Manseau, E., Dvorak, H., and Colvin, R.,** Fibronectin and fibrin provide a provisional matrix for epidermal cell migration during wound re-epithelialization, *J. Invest. Dermatol.,* 79, 264, 1982.

10. **Clark, R. and Colvin, R.,** The significance of fibronectin in wound repair, in *Fibronectin: Its Role in Coagulation and Fibrinolysis,* McDonagh, Ed., Marcel Dekker, New York, 1985.

11. **Akiyama, S. and Yamada, K.,** Fibronectin in disease, in *Connective Tissue Diseases,* Wagner, Fleishmajer, and Kaufman, Williams & Wilkins, Baltimore, 1983, 55.

12. **Postlethwaite, A. E., Seyer, J. M., and Kang, A. H.,** Chemotactic attraction of human fibroblast to type I, II, III collagens and collagen derived peptides, *Proc. Natl. Acad. Sci. U.S.A.,* 75, 871, 1977.

13. **Chiang, T. M., Postlethwaite, A. E., Beachey, E. H., Seyer, J. M., and Kang, A. H.,** Binding of chemotactic collagen-derived peptides to fibroblasts: the relationship to fibroblast chemotaxis, *J. Clin. Invest.,* 62, 916, 1978.

14. **Singer, I. I., Kawka, D. W., Scott, S., Mumford, R. A., and Lark, W.,** The fibronectin cell attachment sequence Arg-Gly-Asp-Ser promotes focal contact formation during early fibroblast attachment and spreading, *J. Cell. Biol.,* 104, 573, 1987.

15. **Dedhar, S., Ruoslahti, E., and Pierschbacher, M.,** A cell surface receptor complex for collagen type I recognizes the Arg-Gly-Asp sequence, *J. Cell. Biol.,* 104, 585, 1987.

16. **Leibovich, S. J. and Ross, R.,** The role of the macrophage in wound repair: a study with hydrocortisone and antimacrophage serum, *Am. J. Pathol.,* 78, 71, 1975.

17. **Leibovich, S. J. and Ross, R.,** A macrophage dependent factor that stimulates the proliferation of fibroblasts *in vitro, Am. J. Pathol.,* 84, 501, 1976.

18. **Castor, C. W. and Lewis, R. B.,** Connective tissue activation. X. Current studies of the process and its mediators, *Scand. J. Rheumatol.,* 5(Suppl. 12), 41, 1975.

19. **Spielvogel, R. L., Kersey, J. H., and Goltz, R. W.,** Mononuclear cell stimulation of fibroblast collagen synthesis, *Clin. Exp. Dermatol.,* 3, 25, 1978.

20. **Johnson, R. L. and Ziff, M.,** Lymphokine stimulation of collagen accumulation, *J. Clin. Invest.,* 58, 240, 1976.

21. **Green, J. A., Cooperband, S. R., Rutstein, J. A., and Kibrick, S.,** Inhibition of target cell proliferation by supernatants of human peripheral lymphocytes, *J. Immunol.,* 105, 48, 1970.

22. **Martinet, Y., Bittermann, P. B., Mornex, J. F., Grotendorst, G. R., Martin, G. R., and Crystal, R. G.,** Activated human monocytes express the c-sis proto-oncogene and release a mediator showing PDGF-like activity, *Nature,* 319, 158, 1986.

23. **Grotendorst, G. R., Seppa, H. E. J., Kleinman, H. K., and Martin, G. R.,** Attachment of smooth muscle cells to collagens and their migration toward platelet-derived growth factor, *Proc. Natl. Acad. Sci. U.S.A.,* 78, 3669, 1981.

24. **Stiles, C. D.,** The molecular biology of platelet-derived growth factor, *Cell,* 33, 653, 1983.

25. **Mizel, S. B.,** Interleukin 1 and T cell activation, *Immunol. Rev.,* 63, 51, 1982.

26. **Lomedico, P., Gubler, V., Hellmann, C., Dulovich, M., Giri, J., Pan, Y-C., Collier, K., Seminow, R., Chua, A., and Mizel, S.,** Cloning and expression of murine interleukin-1 cDNA in *Escherichia coli, Nature,* 312, 458, 1984.

27. **Rupp, E. A., Cameron, P. M., Ranawat, C. S., Schmidt, J. A., and Bayne, E. K.,** Specific bioactivities of monocyte-derived interleukin-1-alpha and interleukin-1-beta are similar to each other on cultured murine thymocytes and on cultured human connective tissue cells, *J. Clin. Invest.,* 78, 836, 1986.

28. **Chin, J., Cameron, P. M., Rupp, E., and Schmidt, J. A.,** Identification of a high-affinity receptor for native human interleukin-1-beta and interleukin-1-alpha on normal human lung fibroblasts, *J. Exp. Med.,* 165, 70, 1987.

29. **Schmidt, J. A., Mizel, S. B., Cohen, D., and Green, I.,** Interleukin 1, a potential regulator of fibroblast proliferation, *J. Immunol.,* 128, 2177, 1982.

30. **Wang, A. M., Creasy, A. A., Ladner, M. B., Lin, L. S., Strickler, J., VanArsdell, J. N., Yamamoto, R., and Mark, D. F.,** Molecular cloning of the complementary DNA for human tumor necrosis factor, *Science,* 228, 149, 1985.

31. **Shirai, T., Yamaguchi, H., Ito, H., Todd, C. W., and Wallace, R. B.,** Cloning and expression in *Escherichia coli* of the gene for human tumor necrosis factor, *Nature,* 313, 803, 1985.

32. **Vilcek, J., Palombella, V. J., Henriksen-Destefano, D., Swenson, C., Feinman, R., Hirai, M., and Tsujimoto, M.,** Fibroblast growth enhancing activity of tumor necrosis factor and its relationship to other polypeptide growth factors, *J. Exp. Med.,* 163, 632, 1986.

33. **Sugarman, B. J., Aggarwal, B. B., Hass, P. E., Figari, I. S., Palladino, M. A., Jr., and Shepard, H. M.,** Recombinant human tumor necrosis factor-alpha: effects on proliferation of normal and transformed cells *in vitro, Science,* 230, 943, 1985.

34. **Bohlen, P., Esch, F., Baird, A., and Gospodarowicz, D.,** Acidic fibroblast growth factor (FGF) from bovine brain: amino terminal sequence and comparison with basic FGF, *EMBO J.,* 4, 1951, 1985.

35. **Neufeld, G. and Gospodarowicz, D.,** Basic and acidic fibroblast growth factors interact with the same cell surface receptors, *J. Biol. Chem.,* 261, 5631, 1986.

36. **Gospodarowicz, D.,** Purification of a fibroblast growth factor from bovine pituitary, *J. Biol. Chem.,* 250, 2515, 1975.

37. **Gospodarowicz, D., Bialecki, H., and Greenburg, G.,** Purification of the fibroblast growth factor activity from bovine brain, *J. Biol. Chem.,* 253, 3736, 1978.

38. **Thomas, K. A., Rios-Candelore, M., and Fitzpatrick, S.,** Purification and characterization of acidic fibroblast growth factor from bovine brain, *Proc. Natl. Acad. Sci. U.S.A.,* 81, 357, 1984.

39. **Thomas, K. A., Rios-Candelore, M., Giminez-Gallego, G., DiSalvo, J., Bennett, C., Rodkey, J., and Fitzpatrick, S.,** Pure brain-derived acidic fibroblast growth factor is a potent angiogenic vascular endothelial cell mitogen with sequence homology to interleukin 1, *Proc. Natl. Acad. Sci. U.S.A.,* 82, 6409, 1985.

40. **Roberts, A. B., Frolick, C. A., Anzano, M. A., and Sporn, M. B.,** Transforming growth factors from neoplastic and non-neoplastic tissues, *Fed. Proc.,* 42, 2621, 1983.

41. **Anzano, M. A., Roberts, A. B., Smith, J. M., Sporn, M. B., and DeLarco, J. E.,** Sarcoma growth factor from conditioned medium of virally transformed cells is composed of both type-alpha and type-beta transforming growth factors, *Proc. Natl. Acad. Sci. U.S.A.,* 80, 6264, 1983.

42. **Cheifetz, S., Like, B., and Massague, J.,** Cellular distribution of Type I and Type II receptors for transforming growth factor-beta, *J. Biol. Chem.,* 261, 9972, 1986.

43. **Derynck, R., Jarrett, J. A., Chen, E. Y., Eaton, D. H., Bell, J. R., Assoian, R. K., Roberts, A. B., Sporn, M. B., and Goeddel, D. V.,** Human transforming growth factor beta complementary DNA sequence and expression in normal and transformed cells, *Nature,* 316, 701, 1985.

44. **Assoian, R. K., Komoriya, C. A., Meyers, D. M., Miller, D. M., and Sporn, M. B.,** Transforming growth factor beta in human platelets: identification of major storage site, purification, and characterization, *J. Biol. Chem.,* 258, 7155, 1983.

45. **Frolik, C. A., Dart, L. L., Meyers, C. A., Smith, D. M., and Sporn, M. B.,** Purification and initial characterization of a type beta transforming growth factor from human placenta, *Proc. Natl. Acad. Sci. U.S.A.,* 80, 3676, 1983.

46. **Keski-Oja, J., Leof, E. B., Lyons, R. M., Coffey, R. J., Jr., and Moses, H. L.,** Transforming growth factors and control of neoplastic cell growth, *J. Cell. Biochem.,* 33, 95, 1987.

47. **Tucker, R. F., Branum, E. L., Shipley, G. D., Ryan, R. J., and Moses, H. L.,** Specific binding to cultured cells of I^{125}-labeled type beta transforming growth factor from human platelets, *Proc. Natl. Acad. Sci. U.S.A.,* 81, 6757, 1984.

48. **Kehrl, J. H., Roberts, A. B., Wakefield, L. M., Jakowlew, S., Sporn, M. B., and Fauci, A. S.,** Transforming growth factor beta is an important immunomodulatory protein for human B lymphocytes, *J. Immunol.,* 137, 3855, 1986.

49. **Postlethwaite, A. E., Keski-Oja, J., Moses, H. L., and Kang, A. H.,** Stimulation of the chemotactic migration of human fibroblasts by transforming growth factor beta, *J. Exp. Med.,* 165, 251, 1987.

50. **Roberts, A. B., Anzano, M. A., Lamb, L. C., Smith, J. M., and Sporn, M. B.,** New class of transforming growth factors potentiated by epidermal growth factor: isolation from non-neoplastic tissues, *Proc. Natl. Acad. Sci. U.S.A.,* 78, 5339, 1981.

51. **Schultz, G. S., White, M., Mitchell, R., Brown, G., Lynch, J., Twardzik, D. R., and Todaro, G. J.,** Epithelial wound healing enhanced by transforming growth factor-alpha and vaccinia growth factor, *Science,* 235, 350, 1987.

52. **Sporn, M. B., Roberts, A. B., Shull, J. H., Smith, J. M., Ward, J. M., and Sodek, J.,** Polypeptide transforming growth factors isolated from bovine sources and used for wound healing *in vivo, Science,* 219, 1329, 1983.

53. **Anderson, P., Yip, Y. K., and Vilcek, J.,** Human interferon-gamma is internalized and degraded by cultured fibroblasts, *J. Biol. Chem.,* 258, 6497, 1983.

54. **Brouty-Boye, D.,** Inhibitory effects of interferons on cell multiplication, *Lymphokine Rep.,* 1, 99, 1980.

55. **Pfeffer, L. M., Murphy, J. S., and Tamm, I.,** Interferon effects on the growth and division of human fibroblasts, *Exp. Cell Res.,* 121, 111, 1980.

56. **Duncan, M. R. and Berman, B.,** Gamma-interferon is the lymphokine and beta-interferon the monokine responsible for inhibition of fibroblast collagen production and late but not early fibroblast proliferation, *J. Exp. Med.,* 162, 516, 1985.

57. **Neilson, E. G., Phillips, S. M., and Jimenez, S.,** Lymphokine modulation of fibroblast proliferation, *J. Immunol.,* 128, 1484, 1982.

58. **Neilson, E. G., Phillips, S. M., and Jimenez, S. A.,** Cell-mediated immunity in interstitial nephritis. III. T-lymphocyte mediated fibroblast proliferation and collagen synthesis: an immune mechanism for renal fibrogenesis, *J. Immunol.,* 125, 1708, 1980.

59. **Korn, J. H., Halushka, P. V., and LeRoy, E. C.,** Mononuclear cell modulation of connective tissue function. Suppression of fibroblast growth by stimulation of endogenous prostaglandin production, *J. Clin. Invest.,* 65, 543, 1980.

60. **Clark, J. G., Kostal, K. M., and Marino, B. A.,** Bleomycin induced pulmonary fibrosis in hamsters. An alveolar macrophage product increases fibroblast prostaglandin E_2 and cyclic adenosine monophosphate and suppresses fibroblast proliferation and collagen production, *J. Clin. Invest.,* 72, 2082, 1983.

61. **Mizel, S. B., Dayer, J. M., Krane, S. M., and Mergenhagen, S. E.,** Stimulation of rheumatoid synovial cell collagenase and prostaglandin production by partially purified lymphocyte-activating factor (interleukin-1), *Proc. Natl. Acad. Sci. U.S.A.,* 78, 2474, 1981.

62. **Elias, J. A., Rossman, M. D., and Daniele, R. P.,** Inhibition of human lung fibroblast growth by mononuclear cells, *Am. Rev. Resp. Dis.,* 125, 701, 1982.

63. **Brinckerhoff, C. E. and Guyre, P.,** Increased proliferation of human synovial fibroblasts treated with recombinant immune interferon, *J. Immunol.,* 134, 3142, 1985.

64. **Boraschi, D., Censini, S., and Tagliabue, A.,** Interferon-gamma reduces macrophage-suppressive activity by inhibiting prostaglandin E_2 release and inducing IL-1 production, *J. Immunol.,* 133, 764, 1984.

65. **Arenzana-Seisdedos, F., Virelizier, J. L., and Fiers, W.,** Interferons as macrophage-activating factors. III. Preferential effects of interferon-gamma on the interleukin-1 secretory potential of fresh or aged human monocytes, *J. Immunol.,* 134, 2444, 1985.

66. **Johnson, H. M. and Torres, B. A.,** Peptide growth factors PDGF, EGF, and FGF regulate interferon-gamma production, *J. Immunol.,* 134, 2824, 1985.

67. **Kirchhofer, D., Reinhardt, C. A., and Zbinden, G.,** Collagen synthesis in growing human skin fibroblasts, *Exp. Cell. Biol.,* 54, 177, 1986.

68. **Postlethwaite, A. E., Smith, G. N., Jr., Mainardi, C. L., Seyer, J. M., and Kang, A. H.,** Characterization of a human lymphokine that stimulates fibroblasts to produce collagen, *Arthritis Rheum.,* 24, 61a, 1981.

69. **Wahl, S. M., Wahl, L. M., and McCarthy, J. B.,** Lymphocyte-mediated activation of fibroblast proliferation and collagen production, *J. Immunol.,* 121, 942, 1978.

70. **Jimenez, S. A., McArthur, W., and Rosenbloom, J.,** Inhibition of collagen synthesis by mononuclear cell supernatants, *J. Exp. Med.,* 150, 1421, 1979.

71. **Krane, S. M., Dayer, J. M., Simon, L. S., and Byrne, M. S.,** Mononuclear cell-conditioned medium containing mononuclear cell factor (MCF), homologous with interleukin 1, stimulates collagen and fibronectin synthesis by adherent synovial cells: effects of prostaglandin E_2 and indomethacin, *Collagen Rel. Res.,* 5, 99, 1985.

72. **Rosenbloom, J., McArthur, W., Malamud, D., and Jimenez, S.,** Characterization of a lymphokine produced by human T cells which inhibits collagen synthesis, *Cell. Immunol.,* 81, 192, 1983.

73. **Postlethwaite, A. E., Smith, G. N., Mainardi, C. L., Seyer, J. M., and Kang, A. H.,** Lymphocyte modulation of fibroblast function *in vitro*: stimulation and inhibition of collagen production by different effector molecules, *J. Immunol.,* 132, 2470, 1984.

74. **Jimenez, S. A., Freundlich, B., and Rosenbloom, J.,** Selective inhibition of human diploid fibroblast collagen synthesis by interferons, *J. Clin. Invest.,* 74, 1112, 1984.

75. **Rosenbloom, J., Feldman, G., Freundlich, B., and Jimenez, S. A.,** Transcriptional control of human diploid fibroblast collagen synthesis by gamma-interferon, *Biochem. Biophys. Res. Commun.,* 123, 365, 1984.

76. **Stephenson, M. L., Krane, S. M., Amento, E. P., McCroskery, P. A., and Byrne, M.,** Immune interferon inhibits collagen synthesis by rheumatoid synovial cells associated with decreased levels of the procollagen mRNAs, *FEBS Lett.,* 180, 43, 1985.

77. **Granstein, R. D., Murphy, G. F., Margolis, R. J., Byrne, M. H., and Amento, E. P.,** Gamma-interferon inhibits collagen synthesis *in vivo* in the mouse, *J. Clin. Invest.,* 79, 1254, 1987.

78. **Raghow, R., Postlethwaite, A. E., Keski-Oja, J., Moses, H. L., and Kang, A. H.,** Transforming growth factor-beta increases steady state levels of type 1 procollagen and fibronectin messenger RNAs post-transcriptionally in cultured human dermal fibroblasts, *J. Clin. Invest.,* 79, 1285, 1987.

79. **Centrella, M. C., McCarthy, T. L., and Canalis, E.,** Transforming growth factor beta is a bifunctional regulator of replication and collagen synthesis in osteoblast-enriched cell cultures from fetal rat bone, *J. Biol. Chem.,* 262, 2869, 1987.

80. **Roberts, A. B., Sporn, M. B., Assoian, R. K., Smith, J. M., Roche, N. S., Wakefield, L. M., Heine, U. I., Liotta, L. A., Falanga, V. A., Kehrl, J. H., and Fauci, A. S.,** Transforming growth factor type-beta: rapid induction of fibrosis and angiogenesis *in vivo* and stimulation of collagen formation *in vitro*, Proc. Natl. Acad. Sci. U.S.A., 83, 4167, 1986.

81. **Hammerman, D., Sasse, J., and Klagburn, M.,** A cartilage derived growth factor enhances hyaluronate synthesis and diminishes sulfated glycosaminoglycan synthesis in chondrocytes, *J. Cell. Physiol.,* 127, 317, 1986.

82. **Whiteside, T. L., Worrall, J. G., Prince, R. K., Buckingham, R. B., and Rodman, G. P.,** Soluble mediators from mononuclear cells increase the synthesis of glycosaminoglycans by dermal fibroblasts from normal subjects and progressive systemic sclerosis patients, *Arthritis Rheum.,* 28, 188, 1985.

83. **Yaron, I., Meyer, F. A., Dayer, J. M., and Yaron, M.,** Human recombinant interleukin-1-beta stimulates glycosaminoglycan production in human synovial fibroblast cultures, *Arthritis Rheum.,* 30, 424, 1987.

84. **Mizel, S. B., Dayer, J. M., Krane, S. M., and Mergenhagen, S. E.,** Stimulation of rheumatoid synovial cell collagenase and prostaglandin production by a partially purified lymphocyte-activating factor (interleukin-1), *Proc. Natl. Acad. Sci. U.S.A.,* 78, 2474, 1980.

85. **Postlethwaite, A. E., Lachman, L. B., Mainardi, C. L., and Kang, A. H.,** Interleukin-1 stimulation of collagenase production by cultured fibroblasts, *J. Exp. Med.,* 157, 801, 1983.

86. **Dayer, J. M., Breard, J., Chess, L., and Krane, S. M.,** Participation of monocyte-macrophages and lymphocytes in the production of a factor that stimulates collagenase and prostaglandin release by rheumatoid synovial cells, *J. Clin. Invest.,* 64, 1386, 1979.

87. **Murphy, G., Reynolds, J. J., and Werb, Z.,** Biosynthesis of tissue inhibitor of metalloproteinases by human fibroblasts in culture, *J. Biol. Chem.,* 260, 3079, 1985.

88. **Dayer, J. M., Beutler, B., and Cerami, A.,** Cachectin/tumor necrosis factor stimulates collagenase and prostaglandin E_2 production by human synovial cells and dermal fibroblasts, *J. Exp. Med.,* 162, 2163, 1985.

89. **Wahl, L. M.,** Collagenase production by human monocytes, *J. Dent. Res.,* 63, 338a, 1984.

90. **Wahl, L. M., Olsen, C. E., Sandberg, A. L., and Mergenhagen, S. E.,** Prostaglandin regulation of macrophage collagenase production, *Proc. Natl. Acad. Sci. U.S.A.,* 74, 4955, 1977.

91. **Nathan, C. F., Murray, H. W., and Cohn, Z. A.,** The macrophage as an effector cell, *N. Engl. J. Med.,* 303, 622, 1980.

92. **Korn, J. H.,** Fibroblast prostaglandin E_2 synthesis. Persistence of an abnormal phenotype after short term exposure to mononuclear cell products, *J. Clin. Invest.,* 71, 1240, 1983.

93. **Worrall, J. G., Whiteside, T. L., Prince, R. K., Buckingham, R. B., Stachura, I., and Rodman, G.,** Persistence of scleroderma-like phenotype in normal fibroblasts after prolonged exposure to soluble mediators from mononuclear cells, *Arthritis Rheum.,* 29, 54, 1986.

94. **Duncan, M. R. and Berman, B.,** Persistence of a reduced-collagen-producing phenotype in cultured scleroderma fibroblasts after short-term exposure to interferons, *J. Clin. Invest.,* 79, 1318, 1987.

95. **Korn, J. H., Brinckerhoff, C. E., and Edwards, R. L.,** Synthesis of PGE_2, collagenase, and tissue factor by fibroblast substrains: substrains are differentially activated for different metabolic products, *Collagen Rel. Res.,* 5, 437, 1985.

96. **Korn, J. H., Torres, D., and Downie, E.,** Clonal heterogeneity in the fibroblast response to mononuclear cell-derived mediators, *Arthritis Rheum.,* 27, 174, 1984.

97. **Hibbs, M. S., Postlethwaite, A. E., Mainardi, C. L., Seyer, J. M., and Kang, A. H.,** Alterations in collagen production in mixed mononuclear leukocyte-fibroblast cultures, *J. Exp. Med.,* 157, 47, 1983.

98. **Korn, J. H.,** Modulation of lymphocyte mitogen responses by co-cultured fibroblasts, *Cell. Immunol.,* 63, 374, 1981.

99. **Steeg, P. S., Moore, R. N., Johnson, H. M., and Oppenheim, J. J.,** Regulation of murine macrophage Ia antigen expression by a lymphokine with immune interferon activity, *J. Exp. Med.,* 156, 1780, 1982.

100. **Pober, J. S., Collins, T., Gimbrone, M. A., Jr., Cotran, R. S., Gitlin, J. D., Fiers, W., Clayberger, C., Krensky, A. M., Burakoff, S. J., and Reiss, C. S.,** Lymphocytes recognize human vascular endothelial and dermal fibroblast Ia antigens induced by recombinant immune interferon, *Nature,* 305, 726, 1983.

101. **Collins, T., Korman, A. J., Wake, C. T., Boss, J. M., Kappes, D. J., Fiers, W., Ault, K. A., Gimbrone, M. A., Jr., Strominger, J. L., and Pober, J. S.,** Immune interferon activates multiple class II major histocompatibility complex genes and the associated invariant chain gene in human endothelial cells and dermal fibroblasts, *Proc. Natl. Acad. Sci. U.S.A.,* 81, 4917, 1984.

102. **Geppert, T. D. and Lipsky, P. E.,** Dissection of defective antigen presentation by interferon-gamma treated fibroblasts, *J. Immunol.,* 138, 385, 1987.

103. **Umetsu, D. T., Katzen, D., Jabara, H. H., and Geha, R. S.,** Antigen presentation by human dermal fibroblasts: activation of resting T lymphocytes, *J. Immunol.,* 136, 440, 1986.

104. **Hayry, P., Von Willebrand, E., and Anderson, L. C.,** Expression of HLA-ABC and DR locus antigens on human kidney endothelial tubular and glomerular cells, *Scand. J. Immunol.,* 11, 305, 1980.

105. **Benson, E. M., Colvin, R. B., and Russell, P. S.,** Induction of Ia antigens in murine renal transplants, *J. Immunol.,* 134, 7, 1985.

106. **Janeway, C. A., Bottomly, K., Babich, J., Conrad, P., Conzen, S., Jones, B., Katz, M., McVay, L., Murphy, D. B., and Tite, J.,** Quantitative variation in antigen expression plays a central role in immune regulation, *Immunol. Today,* 5, 99, 1984.

107. **Chervenick, P. A. and LoBuglio, A. F.,** Human blood monocytes: stimulation of granulocyte and mononuclear colony formation *in vitro, Science,* 178, 164, 1972.

108. **Golde, D. W. and Cline, M. J.,** Identification of colony-stimulating cells in human peripheral blood, *J. Clin. Invest.,* 51, 2981, 1972.

109. **Zuckerman, K. S.,** Human erythroid burst-forming units. Growth *in vitro* is dependent on monocytes, but not T lymphocytes, *J. Clin. Invest.,* 67, 702, 1981.

110. **Bagby, G. C., Jr., McCall, E., and Layman, D. L.,** Regulation of colony stimulating activity production. Interactions of fibroblasts, mononuclear phagocytes, and lactoferrin, *J. Clin. Invest.,* 71, 340, 1982.

111. **Zucali, J. R., Dinarello, C. A., Oblon, D. J., Gross, M. A., Anderson, L., and Weiner, R. S.,** Interleukin-1 stimulates fibroblasts to produce granulocyte-macrophage colony stimulating activity and prostaglandin E_2, *J. Clin. Invest.,* 77, 1857, 1986.

112. **Bagby, G. C., Dinarello, C., and McCall, E.,** Monocyte-derived GM-CSF recruiting activity is IL-1, *Clin. Res.,* 34(Abstr.), 654a, 1986.

113. **Munker, R., Gasson, J., Ogawa, M., and Koeffler, H. P.,** Recombinant human TNF induces production of granulocyte-monocyte colony-stimulating factor, *Nature,* 323, 79, 1986.

114. **Kohase, M., Henriksen-Destefano, D., May, L. T., Vilcek, J., and Sehgal, P. B.,** Induction of beta-2-interferon by tumor necrosis factor: a homeostatic mechanism in the control of cell proliferation, *Cell,* 45, 659, 1986.

115. **Zilberstein, A., Ruggieri, R., Korn, J. H., and Revel, M.,** Structure and expression of cDNA genes for human interferon beta-2, a distinct species inducible by growth stimulatory cytokines, *EMBO J.,* 5, 2529, 1986.

116. **Sehgal, P. B., May, L. T., Tamm, I., and Vilcek, J.,** Human beta-2 interferon and B-cell differentiation factor BSF-2 are identical, *Science,* 235, 731, 1987.

117. **Bevilacqua, M. P., Pober, J. S., Wheeler, M. E., Cotran, R. S., and Gimbrone, M. A.,** Interleukin-1 activation of vascular endothelium. Effects on procoagulant activity and leukocyte adhesion, *Am. J. Pathol.,* 121, 394, 1985.

118. **Gamble, J. R., Harlan, J. M., Klebanoff, S. J., and Vadas, M. A.,** Stimulation of the adherence of neutrophils to umbilical vein endothelium by human recombinant tumor necrosis factor, *Proc. Natl. Acad. Sci. U.S.A.,* 82, 8667, 1985.

119. **Yu, C. L., Haskard, D. O., Cavender, D., Johnson, A. R., and Ziff, M.,** Human gamma-interferon increases the binding of T lymphocytes to endothelial cells, *Clin. Exp. Immunol.,* 62, 554, 1985.

120. **Piela, T. H. and Korn, J. H.,** Lymphocyte-fibroblast adhesion induced by interferon gamma, *Cell. Immunol.,* 114, 149, 1988.

121. **Dustin, M. L., Rothlein, R., Bhan, A. K., Dinarello, C. A., and Springer, T. A.,** Induction by IL-1 and interferon-gamma: tissue distribution, biochemistry and function of a natural adherence molecule (ICAM-1), *J. Immunol.,* 137, 245, 1986.

122. **Maciag, T., Mehlman, T., Friesel, R., and Schreiber, A. B.,** Heparin binds endothelial cell growth factor, the principal endothelial cell mitogen in bovine brain, *Science,* 225, 932, 1984.

123. **Folkman, J. and Klagsburn, M.,** Angiogenic factors, *Science,* 235, 442, 1987.

124. **Zetter, B. R.,** Migration of capillary endothelial cells is stimulated by tumor-derived factors, *Nature,* 285, 41, 1980.

125. **Castellot, J. J., Karnovsky, M. J., and Spiegelman, B. M.,** Differentiation-dependent stimulation of neovascularization and endothelial cell chemotaxis by 3T3 adipocytes, *Proc. Natl. Acad. Sci. U.S.A.,* 79:5597, 1982.

126. **Banda, M. J., Knighton, D. R., Hunt, T. K., and Werb, Z.,** Isolation of a non-mitogenic angiogenesis factor from wound fluid, *Proc. Natl. Acad. Sci. U.S.A.,* 79, 7773, 1982.

127. **Cohen, M. C., Picciano, P. T., Douglas, W. J., Yoshida, T., Kreutzer, D. L., and Cohen, S.,** Migration inhibition of endothelial cells by lymphokine-containing supernatants, *Science,* 215, 301, 1982.

128. **Ooi, B. S., MacCarthy, E. P., Hsu, A., and Ooi, Y. M.,** Human mononuclear cell modulation of endothelial cell proliferation, *J. Lab. Clin. Med.,* 102, 428, 1983.

129. **Martin, B. M., Gimbrone, M. A., Jr., Unanue, E. R., and Cotran, R. S.,** Stimulation of non-lymphoid mesenchymal cell proliferation by a macrophage-derived growth factor, *J. Immunol.,* 126, 1510, 1981.

130. **Friesel, R., Komoriya, A., and Maciag, T.,** Inhibition of endothelial cell proliferation by gamma-interferon, *J. Cell. Biol.,* 104, 689, 1987.

131. **Barrett, T. B., Gajdusek, C. M., Schwartz, S. M., McDougall, J. K., and Benditt, E. P.,** Expression of the sis gene by endothelial cells in culture and *in vivo, Proc. Natl. Acad. Sci. U.S.A.,* 81, 6772, 1984.

132. **Collins, T., Ginsburg, D., Bass, J. M., Orkin, S. H., and Pober, J. S.,** Cultured human endothelial cells express platelet-derived growth factor beta chain: cDNA cloning and structural analysis, *Nature,* 316, 748, 1985.

133. **DiCorleto, P. E. and Bowen-Pope, D. F.,** Cultured endothelial cells produce a platelet-derived growth factor-like protein, *Proc. Natl. Acad. Sci. U.S.A.,* 80, 1919, 1983.

134. **Harlan, J. M., Thompson, P. J., Ross, R. R., and Bowen-Pope, D. F.,** Alpha-thrombin induces release of platelet-derived growth factor-like molecule(s) by cultured human endothelial cells, *J. Cell. Biol.,* 103, 1129, 1986.

135. **Stern, D. M., Bank, I., Nawroth, P. P., Cassimeris, J., Kisiel, W., Fenton, J. W., II, Dinarello, C., Chess, L., and Jaffe, E. A.,** Self-regulation of procoagulant events on the endothelial cell surface, *J. Exp. Med.,* 162, 1223, 1985.

136. **Libby, P., Ordovas, J. M., Auger, K. R., Robbins, A. H., Birinyi, L. K., and Dinarello, C. A.,** Endotoxin and tumor necrosis factor induce interleukin-1 gene expression in adult human vascular endothelial cells, *Am. J. Pathol.,* 124, 179, 1986.

137. **Miossec, P. and Ziff, M.,** Immune interferon enhances the production of interleukin 1 by human endothelial cells stimulated with lipopolysaccharide, *J. Immunol.,* 137, 2848, 1986.

138. **Ascensao, J. L., Vercellotti, G. M., Jacob, H. S., and Zanjani, E. D.,** Role of endothelial cells in human hematopoiesis: modulation of mixed colony growth *in vitro, Blood,* 63, 553, 1984.

139. **Knutson, S. and Mortensen, B. T.,** Growth stimulation of human bone marrow cells on agar culture by vascular cells, *Blood,* 46, 937, 1975.

140. **Quesenberry, P. J. and Gimbrone, M. A.,** Vascular endothelium as a regulator of granulopoiesis: production of colony stimulating activity by cultured human endothelial cells, *Blood,* 56, 1060, 1980.

141. **Bagby, G. C., McCall, E., Bergstrom, K. A., and Burger, D.,** A monokine regulates colony-stimulating activity production by vascular endothelial cells, *Blood,* 62, 663, 1983.

142. **Babgy, G. C., Dinarello, C. A., Wallace, P., Wagner, C., Hefeneider, S., and McCall, E.,** Interleukin-1 stimulates granulocyte macrophage colony-stimulating activity release by vascular endothelial cells, *J. Clin. Invest.,* 78, 1316, 1986.

143. **Sieff, C. A., Tsai, S., and Faller, D.,** Interleukin-1 induces cultured human endothelial cell production of granulocyte-macrophage colony-stimulating factor, *J. Clin. Invest.,* 79, 48, 1987.

144. **Sieff, C. A., Emerson, S. G., Donahue, R. E., Nathan, D. G., Wang, E. A., Wong, G. C., and Clark, S. C.,** Human recombinant granulocyte macrophage colony stimulating factor: a multilineage hematopoietin, *Science,* 230, 1171, 1985.

145. **Broudy, V. C., Kaushansky, K., Segal, G. M., Harlan, J. M., and Adamson, J. W.,** Tumor necrosis factor type alpha stimulates human endothelial cells to produce granulocyte/macrophage colony-stimulating factor, *Proc. Natl. Acad. Sci. U.S.A.,* 83, 7467, 1986.

146. **Schorer, A. E., Kaplan, M. E., Rao, G. H. R., and Moldow, C. F.,** Interleukin-1 stimulates endothelial cell tissue factor production and expression by a prostaglandin-independent mechanism, *Thromb. Haematol.,* 56, 256, 1986.

147. **Moore, K. L., Andreoli, S. P., Esmon, N. L., Esmon, C. T., and Bang, N. U.,** Endotoxin enhances tissue factor and suppresses thrombomodulin expression of human vascular endothelium *in vitro, J. Clin. Invest.,* 79, 124, 1987.

148. **Pober, J. S., Gimbrone, M. A., Cotran, R. S., Reiss, C. S., Burakoff, S. J., Fiers, W., and Ault, K. A.,** Ia expression by vascular endothelium is inducible by activated T cells and by human interferons, *J. Exp. Med.,* 157, 1339, 1983.

149. **Burger, D. R. and Vetto, R. M.,** Hypothesis: vascular endothelium as a major participant in T-lymphocyte immunity, *Cell. Immunol.,* 70, 357, 1982.

150. **Ashida, E. R., Johnson, A. R., and Lipsky, P. E.,** Human endothelial cell-lymphocyte interaction. Endothelial cells function as accessory cells necessary for mitogen-induced human T lymphocyte activation *in vitro, J. Clin. Invest.,* 67, 1490, 1981.

151. **Shore, A., Leary, P., and Teitel, J. M.,** Comparison of accessory cell functions of endothelial cells and monocytes: IL-2 production by T cells and PFC generation, *Cell. Immunol.,* 100, 210, 1986.

152. **Schleimer, R. P. and Rutledge, B. K.,** Cultured human vascular endothelial cells acquire adhesiveness for neutrophils after stimulation with interleukin-1, endotoxin, and tumor promoting phorbol diesters, *J. Immunol.,* 136, 649, 1986.

153. **Bevilacqua, M. P., Pober, J. S., Wheeler, M. E., Cotran, R. S., and Gimbrone, M. A., Jr.,** Interleukin-1 acts on cultured human vascular endothelium to increase the adhesion of polymorphonuclear leukocytes, monocytes and related leukocyte cell lines, *J. Clin. Invest.,* 76, 2003, 1985.

154. **Gowans, J. L. and Knight, E. J.,** The route of re-circulation of lymphocytes in the rat, *Proc. R. Soc. London (Biol.),* 159, 257, 1964.

155. **Gallatin, M., St. John, T. P., Siegelman, M., Reichert, R., Butcher, E. C., and Weissman, I. R.,** Lymphocyte homing receptors, *Rev. Cell.,* 44, 673, 1986.

156. **Irvin, T. T., Chattopadhyay, D. K., and Smythe, A.,** Ascorbic acid requirements in post-operative patients, *Surg. Gynecol. Obstet.,* 147, 49, 1978.

157. **Barnes, M. J. and Kodicek, E.,** Biological hydroxylations and ascorbic acid with special regard to collagen metabolism, *Vitamins Hormones,* 30, 1, 1972.

158. **Murad, S., Sivarajah, A., and Pinnell, S. R.,** Regulation of prolyl and lysyl hydroxylase activities in cultured human skin fibroblasts by ascorbic acid, *Biochem. Biophys. Res. Commun.,* 101, 868, 1981.

159. **Ouitto, J., Tan, E. M. L., Ryhanen, L.,** Inhibition of collagen accumulation in fibrotic processes: review of pharmacologic agents and new approaches with amino acids and their analogues, *J. Invest. Dermatol.,* 79, 113s, 1982.

160. **Russell, J. D., Russell, S. B., and Trupin, K. M.,** Differential effects of hydrocortisone on both growth and collagen metabolism of human fibroblasts from normal and keloid tissue, *J. Cell. Physiol.,* 97, 221, 1978.

161. **Padula, S. J., Clark, R. B., and Korn, J. H.,** Cell-mediated immunity in the rheumatic diseases, *Hum. Pathol.,* 17, 254, 1986.
162. **Agelli, M. and Wahl, S. M.,** Cytokines and fibrosis, *Clin. Exp. Rheumatol.,* 4, 379, 1986.
163. **Postlethwaite, A. E., Snyderman, R., and Kang, A. H.,** Generation of a fibroblast chemotactic factor in serum by activation of complement, *J. Clin. Invest.,* 64, 1379, 1979.

INDEX